Retinal Detachment Surgery and Proliferative Vitreoretinopathy

Ulrich Spandau • Zoran Tomic •
Diego Ruiz-Casas
Editors

Retinal Detachment Surgery and Proliferative Vitreoretinopathy

From Scleral Buckling to Small Gauge Vitrectomy

Second Edition

Springer

Editors
Ulrich Spandau
St Eriks Hospital
University of Stockholm
Stockholm, Sweden

Zoran Tomic
Milos Klinika
Belgrade, Serbia

Diego Ruiz-Casas
Retina Department
Hospital Ramón y Cajal
Madrid, Spain

ISBN 978-3-031-11945-3 ISBN 978-3-031-11946-0 (eBook)
https://doi.org/10.1007/978-3-031-11946-0

This Springer imprint is published by the registered company Springer Nature Switzerland AG
The registered company address is: Gewerbestrasse 11, 6330 Cham, Switzerland

This book is dedicated to all VR surgeons who strive to give their patients good treatment through excellent surgery and dedicated care.

Preface

The retinal detachment is the most important surgery for a vitreoretinal surgeon. Its broad pathological spectrum presents a never-ending challenge.

Ophthalmology is a specialized handcraft. But in contrast to a handyman, we do not work with dead objects but with a living organ, which wants to be treated like a raw egg.

The best situation for an ocular surgeon would be to operate one eye as an exercise and the second eye for real. Especially in PVR detachment, such a situation would be a dream. The pathology is extremely difficult and we have a broad choice of surgical options: Vitrectomy, episcleral buckling, intraoperative gases and liquids.

If you want to become a good VR surgeon you need:

1. Theoretical knowledge: The retina behaves logically in a detachment. Retinal detachment requires knowledge about Lincoff rules and where to find the primary hole.
2. Practical knowledge of many different *surgical techniques* (binocular ophthalmoscopy, scleral buckling, vitrectomy, retinectomy, phacoemulsification, secondary IOL implantation). A surgeon needs many different weapons to succeed against retinal pathologies.
3. *Experience*, because experience results in correct assessment. An important part of experience is a tight and complete follow-up of your patients which results in valuable feedback about your surgery.
4. *Visit* other vitreoretinal clinics in order to learn tips and tricks and to be able to assess the quality of your surgery within the surgical world.
5. Modern *equipment* and qualified *staff*. A microscope with a good viewing system is essential for a successful surgery. Vitreoretinal surgery requires well-educated staff.
6. And finally, last but not least and maybe the most important point: *Motivation* and *passion* for ophthalmology and surgery.

Retinal detachment surgery requires theoretical and practical knowledge. Easy retinal detachments can be learned within 1 year but complicated retinal detachments require 5 years of training. Avoid being ideological about the best method to attach the retina. Be pragmatic. The simplest method which reattaches the retina is the best. And the best method for one eye may not be the best method for another eye.

What is the difference between theory and praxis? Theory means that you know everything, but nothing works. Praxis means that everything works, but you do not know why. So try to acquire as a vitreoretinal surgeon a good mixture of practical and theoretical knowledge.

In this book, all surgical techniques to reattach the retina are demonstrated in detail. The surgery is described like a cookbook: First the instruments and material and then the surgery step-by-step. The surgery is illustrated with pictures, drawings and many videos.

Additional videos can be viewed on the youTube channel of Ulrich Spandau and Diego Ruiz-Casas.

Uppsala, Sweden — Ulrich Spandau
Madrid, Spain — Diego Ruiz-Casas
Belgrade, Serbia — Zoran Tomic

Acknowledgements I want to thank my wife, Katrin, for her non-ending patience regarding her book-writing husband and I want to thank my children, Maximilian, Moritz and Oskar, for showing me that there is a world outside my beloved ophthalmology.

Introduction

Proliferative vitreoretinopathy (PVR) is the biggest surgical challenge within surgical ophthalmology. Small gauge vitrectomy offers new possibilities to tackle with this difficult pathology. The trocars and the small instruments are less traumatic than the old 20G vitrectomy resulting in improved postoperative results.

The book is divided in several parts. It starts with an historical introduction from the father of modern vitreoretinal surgery, Relja Zivojnovic, from Rotterdam. The first part explains the theoretical knowledge for retinal detachment including the four Lincoff rules. All devices and instruments for detachment surgery are then demonstrated. In the next part all surgical techniques for an easy retinal detachment are demonstrated. It includes pneumatic retinopexy (Toronto technique), cryopexy and vitrectomy (Moorfield technique), combined phaco/vitrectomy (Frankfurt technique), encircling band with vitrectomy (Stockholm technique) and much more. The following parts show the surgical management of PVR detachment, ora dialysis, choroidal detachment and even pediatric detachment. In the next part well-known surgeons from all over the world demonstrate their specific surgical techniques with interesting video cases. Finally,all postoperative aspects including complications and follow-up are explained.

The whole textbook is practical, down to earth and hands on. The surgery is described in great detail so you can reproduce it the next day in your OR.

Editors
Ulrich Spandau
Diego Ruiz-Casas
Zoran Tomic

Contents

List of Videos

All videos can be found in a playlist on my YouTube channel:
https://youtube.com/playlist?list=PL0dKYclPD7yMn861X0g-aHCS6KZ5NcH1N

Chapter 3: Basics of Small Gauge Vitrectomy
Left old vitreous cutter and right novel TDC cutter with 6000 cpm and 450 mmHg
Regular cutter Video courtesy DORC
Flow regular cutter Video courtesy DORC
TDC cutter Video courtesy DORC
Flow TDC cutter Video courtesy DORC

Chapter 7: Biometry and Anaesthesia
Biometry

Chapter 10: Pneumatic Retinopexy (Toronto Technique)
Pneumatic retinopexy with Biom

Chapter 12: Combined Phaco/Vitrectomy (Frankfurt Technique)
Retinal detachment for dummies
27G-retinal detachment without PFCL
Retinal detachment high myopia with PFCL

Chapter 15: Episcleral Buckling for Detachment Surgery with BIOM
Episcleral buckling with BIOM 1
Episcleral buckling with BIOM 2
Complication during episcleral buckling
27G vitrectomy and episcleral buckling. How would you operate this case?
Scleral buckling for PVR C2

Chapter 17: Recurrent Retinal Detachment
Recurrent retinal detachment operated with 27G
Aphakia and inferior redetachment: Inferior buckle and Artisan IOL
Traumatic PVR redetachment

Chapter 19: Rhegmatogenous Retinal Detachment in Children
Retinal detachment secondary to Stickler syndrome (1)
Retinal detachment secondary to Stickler syndrome (2)

Chapter 21: Vitrectomy for PVR Detachment Stage C
PVR detachment
Membrane peeling in ARN
Cerclage
Cerclage removal
Extraction of a sponge and cerclage
Phacoemulsification
Iris retractors
Core vitrectomy
Vitreous base shaving
Staining with trypan blue
PVR peeling short
PVR peeling detailed
Peeling techniques for PVR detachment
Removal of peripheral membranes
Subretinal peeling
Removal of Subretinal membranes
PFCL injection
Ando iridectomy
Silicone oil injection
Dislocated IOL and one-year-old retinal detachment
Chronic PVR detachment

Chapter 22: Vitrectomy for PVR Stage D
PVR stage D
Retinotomy
Laser for retinotomy
Vitrectomy for total retinal detachment secondary to morning glory

Chapter 23: Special Surgical Techniques for PVR Detachment
180° retinotomy

Chapter 24: Vitreous Anatomy, Anterior PVR and Hypotony
Anterior PVR Hypotony
PVR Prevention

Chapter 25: Surgical Management of Anterior PVR
Anterior retinal displacement
Anterior PVR secondary morning glory syndrome

Chapter 27: Surgical Management of Intraretinal PVR
27G vitrectomy and episcleral buckling
27G ppV and segmental buckle for primary RD with PVR at 9 o'clock
Inferior PVR detachment part 1
Inferior PVR detachment part 2
Inferior PVR detachment operated with scleral buckle
Failed RD surgery

Chapter 28: Traumatic Retinal Detachment Secondary to Open Globe
Surgical management of a corneal and scleral perforation
Implantation of an iris-IOL (Ophtec) for traumatic aniridia and aphakia
Napkin ring
Trauma with kick scooter with Napkin ring
Trauma with snowblower
PVR detachment secondary to trauma

Chapter 29: Choroidal Detachment: Surgical Management of a Serous Choroidal Detachment
Choroidal detachment for dummies

Chapter 30: Suprachoroidal Haemorrhage
Suprachoroidal haemorrhage after dry vitrectomy

Chapter 31: Surgical Techniques for Silicone Oil and PFCL
27G silicone oil removal
Densiron 68 removal with 25G

Chapter 32: Video Case Reports
Armada, Spain
Cabrera, Spain
Calzada, USA
Cubero
Elgohary, Kingston Hospital
Espejo
Faus
Fernandez-Sanz
García-Martinez
Ghasemi, Iran
Gonzalez
John Kitchens, USA
Kazaikin, Russia
Kusaka, Japan
Koch, France
Lara, Spain
Marticorena
Nadal, Spain
Relimpio
Ruiz-Casas, Spain
Tomic, Serbia
Veckeneer, Belgium
Zarranz

Chapter 33: After Surgery and Complications
Iridectomy
Iris-IOL capture
Complication lasernecrosis
Managing Dry Macular Folds after Vitreoretinal Surgery Dr. Mateo

All videos of chapter 31 (International VR surgeons) can be found in a playlist on my YouTube channel:
https://www.youtube.com/playlist?list=PL0dKYclPD7yNSVWL4zlBcgvrDlWUCyCv9

Contributors

Antonella D'Aponte Wilmer Eye Institute, Johns Hopkins University, Baltimore, MD, USA

Zora Ignjatović Director of Milos Clinic Eye Hospital, Belgrade, Serbia

Marco Mura The King Khaled Eye Specialist Hospital, Riyadh, Kingdom of Saudi Arabia

J. C. Pastor IOBA-Eye Institute, University of Valladolid, Valladolid, Spain

Diego Ruiz-Casas Retina Department, Hospital Ramón Y Cajal, Madrid, Spain;
Ramón y Cajal Hospital, University of Alcalá de Henares, Madrid, Spain

Ulrich Spandau St. Eriks Hospital, University of Stockholm, Stockholm, Sweden;
Department of Ophthalmology, Uppsala University Hospital, Uppsala, Sweden

Zoran Tomic Milos Klinika, Belgrade, Serbia;
Department of Ophthalmology, Uppsala University Hospital, Uppsala, Sweden

Relja Živojnović Stjepe Sarenca, Herceg Novi, Montenegro

Part I

Basics of Retinal Detachment Surgery

All videos of this part are found in a playlist on my youTube channel:
https://youtube.com/playlist?list=PL0dKYclPD7yMn861X0g-aHCS6 KZ5NcH1N
Chapter 1: No video
Chapter 2: No video
Chapter 3: **Basics of Small Gauge Vitrectomy**
Left Old vitreous cutter and right novel TDC cutter with 6000 cpm and 450 mmHg
Regular cutter Video courtesy DORC
Flow regular cutter Video courtesy DORC
TDC cutter Video courtesy DORC
Flow TDC cutter Video courtesy DORC
Chapter 4: No video
Chapter 5: No video
Chapter 6: No video
Chapter 7: **Biometry and Anaesthesia**
Biometry.

Surgery of Vitreoretinal Disorders—Past, Present, and Future

1

Relja Živojnović

Pre-Gonin era: Retinal detachment has always been a dramatic and terrifying experience for the patient, and for the surgeon, a source of frustration for a long time. Practical knowledge in the nineteenth century was based on pathoanatomical observations, and the therapy consisted of drainage and bed rest. The invention and introduction of ophthalmoscopy by Helmholtz in 1851, enabling fundus visualization in vivo for the first time marked the decisive step in understanding and treatment of retinal detachment. Nevertheless, it took 70 long years to totally comprehend the course and dynamics of the pathological process. The main components of this process—traction, fluid, current in the eye as well as the hole in the retina were observed separately, but were not causally connected. The importance of particular components of the pathological process was either over- or underestimated, while the therapy itself relied on the surgeon's assumptions. Cutting of the» vitreous strands« Deutschmann, Graefe; Intraocular injection of various substitutes with or without drainage of subretinal fluid; extensive diathermy—Lagrange; shortening of the eyeball—Müller, combined with strict bed rest and positioning are some of many futile attempts whose rare positive results were at the most only temporary.

R. Živojnović (✉)
Stjepe Sarenca, 285340 Herceg Novi, Montenegro
e-mail: info@milosklinika.com

1.1 The Beginning of Retinal Surgery—Jules Gonin

In the early twentieth century, after extensive studies of pathological specimens, ophthalmoscopic observation of the dynamics of the pathological process and looking for holes in the retina, trying all the hitherto applied surgical methods in the treatment of retinal detachment, Jules Gonin, Lausanne, Switzerland, came to the epochal conclusion that a hole in the retina is the cause of detachment. Using Paquelin's thermocautery to perforate the eyeball on the spot of the defect and incarcerating its edges by the withdrawal of the needle, he achieved retinal reattachment. Using this method, he successfully reattached the retina in 40–50% of cases. After long years of disbelief and dismissal, he finally got recognition for his work at the international congress in Amsterdam in 1929. His enthusiastic followers were Arruga in Spain, Amsler in Switzerland, and Wewe in the Netherlands. However, in spite of the 40–50% success rate in the previously inoperable cases, a large number of patients still could not be treated successfully. The reason was that the treatment did not comprise the other two components of the pathological process, vitreoretinal traction and fluid current in the eye. Shortening of the eyeball to reduce its volume as introduced by Lindner and later by Wewe, based on earlier attempts by Müller, resulted in certain improvements.

U. Spandau et al. (eds.), *Retinal Detachment Surgery and Proliferative Vitreoretinopathy*,
https://doi.org/10.1007/978-3-031-11946-0_1

Ophthalmoscopy. As it was said before, in 1850, Helmholtz introduced ophthalmoscopy, which technically consisted of a strong source of light near the patient's head, a concave mirror with a hole in the middle through which the surgeon—by means of reflected light via convex lens—could see the lightened fundus. In the 1950s, that system was developed into a sophisticated ophthalmoscope with light and a system of lenses, which was used as both direct and indirect ophthalmoscope. Development of visualization was of crucial importance for the development of vitreoretinal surgery and had a curious course. In the early 1950s, Schepens, Boston, USA, and the Fison in London, UK, designed the binocular indirect ophthalmoscope, which was accepted and used in these countries at the time. In Germany, the Zeiss ophthalmoscope for direct and indirect ophthalmoscopy came into use very early. In the 1960s, it was replaced by the bonoscope, an indirect monocular ophthalmoscope with extra strong light. In France, indirect ophthalmoscopy was as good as unknown and direct ophthalmoscope was used in surgery, which culminated in the use of Goldmann′s three-mirror glass under the microscope. The superiority of the binocular indirect ophthalmoscope with the possibility of indentation of the periphery was obvious, so in the 1980s, it was eventually generally accepted. For diagnostic purposes, besides the ophthalmoscope, Goldmann's three-mirror glass and panfundoscope for its panoramic picture were used. In the 1990s, they were all replaced by 90D lens.

1.2 Scleral Indentation

The introduction of scleral indentation was a capital contribution to this surgery, as it simultaneously treated all three components of the pathological process: vitreoretinal traction, fluid current, and their consequence—the retinal hole. The first attempt at indentation—»buckle«—was reported in 1937, when Jess sutured a gauze tampon under Tenon's capsule. Although basically logical, this attempt did not find followers. The father of the»buckle« surgery was undoubtedly Ernst Custodis, Duesseldorf, Germany, who used a plastic "egzoplant" sutured on the sclera. This technique was soon accepted and increased positive results in the surgery to 80%. However, frequent complications of globe perforation due to the hardness of the plastic material, combined with surface diathermy, inspired surgeons in many countries to look for other solutions. For detachments with multiple holes in the periphery, Arruga introduced *cerclage equatorial*—circumferential buckle—by suturing a nylon thread through the sclera on the equator of the eyeball. The logic and simple use of this method were appealing. Perhaps that is why perforation of the globe during surgery and ischemia of the anterior segment postoperatively were rather frequent complications. The idea itself was perfected by Schepens, Boston, USA, who used softer material, i.e., silicone. An encircling band with or without a radial buckle, combined with diathermy replaced finally Arruga's cerclage. Complications with plastic material inspired Pofique and Spira Lyon, France to use biological material—human sclera. Lamellar scleral pocket—*poche scleral*—filled with pieces of the human sclera or sutured upon the sclera—*poche apportee*—filled with the same material were frequently used in the 1960s. At the same time, Kloeti, Zuerich, Switzerland, propagated the use of fascia lata as cerclage material. Naturally, biological materials did not cause any complications, but the effect of indentation was short-lived, and in some cases caused redetachment. Looking for new materials more or less ended, when Lincoff, New York, USA, introduced silastic sponge and replaced diathermy with cryocoagulation. In the early 1970s, this became the method of choice in the treatment of detachment and has been sustained as such up to the present time. Recently hydrogel as the material for indentation has not brought much change.

Retinopexy: The purpose of retinopexy is to create a chorioretinal scar and it has no impact on vitreoretinal traction. After the use of thermocautery in Gonin's time, surgery moved on to non-perforative diathermy as introduced by Pischel. Diathermy coagulation, technically improved by Wewe, was applied for many years. In the 1970s, Lincoff, following Bietti's (Rome, Italy) experience, combined the silastic buckle with cryocoagulation, which, properly used, did not damage the sclera. It should be mentioned that extensive use of diathermy but also of cryocoagulation, may have very serious consequences and provoke proliferative process in the eye. At the beginning of the 1960s, Meyer Schwickerath, Essen, Germany, introduced xenon photocoagulation, which opened a new chapter in retinopexy. Laser coagulation based on the same principle and introduced by Zweng and Little, USA, was technically much easier to use and replaced completely xenon photocoagulation. In this way, the chapter of retinopexy has been completed.

1.3 Intraocular Tamponade

Owing to his attempt in 1911 to treat retinal detachment by means of intravitreal air injection, Ohm can be regarded as the forerunner of tamponade. With much more understanding of the pathological process, Rosengren, Gothenburg, Sweden, used the air for tamponade in 1938. In the early 1970s, Norton, Miami, USA, introduced SF6, and in the early 1980s, Lincoff pioneered long-lasting gases, which have the advantage of long-lasting tamponade and the disadvantage of expansion under low pressure.

Tamponade is fully effective only when combined with indentation. Without indentation, propagated as fast and cheap surgery, it only has a temporary effect because of the persistence of vitreoretinal traction. From the early 1970s, the»buckle« surgery combined with cryocoagulation, drainage if necessary, with or without tamponade has become the method of choice in the treatment of retinal detachment and it is successful in 90–95% of detachments with the mobile retina. But it failed with detachments complicated by multiple equatorial ruptures, giant tears, and detachments caused by proliferative process.

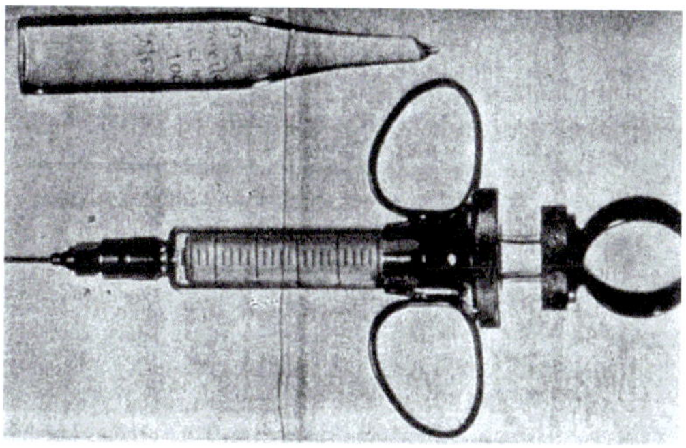

Fig. 1.1 Cibis syringe for injection of silicone oil

Introduction of silicone oil. In the 1970s, Paul Cibis, Saint Louis, USA, introduced silicone oil in retinal detachment surgery (Fig. 1.1). Under control of binocular ophthalmoscope in the reversed picture, using the surface tension of silicone oil and expansion of the silicone bubble, he tried to separate the detached retina from the changed vitreous and fibrotic membranes. At the same time, he tried to attach the retina by evacuating intraocular fluid. With successful results, he left silicone oil in the eye as permanent tamponade. By this extremely difficult technique, he achieved surprisingly good results in some cases that used to be inoperable. Probably owing to its difficult application, this technique had only a few followers in USA (Okun, Watzke). In the mid-1960s attempts of the use of this technique in some European countries were published—Moreau in France, Dufour in Switzerland, Liesenhof, Lund in Germany. Cibis' early death and legal problems concerning the use of silicone oil being an industrial product not registered by the FDA resulted in the restricted spread of this method. In Europe, surgeons did not use binocular ophthalmoscope and were not very familiar with the dynamics and consequences of pathological processes in the eye, which resulted in poor outcomes and the discontinuation of the use of silicone oil in Europe in the late 1960s.

Modern times. In the early 1970s John Scott, Cambridge, UK, impressed by Cibis' results with silicone oil, attempted the treatment of complex cases in which conventional technique was unsuccessful. Trying to separate fibrotic membranes and the changed vitreous body from the contracted retina by means of expansion of the silicone bubble, he also used intraocular instruments. He used the bent pick needle to lift membranes, the blunt flute needle for fluid evacuation, and scissors. The surgery was performed under the control of a binocular ophthalmoscope in the reversed picture. With a positive outcome, the central retina could be reattached and the fibrotic tissue and membranes pushed to the periphery. Silicone oil would stay as permanent tamponade preventing re-contraction of fibrotic tissue. With his skill, insight into the course of the pathological process, as well as by his enormous persistence, John Scott achieved remarkable results. Owing to the difficulty of the procedure itself and his good results, only a small number of surgeons could be compared to him, so Cambridge was the place of reference for patients from all over the world. With this method, John Scott made a huge step forward in the treatment of difficult cases, but even this method had its limitations. Giant tears with PVR, traumatic detachments with the incarcerated retina, diabetic tractional detachment, and others could not be treated successfully in this way. Permanent tamponade with silicone oil also caused complications in the long run.

At the end of the 1960s, David Kasner, Miami, USA, tried a new treatment of prolapse of the vitreous body during cataract surgery and trauma of the eye and called it open sky vitrectomy. Using cellulose sponges and scissors, he removed the prolapsed vitreous body. Through successful surgery, he proved that the vitreous body was not of vital importance to the eye. In 1970, the new technique inspired Robert Machemer, Miami, USA, with the technical assistance of J.M. Parel, to design an instrument that enabled entering the vitreous space through a relatively small opening, and under the microscope to remove the blurred vitreous body. The multifunctional instrument called Vitreous Infusion Suction Cutter was a revolutionary step in the history of vitreoretinal surgery. After a short time, O'Malley introduced a bimanual system with a separate source of light and standardized system of 20 gauge instruments. Pars plana vitrectomy opened new possibilities in vitreous body surgery, but it was not aimed at the treatment of retinal detachment. Even more, the fear of injuring the retina during surgery was great and comparable to the fear of loss of the vitreous body in earlier cataract surgery. In USA, the standard procedure for the treatment of retinal detachment for more than 10 years was the silastic buckle with cryopexy and possible gas tamponade. Complex cases of detachment with proliferative process usually were not operated on. The only kind of detachment in which vitrectomy was implemented was the detachment caused by a hole in the macula, which due to its location used to present a problem. In the past, indentation techniques were applied with modest success, such as the silver ring of Rosengren, the silver plomb of Gloor, Zurich, Switzerland, and others. For this kind of detachment, pars plana vitrectomy with removal of epiretinal membranes, gas tamponade, and positioning was the method of choice then and has remained so ever since. Recently, the relocation of the macula as introduced by Machemer in the 1990s is one more indication of the implementation of vitrectomy.

Pars plana vitrectomy has opened new possibilities for research of proliferative processes which now can also be followed in pathological specimens of the ocular tissue. In the late 1970s, Machemer described the proliferative process in the eye on the basis of acquired specimens and clinical experience, and introduced the familiar name Proliferative Vitreo Retinopathy (PVR), instead of MVR (Massive Vitreous Retraction).

Pars plana vitrectomy was rather hesitantly accepted in Europe by way of pioneers in particular countries: Kloeti in Switzerland, Laqua and Heimann in Germany, and Leaver in the UK. In the 1970s, Jean Haut, Paris, France, was the first to combine vitrectomy with silicone oil.

1.4 The New Concept

In the early 1970s, practicing retinal surgery in Rotterdam, the Netherlands, I was dissatisfied with my results. Visiting other centers in Europe—Zurich, Bonn, Paris—and comparing my work with that of the others, I did not notice major differences in results. After several visits to John Scott, I was convinced that his technique and approach were absolutely superior to anything I had seen before. In the late 1980s, I implemented his technique in surgery of a considerable number of patients and achieved results satisfying for that time. After a year, together with Diane Mertens, I abandoned binocular ophthalmoscopy. I switched to the surgical microscope with a contact lens (Fig. 1.2). Now I had a free hand and a direct image as in reality. For me, the surgical microscope is part of vitrectomy as a surgical technique.

I also abandoned combined vitrectomy with silicone oil, using it only as temporary tamponade. As the admitted patients were increasingly complex, it was soon obvious that this technique also had its limitations. In complex cases, when due to proliferative process the retina was contracted, incarcerated or shortened, removal of all membranes and scarred tissue was not sufficient to produce results we aspired to. The only solution for these cases appeared to be surgical intervention—retinotomy and retinectomy. Initially, only one-eyed patients in a desperate situation were treated in this manner. Nevertheless, I very soon managed to operate a considerable number of the most difficult, previously inoperable cases with favorable results.

I, therefore, established a new concept of treatment, which consisted of vitrectomy, meticulous removal of all epi- and subretinal membranes, retinal surgery, retinotomy, retinectomy, if necessary, laser coagulation, and temporary tamponade with silicone oil. After the first publications and frequent presentations at meetings, the introduction of retinal surgery in the arsenal of surgical measures was soon accepted and adopted.

At the very beginning of the development of this demanding technique, I was confronted with the absence of adequate instruments for this new kind of surgery. The presence of Ger Vijfvinkel, a technician in our hospital, was crucial for the development of new instruments (Fig. 1.3).

His frequent presence in the operating theater and observation of surgery resulted in prompt design and construction of adequate instruments. Besides numerous small instruments, we developed together the foot-driven silicone pump (Fig. 1.4), the back-flush needle with a silicone tip (Fig. 1.5), 4-port system, 25-gauge vitreous cutter and instruments, replaced Ando's plastic tacks with steel ones for perioperative use, etc. Ger Vijfvinkel with his inventiveness contributed considerably to the development of vitreoretinal surgery.

This new, more aggressive concept of vitreoretinal surgery was not associated with many postoperative complications. After the introduction of 6 o'clock iridectomy (Ando, Japan, 1986), the problem of the pupillary block was solved. Other complications could be ascribed to inadequate surgical technique or to the continuation of proliferative process which required frequent reoperations. This proliferative process was also often provoked by careless surgery. It should be mentioned that the pathological basis of all complex cases was the biological process

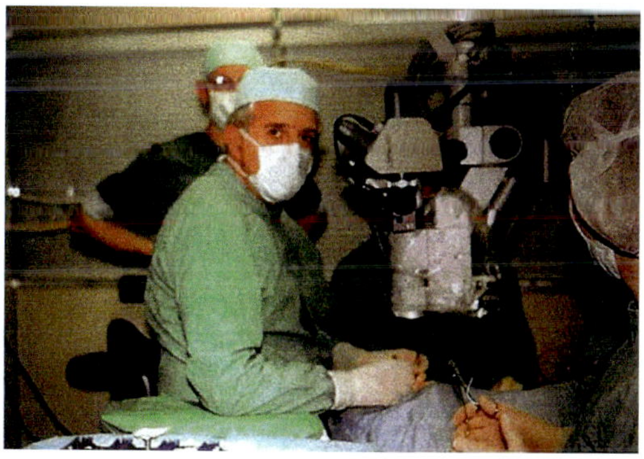

Fig. 1.2 The surgical microscope is an essential part of vitrectomy

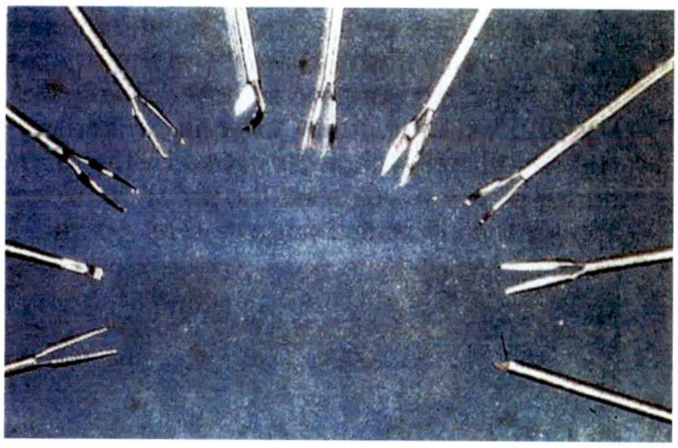

Fig. 1.3 Scissors and forceps

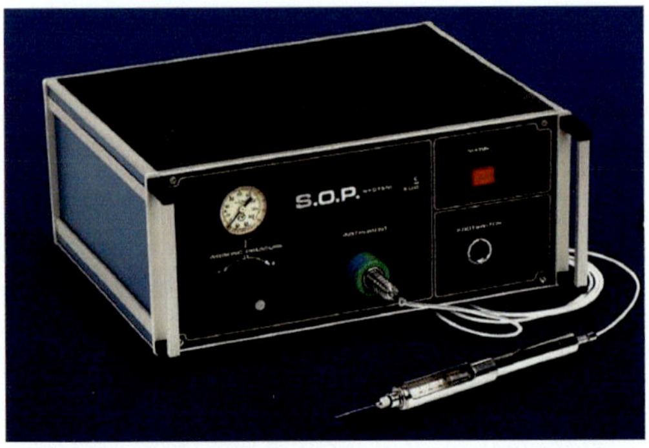

Fig. 1.4 Air driven silicone oil pump

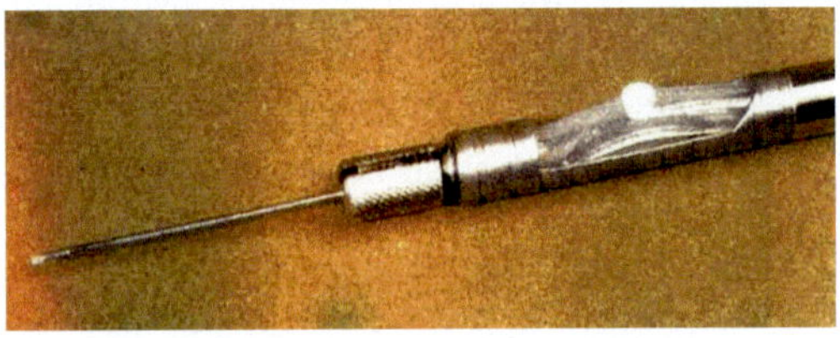

Fig. 1.5 Back-flush needle with silicone tip

and that surgical therapy is only adequate and indicated in absence of better and more appropriate treatment.

In the last 20 years, no radical changes in therapy have taken place. Introducing PFCL (heavy liquid) Stanley Chang greatly simplified the surgical process. Double filling silicone with PFCL as used by Peperkamp, Rotterdam, Netherlands, in the prevention of inferior detachment gave positive results. Improved visualization of membranes by the use of colors—trypan blue—as well as triamcinolone acetonide for better visualization of vitreous cortex, made the surgical process easier and safer. The use of finer instruments, thinner vitreous cutters, as well as sutureless vitrectomy, simplified the course of surgery. Even with all this technical progress, meticulous removal of complete proliferative tissue before retinal surgery and injection of silicone oil remains an absolute must for the success of the operation.

A correctly performed »buckle« surgery with a binocular ophthalmoscope and its success rate of 90–95%, with the mobile retina, is practically complications-free. (Choroidal bleeding at drainage is the complication most frequently mentioned, which we practically reduced to zero by using the blunt lacrimal probe for penetration of the choroid after incision of the sclera.) This conventional surgery is much cheaper than vitrectomy in terms of both personnel and instruments. Pars plana vitrectomy in itself is an invasive method with more possible complications such as endophthalmitis, cataract, etc. However, nowadays there are few people ready to master indirect ophthalmoscopy and I am afraid that in the future, conventional surgery will lose the battle with 90D lens, wide angle microscope, and vitrectomy.

Finally, I would like to add a few comments. Development of the surgery has confirmed an old truth again: Not a single, even the most important step in development can exist alone but only builds on earlier achievements of its predecessors. Still, the development of vitreoretinal surgery was many times slowed down for seemingly incomprehensible reasons. For instance, it took many years before absolutely superior binocular ophthalmoscopy was generally accepted in Europe. Further, more than 10 years after the epochal invention of pars plana vitrectomy, the complex pathology was not treated in USA, while at the same time, such cases were successfully treated in Cambridge. How to explain it? Was it complacency, vanity, conservatism, or arrogance? Perhaps some of it all but the main reason was the poor flow of information. For a long time, retinal surgeons were perceived as curious people, almost nerds, and were isolated. Results of both successful and unsuccessful operations were considered inadequate. For quite a while, the prestigious bi-annual Gonin club meeting was almost the only place for the exchange of ideas and experiences. The presentation technique was weak and unconvincing. Mutual visits were not frequent or common, and learning and transfer of knowledge were not formalized, at least not in Europe.

This situation dramatically changed in the early 1980s. With the introduction of new surgical methods, new technology, and better results, interest in new surgery was on the rise. At numerous meetings, the new surgery was presented by new visual means: film, video, live surgery, in an attractive, instructive, and impressive way. Initially, that advancement was limited to the developed countries, but now, it has covered most countries that can afford it. Vitreoretinal surgery is not restricted to a small number of places. Instead, the number of centers, as well as the number of vitreoretinal surgeons, have multiplied.

2 Lincoff Rules and Surgical Techniques for Retinal Detachment

Zoran Tomic and Ulrich Spandau

2.1 Lincoff Rules for Retinal Detachment

A thorough and correct assessment of the detached retina is essential for surgical success. The retina behaves logically. And you need to understand this logic in order to understand retinal detachment.

What is the anatomical course of a retinal detachment?

Lincoff and Gieser [1] found the following development of a retinal detachment (Fig. 2.1): A retinal detachment spreads first to the ora serrata. The subretinal fluid continues then to the optic disc.

The next most important theoretical knowledge for retinal detachment are the Lincoff rules.

Lincoff rules: Lincoff and Gieser examined 1000 patients with retinal detachments and extracted 4 different shapes of retinal detachments [1]:

(1) The superior detachment is identical to a total detachment. A superior detachment develops/goes over to a total detachment (Fig. 2A, B).
(2) The superotemporal/superonasal detachment (Fig. 2C, D).
(3) The inferior shallow detachment (Fig. 2E).
(4) The inferior highly bullous detachment (Fig. 2F).

The **second finding** of Lincoff and Gieser is that every detachment shape (1–4) has a rupture at a specific location. This rupture (=primary hole) is responsible for the specific shape of detachment. More ruptures are possible but in most cases, there is only one second hole which is within 1 quadrant of the primary hole. The location of the primary hole is as follows (Fig 2.3):

(1) Superotemporal/superonasal detachment: The primary hole lies within 1 ½ clock hours of the highest border.
(2) Superior/total detachment: The primary hole is located within a triangle where the apex is located at 12:00 and the sides at 10:30 and 1:30.
(3) The inferior shallow detachment has a hole on the side with the higher detached edge. The hole is located in an area between the upper edge of the retinal detachment and 6:30.
(4) The inferior highly bullous detachment is the most astounding one. The small hole is not, as one may expect, located in the inferior pole but at 11:00 or 1:00. A peripheral bridge connects the hole with the inferior detachment.

Z. Tomic
Milos Klinika, Belgrade, Serbia

U. Spandau (✉)
St Eriks Hospital, University of Stockholm, Stockholm, Sweden
e-mail: ulrich_spandau@yahoo.de

U. Spandau et al. (eds.), *Retinal Detachment Surgery and Proliferative Vitreoretinopathy*,
https://doi.org/10.1007/978-3-031-11946-0_2

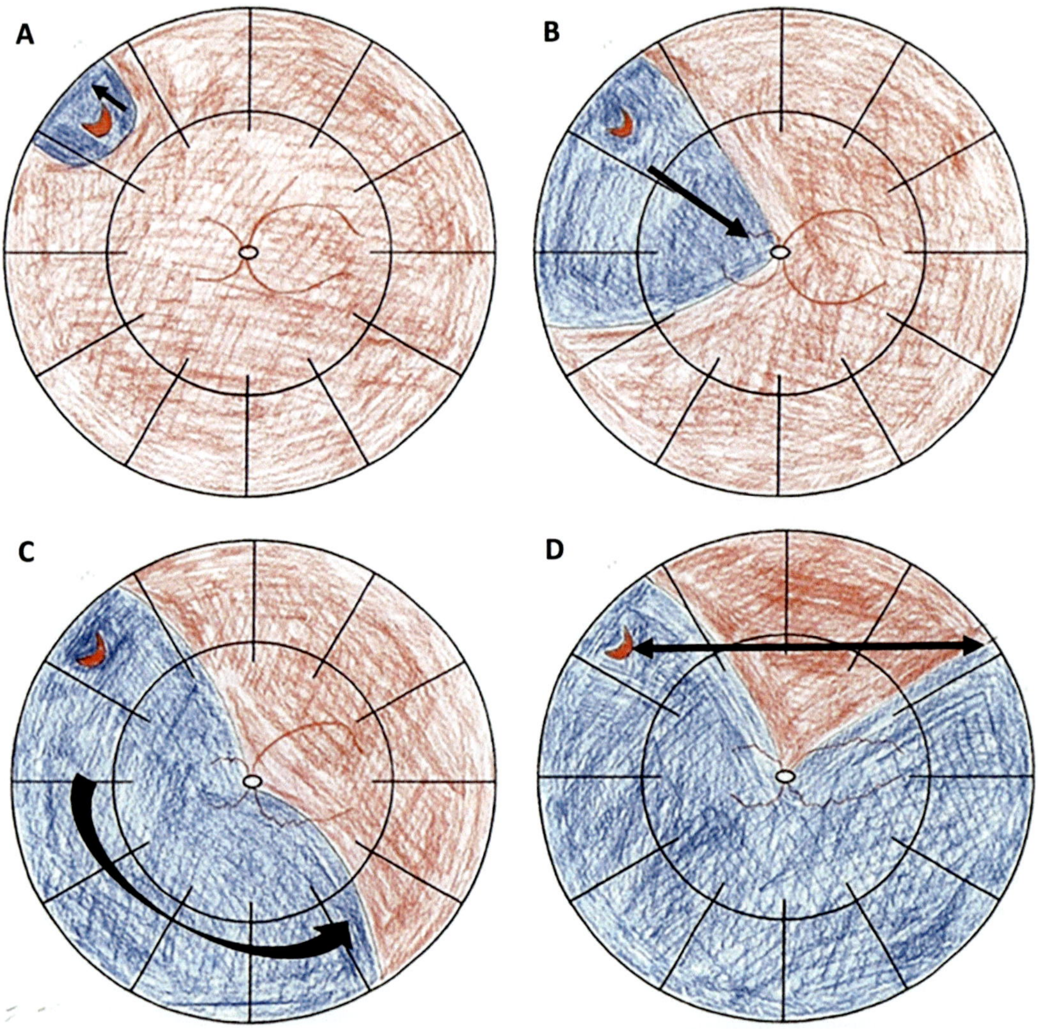

Fig. 2.1 Development of a retinal detachment. A horse shoe tear at 10:30. The detachment spreads first to the ora serrata **A**. Then the subretinal fluid moves towards the optic disc **B**. Then the retinal detachment continues towards the inferior pole **C**. Finally the detachment moves upwards until it reaches the height of the break on the other side **D**. It will not move further, a total retinal detachment is not possible with a hole at 10:30

Frequency of Lincoff 1-4 detachments [1]:
The frequency of the superior detachments is 80%.
The frequency of the inferior detachments is 20%.

We mention always the retinal rupture and the influx of fluid into the subretinal fluid. But we forget that the RPE pumps continuously subretinal fluid out of the eye (Fig 2.4). Why is this important? If the rupture is closed, then the subretinal fluid will be removed by the eye itself. Drainage is NOT necessary. In episcleral buckling surgery, for example, a buckle seals the hole but drainage is not required. The retina will be attached after 1–2 days.

2.2 Short Introduction to Surgical Methods

Retinal detachment surgery is divided into two main techniques: (1) Internal approach with gas injection and (2) External approach with episcleral buckling.

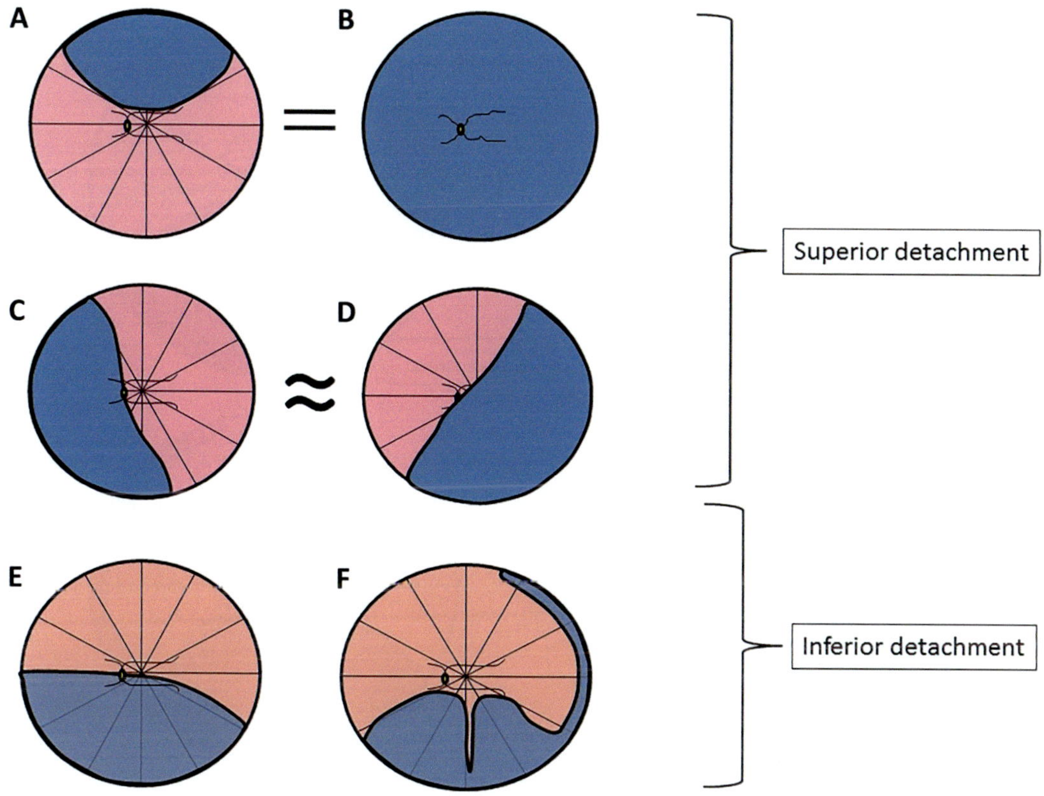

Fig. 2.2 Lincoff and Gieser found two types of superior detachments and two types of inferior detachments. The superior **A** or total detachment **B** is identical. The superonasal **C** detachment is equivalent to the superotemporal **D** detachment. Regarding the inferior detachments a shallow detachment **E** and a highly bullous detachment **F** can be identified

At the University of Stockholm we employ the following surgical methods:

(1) Pneumatic retinopexy
(2) Lenssparing vitrectomy with cryopexy and gas (Moorfield technique)
(3) Combined phaco + vitrectomy with chandelier light and PFCL (Frankfurt technique)
(4) Encircling band + vitrectomy + C_3F_8 (Stockholm technique)
(5) Bimanual peeling + 180–360° retinotomy for PVR detachment
(6) Minimal buckling surgery with chandelier light and microscope

We will give a short introduction to the aforementioned techniques:

(1) Pneumatic retinopexy is very popular in California and has recently experienced a renaissance in Canada. Macula on and off detachments with breaks from 8 o'clock over 12 o'clock to 4 o'clock can be treated with this technique. The retina is reattached with gas injection and one day later laser photocoagulation of the break is performed. The risk for a recurrent RD is increased but the final visual and anatomical outcome is high.

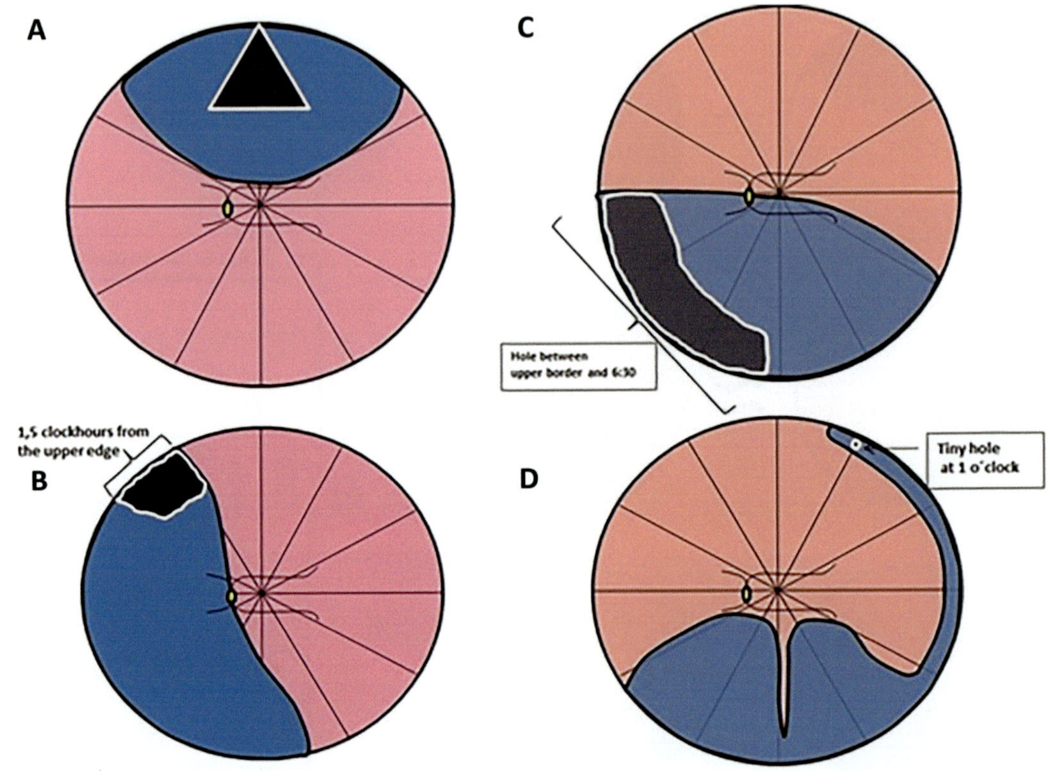

Fig. 2.3 **A: Superior or total detachment**. The primary break is located within a triangle where the apex is located at 12:00 and the sides at 10:30 and 1:30. **B: Superotemporal/superonasal detachment**. The primary break lies within 1 ½ clock hours of the highest border **C: Inferior shallow detachment**. The hole is located in an area between the upper edge of the retinal detachment and 6:30. **D: Inferior highly bullous detachment**. A small hole is located at 11:00 or 1:00

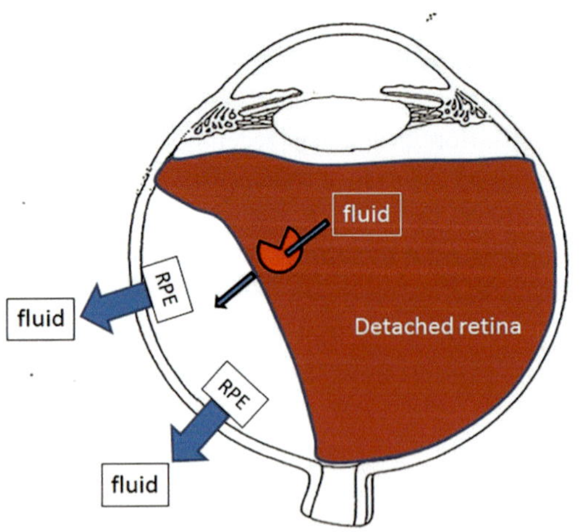

Fig. 2.4 Fluid flows through the rupture into the subretinal space. At the same time, the RPE pumps the subretinal fluid outside. A bullous detachment is attached after 1–2 days

(2) The Moorfield technique is the most common technique at Moorfield hospital, London. A lens sparing vitrectomy is performed, the retinal ruptures are treated with cryopexy and gas is injected. A vitreous base shaving is not performed. The surgical time is short and the required material is limited. This technique is used for all types of RD. Also, macula off techniques are operated with this technique.

(3) The combined phaco/vitrectomy is nowadays the gold standard technique for RD and was developed by Prof Eckardt in Frankfurt, Germany. In patients with an age over 50 years, phacoemulsification is performed and a chandelier light is inserted. A complete vitrectomy with vitreous base shaving is performed. The anterior vitreous

can be removed completely reducing the risk for a PVR redetachment.

(4) The Stockholm technique is the standard technique for all types of detachments at St Eriks hospital in Stockholm. This technique is especially advisable for myopic patients and inferior detachments. The surgery is usually performed without phacoemulsification. An encircling band is placed, and a central and peripheral vitrectomy is performed. The subretinal fluid is removed through a posterior retinotomy. The standard tamponade is C_3F_8.

(5) This method is employed for PVR detachments with intravitreal and retinal PVR. An encircling band is placed, a chandelier light is inserted and the membranes are removed with bimanual peeling. If necessary a 180–360° retinotomy is performed. This technique is surgically very demanding and requires several intravitreal instruments.

(6) Episcleral buckling is still required for RD surgery and is demonstrated in this book with an easier technique. Indirect binocular ophthalmoscopy is not required. For visualization of the fundus, a chandelier light is inserted and a microscope with a viewing system is employed. Cryopexy and suturing of the segmental buckle are done with the microscope.

2.3 Which Technique for Which Detachment

All superior retinal detachments with breaks from 8 over 12 to 4 o'clock including macula off can be operated with pneumatic retinopexy, Moorfield technique and phaco/vitrectomy.

An inferior detachment with breaks from 5 to 7 o'clock can be operated with episcleral buckling, Stockholm technique and Frankfurt technique with Densiron Xtra tamponade.

Ora dialysis and young myopes are excellent indications for episcleral buckling.

2.4 Assessment at the University of Stockholm

The choice of surgical technique for surgical management of retinal detachment differs from clinic to clinic and even from surgeon to surgeon. Here we present the choice of techniques we use at the University of Stockholm.

Attached retinal break versus detached retinal break.

An eye with a retinal detachment has always a detached tear and sometimes also attached tears. We recommend treating all attached breaks *with laser before* surgery. We recommend laser and not cryopexy because the healing time is faster and the PVR risk lower. In contrast, a detached break is treated *during* surgery. A detached break can only be treated with cryopexy. Treatment with laser is only possible after attachment of the tear with PFCL or gas.

Focal detachment: Pneumatic retinopexy technique.

A retinal break with detached edges is a focal detachment. A focal detachment requires treatment with gas or episcleral buckle to attach the break onto the retinal pigment epithelium and then laser photocoagulation or cryopexy of the retinal edges. A focal detachment cannot be treated with laser alone. Figure 2.5 shows an example where a focal detachment was treated with laser photocoagulation. A complete laser barrier was not performed. This focal detachment may spread later to a large detachment, especially when a posterior vitreous detachment (PVD) occurs. *Remember*: A focal detachment is only sufficiently treated when the edge of the break is attached. We treat these focal detachments with pneumatic retinopexy.

Superotemporal, superonasal and superior detachments with ***macula on****: Moorfield technique.*

Retinal detachments with attached macula are best operated with the Moorfields technique (Fig. 2.6A, B). We operate macula on

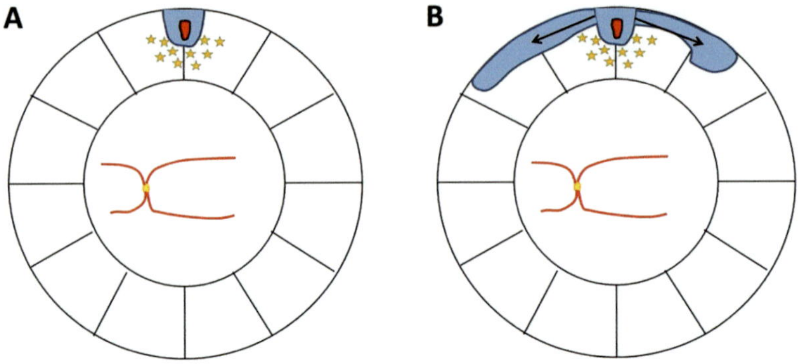

Fig. 2.5 **A**: An eye with a focal detachment at 12 o'clock. The focal detachment was treated with a partial laser barrier. The posterior part could not be treated due to the focal detachment. **B**: An eye with a focal detachment at 12 o'clock. This focal detachment may remain stable for several years but in the case of PVD, the focal detachment may spread to both sides

detachments with detached tears between 8 to 12 and 4 o'clock. We do not use this technique for detached breaks from 4 to 8 o'clock. We do not operate macula off RD´s with this technique because the postoperative posture is strict. Surgery is easy, fast and has low costs. A core and peripheral vitrectomy are performed; shaving is not necessary. The break is treated with cryopexy and then gas is injected.

Superotemporal, superonasal and superior detachments with ***macula off****: Phaco/vitrectomy (Frankfurt technique).*

The huge majority (80%) of retinal detachments are superior, superotemporal and superonasal. Usually, one detached retinal break is present (Figs. 2.7 and 2.8). If the macula is detached we choose the combined phaco/vitrectomy technique. Why? We want to attach the macula during surgery. Pneumatic retinopexy and Moorfield technique attach the macula after surgery with postoperative posture.

Myopic detachments, several break detachment: Stockholm technique.

Myopic detachments with lattice and several breaks are best operated with an encircling band, vitrectomy and gas tamponade. Usually, phacoemulsification is not performed, the subretinal fluid is removed from a posterior retinotomy and tamponade with C_3F_8 is chosen (Fig. 2.9).

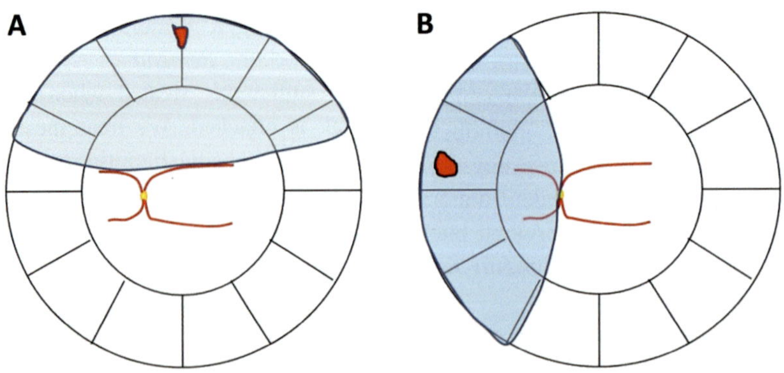

Fig. 2.6 **A**: A superior retinal detachment from 9:00 to 2:30 and one retinal break at 12 o'clock. Macula is attached. **B:** A nasal retinal detachment with the attached macula and one retinal break at 9 o'clock. Macula is attached

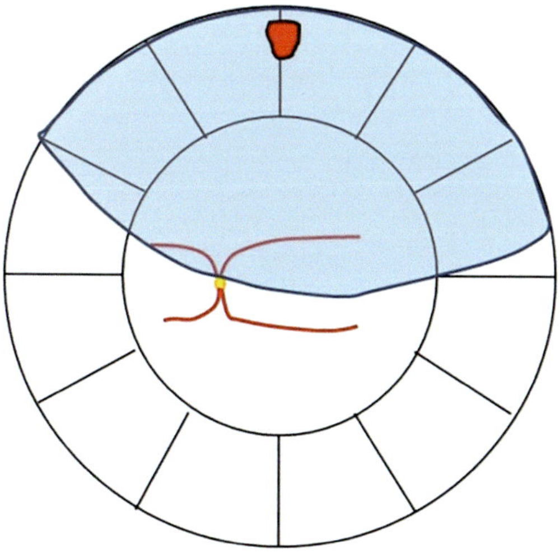

Fig. 2.7 A superior detachment with rupture at 12 o'clock

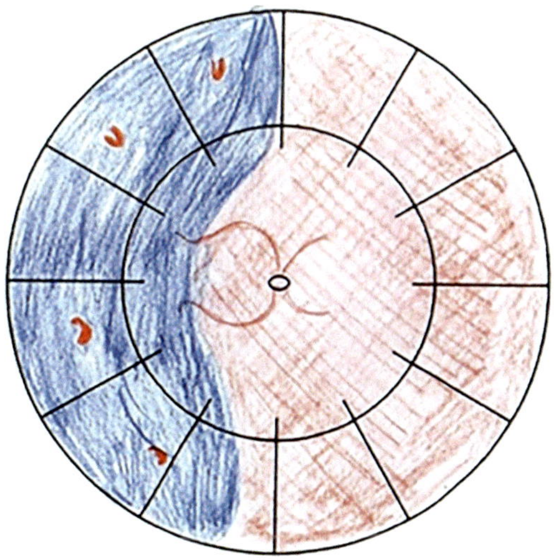

Fig. 2.9 A myopic detachment. A temporal detachment with breaks in 2 quadrants

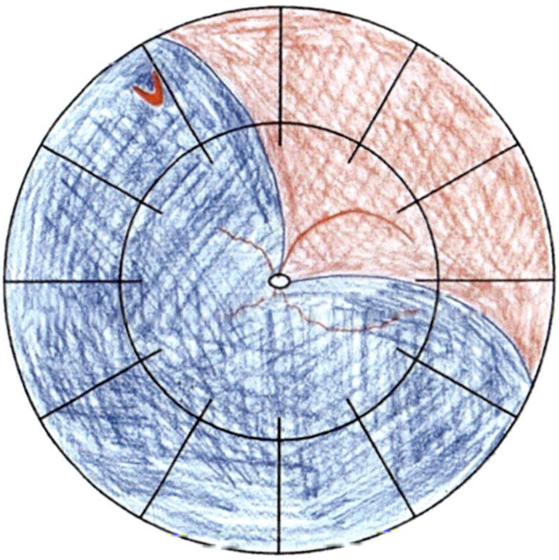

Fig. 2.8 A superotemporal detachment. A suitable surgical technique is a combined phaco/vitrectomy

Inferior detachments: Stockholm technique or Frankfurt technique with Densiron Xtra.
When approaching an inferior detachment the surgery becomes more challenging. In case of an inferior detachment with a break at 4 or 8 o'clock, all techniques can be employed because a long-acting gas and correct postoperative posture cover the break at 4 o'clock (Fig. 2.10A). Even Sf_6 may be used if the patient follows postoperative posture. In case of an inferior break between 5 and 7 o'clock, and especially 6 o'clock (Fig. 2.10B), the choice is limited [4]. In this case, a buckle or a tamponade with Densiron Xtra is required. The Stockholm technique with gas is possible because the encircling band covers inferior breaks. If you want to avoid an encircling band, we recommend the phaco/vitrectomy method with a Densiron Xtra tamponade. Remark: In case of silicone oil, we do not recommend the Moorfield method because the vitreous base is not removed in the Moorfield method which is necessary for a silicone oil tamponade.

Giant tear: Phaco/vitrectomy with silicone oil
For giant tears, vitrectomy is the technique of choice (Fig. 2.11). We recommend the phaco/vitrectomy method with a silicone oil tamponade because the risk for slippage is high. We do not recommend the Stockholm technique because the encircling band is not necessary and gas has a high risk for slippage. The same argument applies to the Moorfield technique. We recommend a vitrectomy with a silicone oil tamponade because the risk for slippage is minimal.

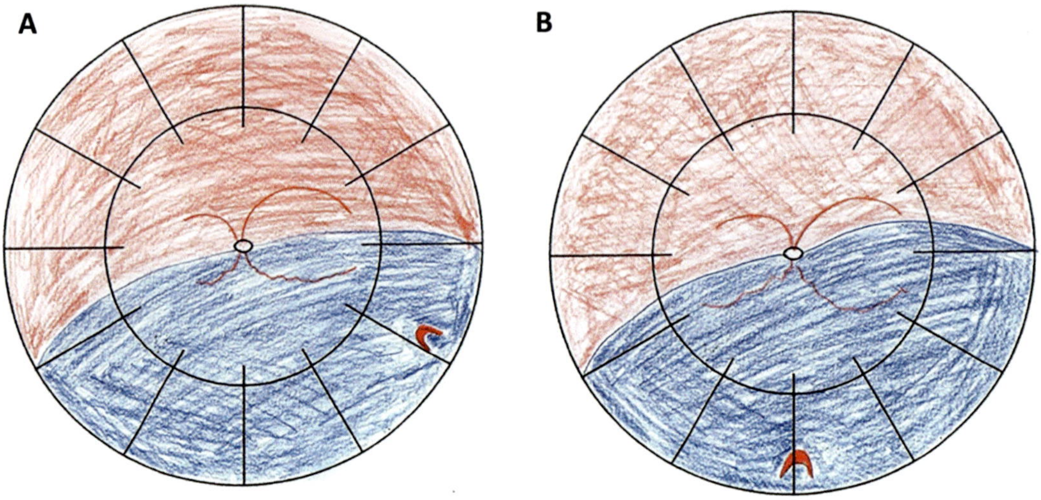

Fig. 2.10 An inferior detachment with a break at 4 o'clock **A** and at 6 o'clock **B**

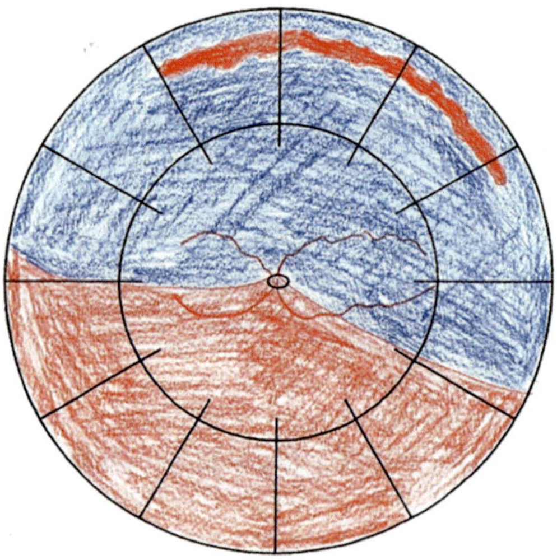

Fig. 2.11 A giant retinal tear has a length of 90 deg and more. A good candidate for vitrectomy

Young myope: Episcleral buckling.
In the United States, there are two remaining indications for episcleral buckling: Young myopic detachment and ora dialysis.

Retinal detachments in patients <40 years we operate with episcleral buckling. The posterior vitreous is attached and the optical media are clear. A typical example is young myopes. Myopic eyes with an inferior RD are a good indication for episcleral buckling surgery. Encircling bands and segmental buckles may be used for this pathology. An encircling band causes a myopic shift of approximately 3D and a segmental buckle causes astigmatism. In both cases, the buckle can be removed after 4 weeks so that the globe can regain its original shape. We prefer segmental buckles in these cases.

Example: A 27 y/o male patient with −3.5sph = 0.4 and an inferior detachment with 6 retinal breaks at 6–7 o'clock. Cryopexy and segmental buckle from 5:30 to 7:30 (under inferior rectus muscle) (Fig. 2.12A, B). One day postoperative the retina was attached.

Ora dialysis: Episcleral buckling.
The ora dialysis is another pathology where an episcleral buckling is recommended because the success rate of reattachment for ora dialysis is 99% with this technique. If you choose to operate an ora dialysis with vitrectomy, you need to achieve the same reattachment rate.

Example: 42 y/o male patient with ora dialysis at 6–7 o'clock and chronic inferior detachment due to trauma. Scleral buckling with a segmental

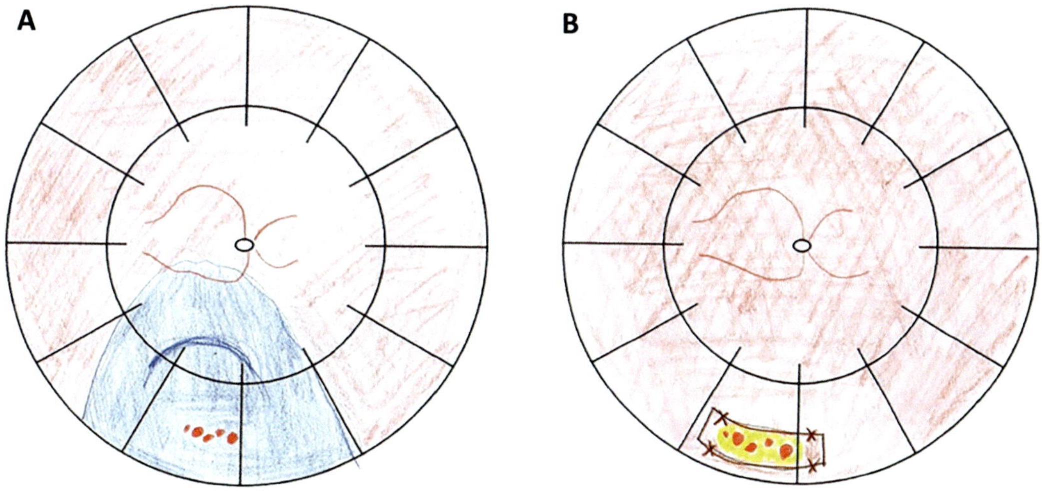

Fig. 2.12 Myopic retinal detachment **A** is an ideal candidate for scleral buckling **B**

buckle from 5 to 8 o'clock (under inferior rectus muscle) was performed (Fig. 2.13A). After 2 months, the subretinal fluid was reduced (Fig. 2.13B) and after 6 months the subretinal fluid had completely disappeared (Fig. 2.13C).

Recurrent retinal detachment (failed RD): Encircling band, vitrectomy

The highest risk for recurrent detachment has eyes with a VA <2/60, a detachment involving more than three quadrants and a previous retinal detachment [3]. The main problem for recurrent detachments is to find the retinal break. The Lincoff rules apply even here but if in the first surgery a 360 ° laser cerclage or extensive cryopexy was performed then the retinal break responsible for the recurrent detachment is now difficult to find. Our treatment algorithm for a recurrent detachment is depicted in Fig. 2.14.

*Chronic retinal detachment **without** PVR: Episcleral buckling*

An old retinal detachment is a complicated retinal detachment. If a clear retinal break is present and no tractive PVR is present, then episcleral buckling is easier than a vitrectomy. Subretinal strands are often present but have no contraindication for episcleral buckling.

A vitrectomy is technically difficult because you may need to remove the lens and then remove subretinal membranes resulting in increased PVR and recurrent detachment risk. If you choose episcleral buckling, things get much easier. The clear optical media in these young patients facilitates working with a binocular indirect ophthalmoscope or microscope and the attached vitreous makes reattachment easy. Place a segmental buckle on the break, external drainage is not necessary and the next day the subretinal fluid will be resorbed.

*Old retinal detachment **with** PVR: Encircling band, removal of membranes and silicone oil*

The PVR stage C is a surgically demanding RD with a high redetachment risk (Fig. 2.15). ZT and US have slightly different approaches. Usually, 2–3 surgeries are required. US would place an encircling band in the first surgery and ZT only in the second or third surgery. Both would do a bimanual peeling and choose a 1000 or 5000 csts silicone oil tamponade. Sometimes an inferior recurrent detachment occurs. In the second surgery, all new membranes are removed with bimanual peeling and a Densiron Xtra tamponade is chosen. Our treatment algorithm for PVR detachment stage C is depicted in Fig. 2.15.

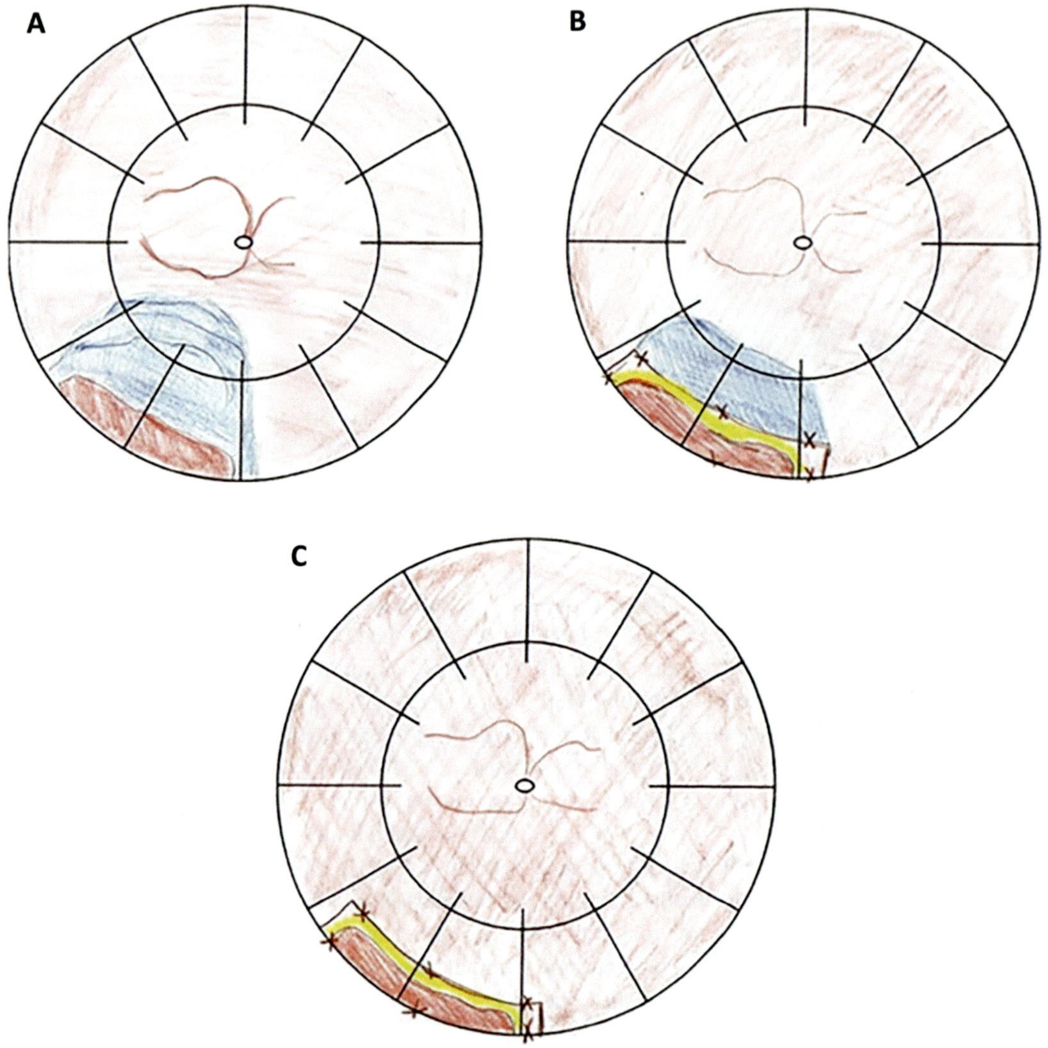

Fig. 2.13 **A, B, C**: chronic ora dialysis after trauma with a plastic ball 1 year ago **A**. A cryopexy with episcleral buckling was performed and after 2 months residual fluid was reduced **B**. After 6 months, the residual fluid was absorbed **C**

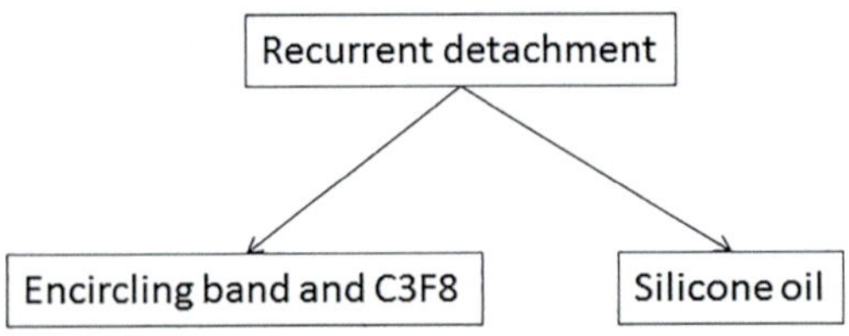

Fig. 2.14 Our treatment algorithm for a recurrent detachment. The two most common methods at our hospital are (1) encircling band with C_3F_8 and (2) silicone oil tamponade

Summary:

In short, we operate retinal detachments with the following techniques:

- Break with focal detachment: Pneumatic retinopexy
- Superior retinal detachment with macula on: Moorfield technique
- Superior retinal detachment with macula off: Phaco/vitrectomy technique

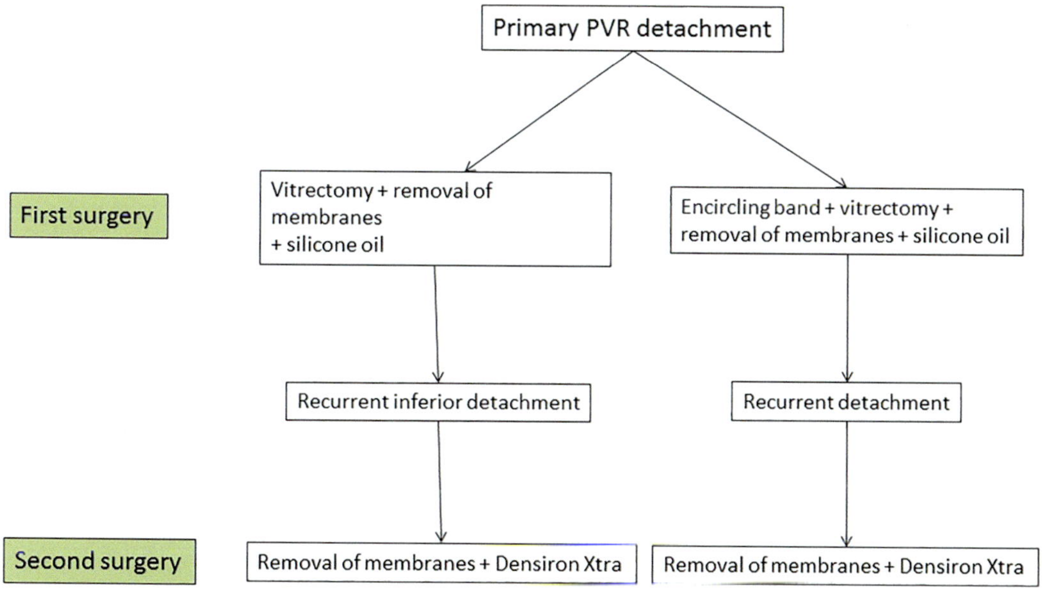

Fig. 2.15 Our treatment algorithm for a primary PVR stage C detachment and a recurrent detachment. Usually, two or even more surgeries are required. The author Ulrich Spandau would place an encircling band and perform a membrane peeling and inject silicone oil. The author Zoran Tomic would not place an encircling band in the first surgery, but remove meticulously all membranes until the retina is mobilized. Sometimes a recurrent detachment occurs at the inferior pole. This is operated with the removal of membranes and or laser and a change of silicone oil

- Inferior retinal detachment: Frankfurt technique with Densiron Xtra or Stockholm technique
- Giant tear: Frankfurt technique with silicone oil
- Myopic RD: Stockholm technique
- Ora dialysis and inferior RD in young myope: Episcleral buckling.

References

1. Lincoff H, Gieser R. Finding the retinal hole. Arch Ophthalmol. 1971;85(5):565–9.
2. Silicone Study Report 1. Vitrectomy with silicone oil or sulfur hexafluoride gas in eyes with severe proliferative vitreoretinopathy: results of a randomized clinical trial. Arch Ophthalmol. 1992;110(6):770–9.
3. Törnquist R, Bodin L, Törnquist P. Retinal detachment. A study of a population-based patient material in Sweden 1971–1981. IV. Prediction of surgical outcome. Acta Ophthalmol (Copenh). 1988;66 (6):637–42.
4. Starr MR, Obeid A, Ryan EH, Ryan C, Ammar M, Patel LG, Forbes NJ, Capone A Jr, Emerson GG, Joseph DP, Eliott D, Gupta OP, Regillo CD, Hsu J, Yonekawa Y. Primary retinal detachment outcomes (PRO) study group. Retinal detachment with inferior retinal breaks: primary vitrectomy versus vitrectomy with scleral buckle (PRO Study Report No. 9). Retina 2021;41(3):525–30. https://doi.org/10.1097/IAE.0000000000002917. PMID: 33600131.

Basics of Small Gauge Vitrectomy

3

Zoran Tomic and Ulrich Spandau

We started to operate vitrectomies with 20G sclerotomies. 20G sclerotomies have a diameter of 0.9 mm; see Table 3.1. In 2006, we switched to 23G trocar vitrectomy. We used trocars with valves from DORC. We were very satisfied and could not imagine at all switching to 25G. Then we started to operate membranes with 25G and had some problems with the softer peeling forceps. We returned to 23G but tried again with 25G for myopic eyes. This was a clear improvement because the globe had an improved postoperative tonus. And successively we switched completely to 25G.

Then 27G came up and again we thought that we would never use 27G. 27G has a diameter of 0.41 mm. But a few ROP cases forced us to use 27G. And then we used 27G for myopic eyes and 27G proved to be superior for myopic eyes compared to 25G. Regarding peeling surgery, we could not see an advantage. But in retinal detachment surgery, 27G was again superior to 25G because in 27G there is no leakage from the sclerotomies. At the end of the surgery, the globe has normal tonus; without sutures and without reinjecting gas. In addition, the lack of leakage results in prolonged gas tamponade.

Z. Tomic
Milos Klinika, Belgrade, Serbia

U. Spandau (✉)
St Eriks Hospital, University of Stockholm, Stockholm, Sweden
e-mail: ulrich_spandau@yahoo.de

Today we operate all our cases with 27G. 27G is in our experience the best gauge for the experienced vitreoretinal surgeon. The soft instruments, however, are a disadvantage that must be solved in the future.

3.1 Does Size Matter?

We are convinced that size does matter. The size was the major motivator to switch from ECCE to phacoemulsification. The small incisions of phacoemulsification are better in almost all aspects than the gaping wound of ECCE: faster postoperative recovery, improved visual results, less astigmatism and a closed and safe globe.

The same principle applies to vitrectomy. 27G trocars create sclerotomies with a size of 25G. 23G trocars, however, create a sclerotomy with a size of 22G (Fig. 3.1). After removing 27G trocars, the globe has normal tonus (without a gas filling). To achieve the same effect for 23G, you need a gas filling. And even with a gas filling, the eye often has low tonus directly after surgery. In 27G, the small sclerotomies induce an improved postoperative gas filling and less leakage which is important for retinal detachment surgery.

Smaller trocars result in smaller instruments. It is obvious that the small 27G instruments induce less intraoperative trauma and result in a faster postoperative recovery.

When talking about small gauge vitrectomy, we mention often sutureless vitrectomy. But 27G

U. Spandau et al. (eds.), *Retinal Detachment Surgery and Proliferative Vitreoretinopathy*,
https://doi.org/10.1007/978-3-031-11946-0_3

Table 3.1 Outer diameter of a needle in gauge and mm

Gauge	Diameter in mm
17	1.4
19	1.07
20	0.9
23	0.64
25	0.51
27	0.41
29	0.34
30	0.30

is the only sutureless vitrectomy; not 25G, not 23G. 27G is the only gauge where sutures are not required. In contrast, 25G and even more 23G sclerotomies require often sutures. If you operate on a myopic patient for retinal detachment then you need no sutures for 27G. And sutures result quite often in conjunctival granulomas, which are very irritating for the patient.

The principle "the smaller the Gauge, the better" is evident; see Table 3.2.

3.2 The Dilemma of the Law of Hagen–Poiseuille

But physics is against small gauge vitrectomy and 27G. The Hagen–Poiseuille equation states that the flow is proportional to the fourth power of the internal diameter of a lumen; see Table 3.3. The flow in 23G is 3.65 times slower than in 20G. The flow in 27G is 12.5 times slower than in 23G.

If the performance of a 23G cutter is 100%, then a 25G cutter has approximately 30% less performance and a 27G cutter approximately 30% less performance (Table 3.4).

This physical obstacle has been overcome with powerful vitrectomy machines and novel vitreous cutters with double cutting frequency and permanent flow. The novel double-cut vitrector has made 27G a fierce competitor of 23G.

3.3 27G and Double-Cut Vitreous Cutter

27G vitrectomy was developed in 2010 by Oshima and colleagues in Japan. The old 27G cutter had lower fluid dynamics and less cutting efficiency than a 25G cutter. The same is applied also for aspiration and infusion rates. These obvious disadvantages of 27G became obsolete after a novel type of vitreous cutter was introduced. The companies DORC (Netherlands) and Geuder (Germany) developed this novel double-cut citreous cutter.

3.4 History of Double-Cut Vitrector

The initial idea for the novel vitreous cutter came from Hayafuji and colleagues from Japan in 1992 (see Table 3.5). After a journey of trial and

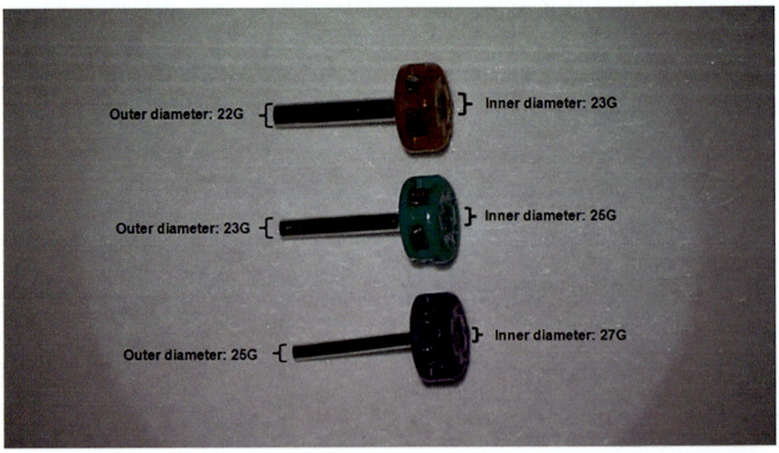

Fig. 3.1 The inner and outer size of the 23G, 25G and 27G trocar (Alcon)

Table 3.2 Advantages and disadvantages of 27G VR surgery

Advantages of 27G
A 27G trocar induces a 25G sclerotomy. A 23G trocar induces a 22G sclerotomy. A 22G sclerotomy is more prone to leakage of fluid and gas than a 25G sclerotomy
no sutures, no suture granuloma
no postoperative irritation and foreign body sensation ⇨ fast healing
less leakage ⇨ less postoperative hypotony ⇨improved gas tamponade
small instruments ⇨atraumatic surgery
Disadvantages of 27G
soft instruments

Table 3.3 Hagen–Poiseuille equation (**Flow** ≈ **diameter**^{4}) and its relevance for vitrectomy

Gauge	Diameter in mm	
23	0.6	3.65 × less flow than 20G
25	0.5	2.8 × less flow than 23G
27	0.42	12.5 × less flow than 23G

Table 3.4 Performance comparison of a regular and TDC cutter in relation to the Gauge. Measured is the aspiration time of artificial vitreous (Courtesy DORC)

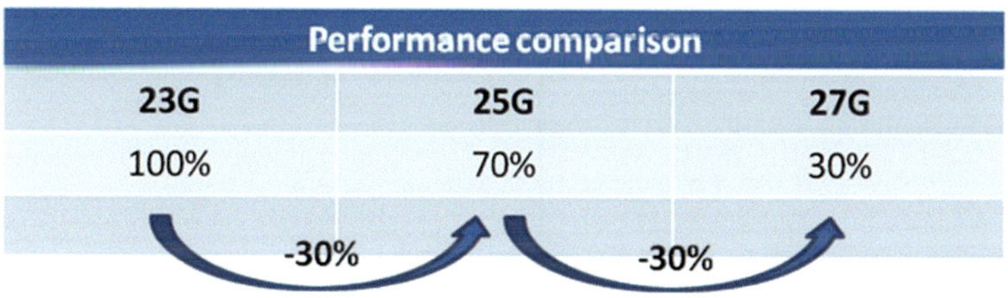

Table 3.5 Historical development of TDC cutter (Photo courtesy DORC)

Year	Description	Image
First idea (1992)	M. Hayafuji Y. Hanamura S. Niimura	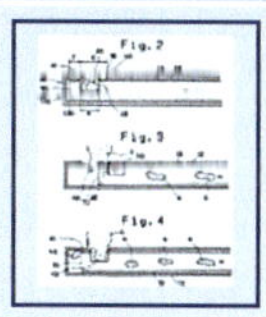
DORC (1996)	Vitreous shaver with 3 adjustable (slit) aspiration ports	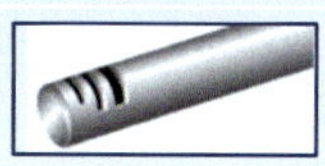

(continued)

Table 3.5 (continued)

Year	Description	Image
Luiz Lima (2010)	New dual port cutter system	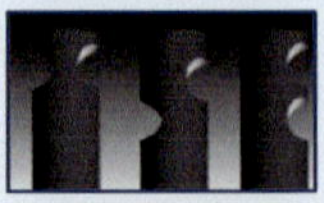
Rizzo (2011)	Extra aspiration port in internal capillary	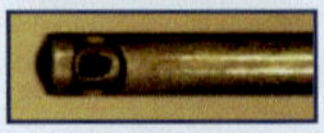
DORC (2013)	Twin duty cycle vitrectome	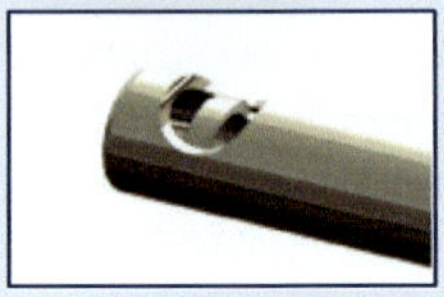

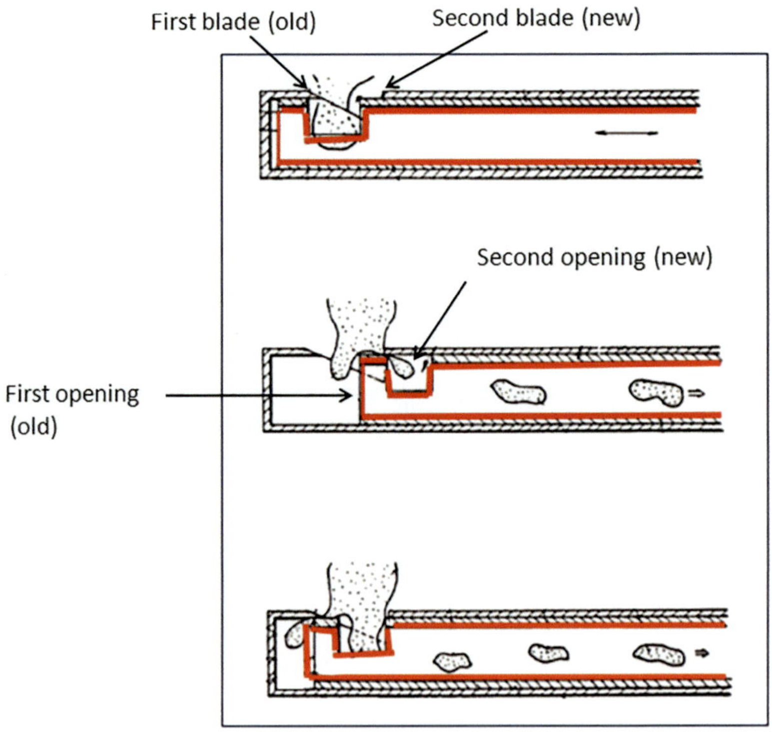

Fig. 3.2 The novel TCC cutter with two blades

errors, the final vitrector was developed in 2013 from DORC. This new vitreous cutter has two open cutting ports and a second cutting blade. It is named Twin Duty cycle (TDC) cutter (Fig. 3.2). This new invention comprises two new features: (1) a permanent flow and (2) two cutting blades.

3.5 The New TDC Cutter is Much Faster Than the Regular Cutter

The two cutting blades have the result that the cutter cuts two times during one movement, effectively doubling the cutting speed. The

Table 3.6 Performance comparison of TDC cutter versus regular cutter (Courtesy DORC)

TDC cutter 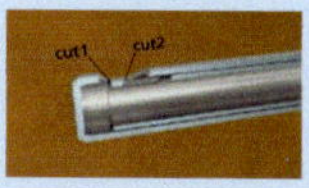	Comparison	Regular cutter 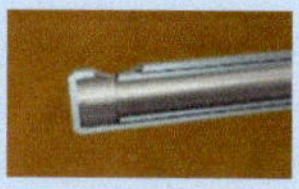
23G TDC	164% faster	23G regular
25G TDC	176% faster	25G regular
27G TDC	150% faster	27G regular

vitreous cutter has a cutting rate of 8000 cuts/min. But the actual cutting rate with two cutting blades is 8000 × 2 = 16,000 cuts/min, which reaches new dimensions. The second novelty is a continuous and even flow due to the two open-cutting ports. This novel technology reduces vitreous traction, decreases surgical time and increases the safety of surgery; see Table 3.6.

3.6 27G and PVR Detachment

Can 27G only be used for easy detachments and not for complicated detachments? Nowadays, all required intravitreal instruments such as scissors, forceps and delamination instruments are available in 27G. Regarding silicone oil removal or silicone oil injection, we insert a 25G trocar for this step. So, there is no hinder to employ 27G for difficult PVR detachments.

27G is *very useful* for the following pathologies:

(1) Children's eyes: No sutures necessary.
(2) Myopic eyes: No sutures necessary, excellent tamponade.
(3) Uveitis eyes: 27G causes minimal postoperative inflammation.
(4) Silicone oil removal: Less postoperative hypotony compared with 23G.
(5) Retinal detachment: Tight globe, less leakage resulting in better tamponade.

= > These are eyes that tend to have a postoperative hypotony and make them, therefore, excellent candidates for 27G.

27G is *less useful* for the following pathologies:

(1) Macular pucker: No advantage to 23G except for faster postoperative recovery.
(2) Macular hole: better tamponade with 27G but clinically no difference.

=> These eyes have a low risk of postoperative hypotony. There is not really a difference between 27G, 25G and 23G regarding this important feature. If you, however, wish a white eye after 1 week follow-up like after phacoemulsification, then you should again choose 27G.

3.7 Conclusion

27G is superior to 25G and 23G for retinal detachment because the small sclerotomies minimize leakage and result in a prolonged gas tamponade. In addition, the small 27G instruments are less traumatic resulting in less surgical trauma and faster postoperative recovery. The disadvantage of 27G is the softness of the instruments making the removal of the peripheral vitreous more difficult.

Devices and Instruments

4

Zoran Tomic and Ulrich Spandau

4.1 Chandelier Light Fiber

A chandelier light (Figs. 4.1, 4.2, 4.3 and 4.4) provides a panoramic light source and illuminates the entire fundus. Chandelier light is either fixated directly in the sclera (Fig. 4.1) or in a trocar (Fig. 4.2). This enables bimanual surgery and allows the surgeon to use a second active instrument in addition to the vitreous cutter. An alternative is the 27G—an Eckardt TwinLight Chandelier with scleral fixation (DORC 3269. MBD27) (Fig. 4.3).

For optimal illumination of chandelier light, an external light source (Photon, Xenon) or a modern vitrectomy machine (Stellaris PC, Constellation, Eva) is required. Old vitrectomy machines such as Accurus (Alcon) or Millenium (B&L) do not give sufficient light for a chandelier light fiber. In our OR we use the chandelier light from Synergetics (Fig. 4.1) and the external Photon illumination (Fig. 4.4).

4.2 Laser Photocoagulation and Cryopexy

Cryopexy A Cryo machine (DORC, ERBE) should be at our disposal in the operating room. The big advantage of cryopexy is that it can be performed on a *detached* retinal break. Laser coagulation can only be performed on an *attached* break. Indications are a cryopexy of a retinal break, the retina or the ciliary body due to neovascular glaucoma. Cryopexy is nowadays performed less frequently during vitrectomies because cryotherapy has been associated with a higher rate of PVR formation in some studies of retinal detachment surgery. Finally, the chorioretinal scar formation appears several days later following cryotherapy compared to laser retinopexy.

Laser photocoagulation One can purchase straight or curved laser probes (Fig. 2.13). The curved laser is particularly suitable for the peripheral retina; the straight laser is easier for the central posterior pole. If you apply a peripheral laser treatment (break, peripheral ischemic retina), the use of a scleral depressor is recommended, which makes the break more accessible and avoids touching the lens. This can be performed either using a chandelier light and a scleral depressor or using the light pipe as a scleral depressor with transscleral illumination. Alternatively, you can use a laser fiber with endoillumination (see below).

Z. Tomic
Milos Klinika, Belgrade, Serbia

U. Spandau (✉)
St Eriks Hospital, University of Stockholm, Stockholm, Sweden
e-mail: ulrich_spandau@yahoo.de

U. Spandau et al. (eds.), *Retinal Detachment Surgery and Proliferative Vitreoretinopathy*,
https://doi.org/10.1007/978-3-031-11946-0_4

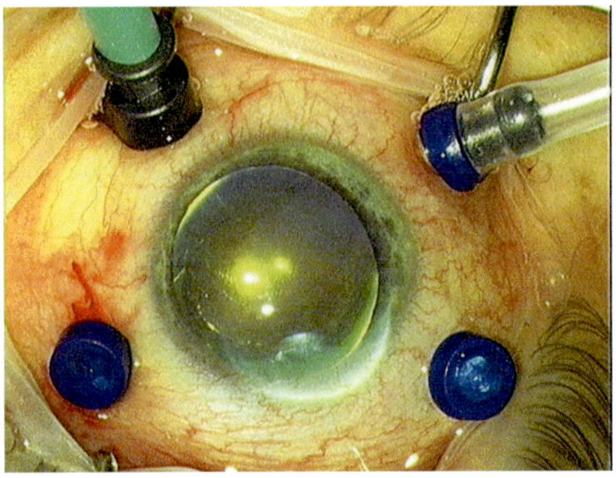

Fig. 4.1 4-port vitrectomy with chandelier light. The chandelier light is fixated into the sclera (Awh, Synergetics, USA)

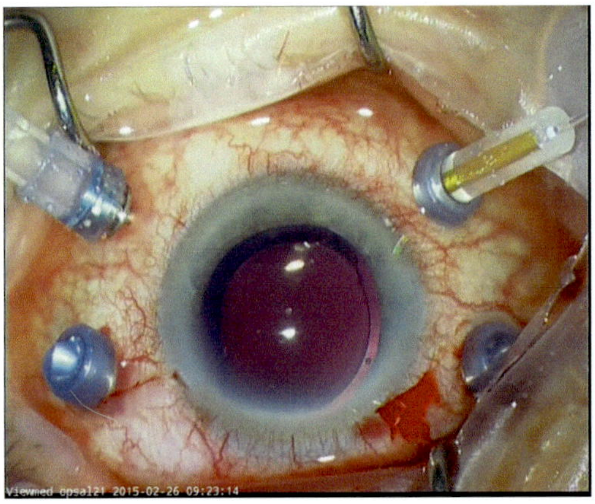

Fig. 4.2 This chandelier light is placed into a trocar which is technically easier (DORC, NL)

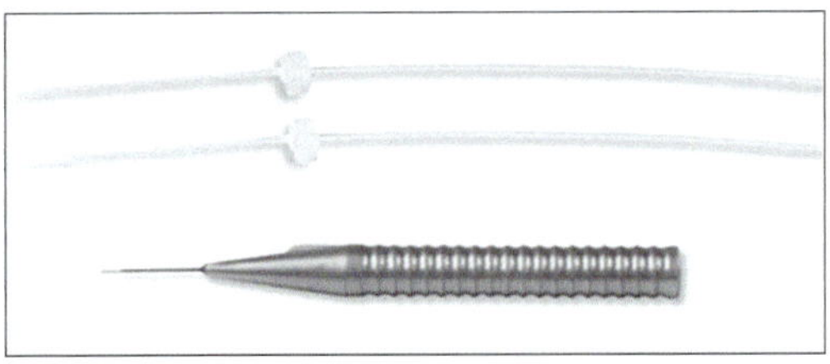

Fig. 4.3 An Eckardt twin chandelier light (DORC, NL)

The use of the laser probe requires some training. A great proportion of intraoperative lens touch is caused by the tip of the endolaser. This is because the surgeon usually focuses on the area of the illuminated retina that requires treatment and may forget about the position of the

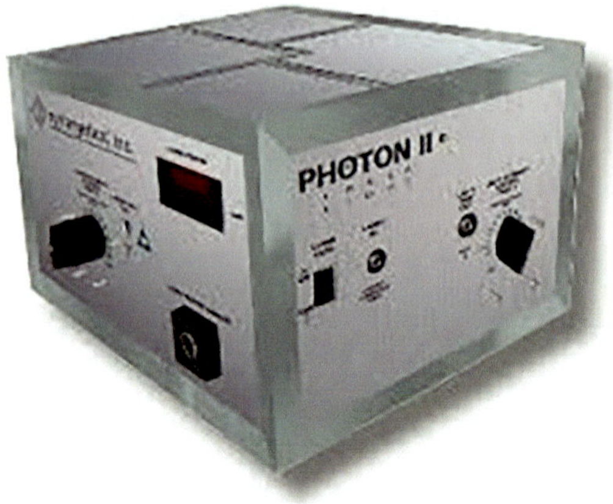

Fig. 4.4 An excellent external illumination for light fibers and especially for chandelier lights (Photon, Synergetics)

laser probe, in particular when indenting the vitreous base. One of the rules of laser treatment is not to cross the midline of the eye with the tip of the instrument when treating the retinal periphery on the opposite side.

Curved laser probes prevent this problem. They can be advanced and retracted through a mechanism within the handpiece. This requires some training before operating safely within the eye. Also, the flexible part of the probe needs to be retracted before removing the instrument from the eye. Otherwise, the probe will get stuck in the trocar and the trocar will be removed with the instrument. Combined laser and light fiber handpiece. This laser handpiece is combined with a light fiber. Indications: Peripheral retinal breaks or ischemic retinopathy. With one hand you can indent the retina with the scleral depressor and treat the break with the other hand (Illuminated Laser Probe, 23G with Iridex adapter. DORC. 7510.IRI).

Remark: Laser photocoagulation and cryopexy can both seal a retinal break. The method of choice is laser photocoagulation. It achieves a faster closure of the retinal break and causes less PVR. There is, however, a big advantage of cryopexy compared to laser photocoagulation: Cryopexy can be performed on a detached break, and laser photocoagulation can only be performed on an attached break.

4.3 Instruments for Dissection of Membranes

Membrane pic (Fig. 4.5)

Indication: To elevate a membrane, which is firmly attached to the retina. DORC 1292.EO4. Recently a 27G membrane pic was introduced from DORC. A dissection with minimal trauma of the retina is possible.

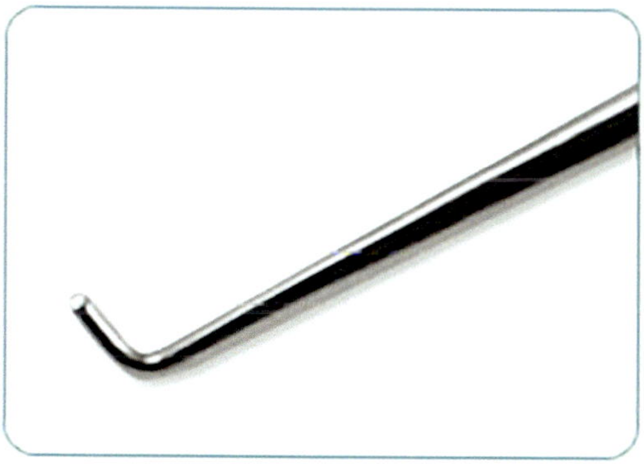

Fig. 4.5 Membrane pic

Retinal scraper (27G retrobulbar cannula Atkinson, Fig. 4.6A, B)

This blunt cannula is suitable for the opening of the posterior hyaloid or delamination of flat membranes (A, B). The membrane can be lifted up with the blunt cannula and then removed with the microforceps. Beaver Visitec, 27G retrobulbar cannula Atkinson.

Knob spatula (Fig. 4.7)

The 23G and 25G knob spatula have a thick knob at their tip. Indication for use is the manipulation of membranes, a retinal massage and hemostasis. For delamination, place the knob spatula between the membrane and the retina and separate both tissues from each other. A retinal massage is possible if there are retinal folds. A bleeding vessel can be occluded with a knob spatula and a waiting time of one minute. Alternatively, the vitreous cutter can be used. A wonderful instrument which we recommend warmly (EyeTechnology, UK: VR-2095).

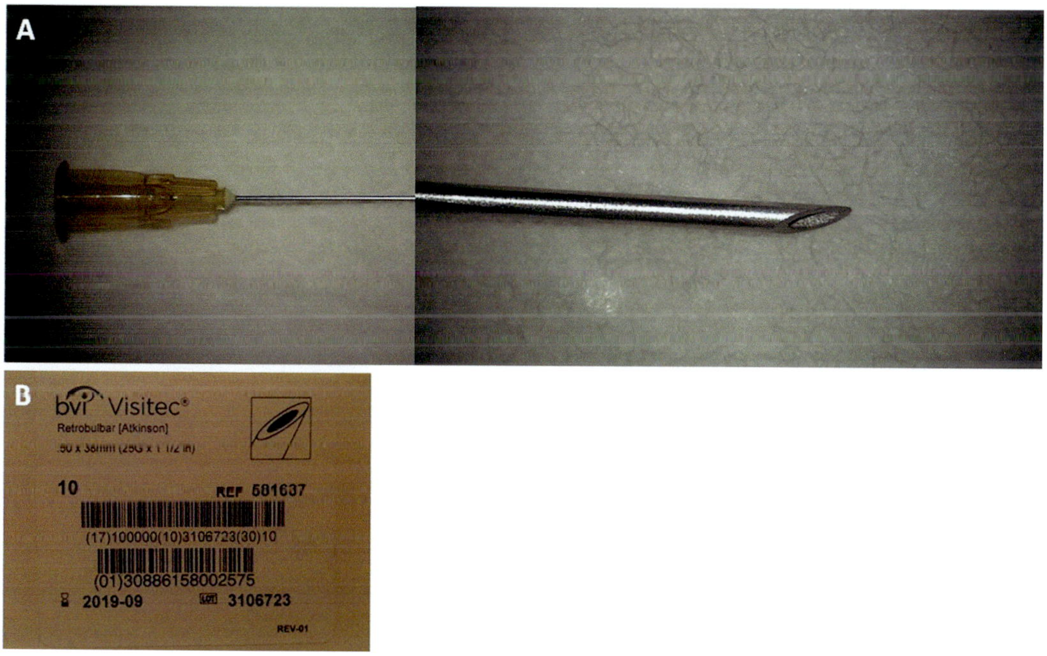

Fig. 4.6 **A, B**: The 25G and 27G retrobulbar cannula is suitable for delamination of epiretinal membranes

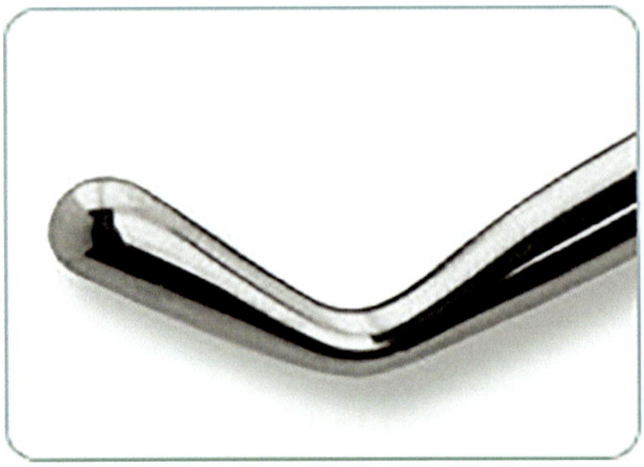

Fig. 4.7 Knob spatula

4.4 Instruments for Removal of Membranes

Eckardt end-gripping forceps (Fig. 4.8A, E)
The 27G end-gripping forceps from DORC is a mix of ILM forceps and end-gripping forceps. It functions well for ILM and membranes. We use the 27G forceps for 27G and 25G surgery. DORC, 27G disposable microforceps.1286. WD04.

Power end-gripping forceps (Fig. 4.8B, E)
The power end-gripping forceps is useful for firmly attached membranes such as in PVR retinal detachment. DORC, 27G disposable microforceps. 1286.WPD04 or DORC, 23G disposable microforceps. 1286.WP06.

Serrated forceps (Fig. 4.8C, E)
The serrated jaws forceps is an alternative to the power end-gripping forceps and is useful for the removal of firmly attached membranes. 23G: DORC. 1286.CO6.

Curved microscissors (Fig. 4.8D, E)
The microscissors are a useful instrument for cutting membranes. DORC, 27G disposable microscissors. Available in 23G (DORC 1286. M06), 25G (DORC 1286.MD05), and 27G (2286.PD04).

Straight microscissors (Fig. 4.9)
Straight microscissors are a useful instrument for cutting membranes. Available in 23G and 25G. Geuder. G-36 578 or DORC, 1286.JO6.

4.5 Instruments for Subretinal Peeling

Subretinal spatula (Fig. 4.10)
The subretinal spatula is only available in 20G. The trocars must be removed before use. The subretinal spatula pierces the retina (retinotomy) and then delaminates the membrane from the retina. Geuder: 20G subretinal spatula,

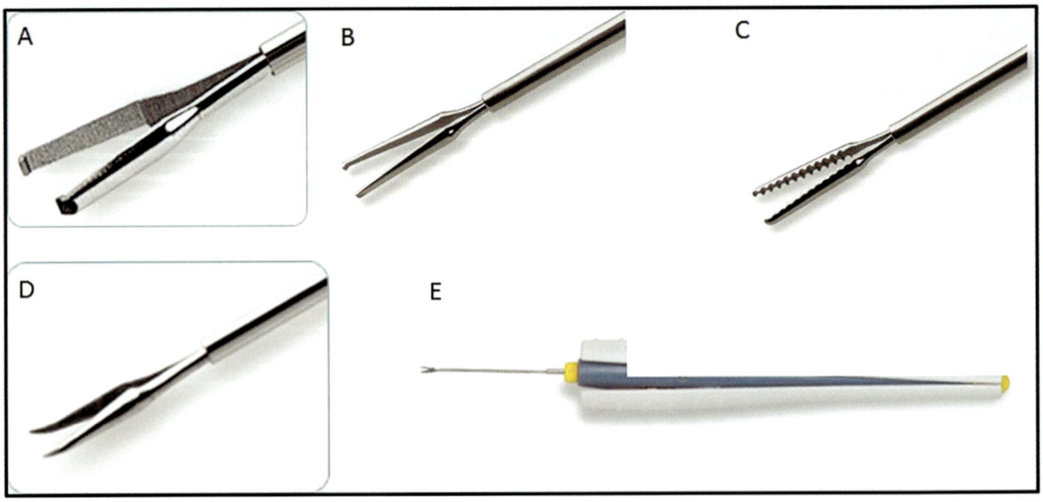

Fig. 4.8 **A–E**: ntravitreal forceps and scissors

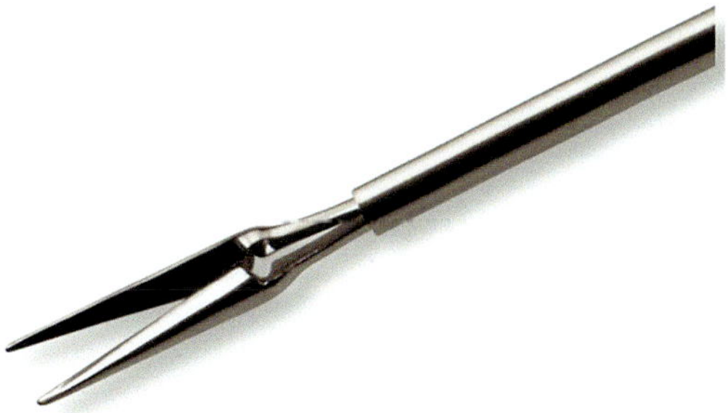

Fig. 4.9 Straight microscissors (25G, Eye Tech, UK)

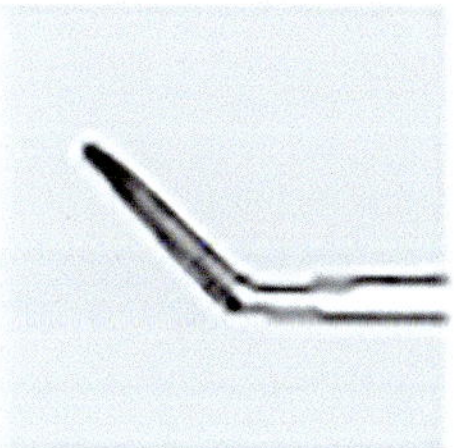

Fig. 4.10 Subretinal spatula (20G, Geuder, Germany)

37,545 and 37,546. DORC: 20G subretinal spatula 1295–1 0995.

Subretinal forceps (Fig. 4.11)

The subretinal forceps is only available in 20G. The subretinal forceps pieces the retina (retinotomy) and then delaminates the membrane from the retina. Geuder: 20G subretinal forceps, 36,236. DORC: 20G subretinal forceps 1286 01 1095.

Serrated forceps (Fig. 4.12)

The serrated jaws forceps is necessary for bimanual removal of the subretinal membranes. DORC. 1286.CO6 (23G).

4.6 Instruments for Retinotomy

Endodiathermy probe (Fig. 4.13)

An endodiathermy probe is required to cauterize the edges of the retinotomy (Alcon, DORC).

Vertical scissors (Fig. 4.14)

The vertical scissors are required for performing a circumferential retinotomy. Vertical scissors are available in 23G (1286.E06) and 25G (1286. ED05) (DORC). Better alternatives are the 25G and 27G cutters which can also be used for a retinotomy.

4.7 Dyes

Triamcinolone

Kenalog (Squibb): Indication: For staining of the vitreous and membranes. We use it only for vitreous staining. We recommend diluting the triamcinolone (1:3) with BSS. It must be injected repeatedly because triamcinolone crystals only stain the outer part of the vitreous cortex.

Combined dye (Trypan Blue and Brilliant Blue G)

Contains two dyes (Trypan Blue and Brilliant Blue G) (Membranc Dual®, DORC): Indication: For staining of epiretinal membranes and ILM.

4.8 Episcleral Buckling

Encircling bands (tyre) (Fig. 4.15)

The encircling band (Fig. 4.15) is placed under all 4 rectus muscles. The sleeve (Fig. 4.16)

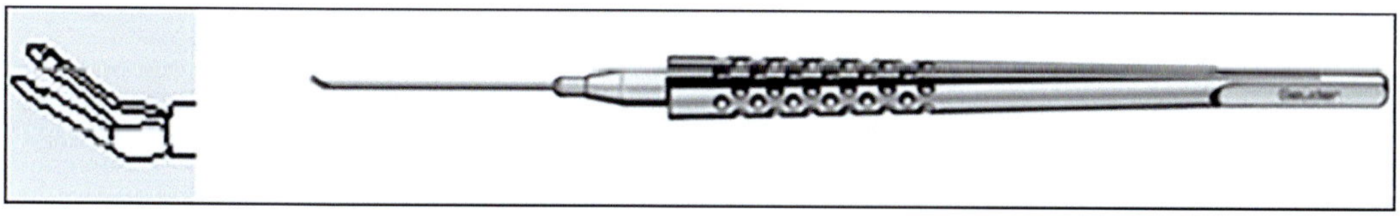

Fig. 4.11 Subretinal forceps (20G, Geuder, Germany)

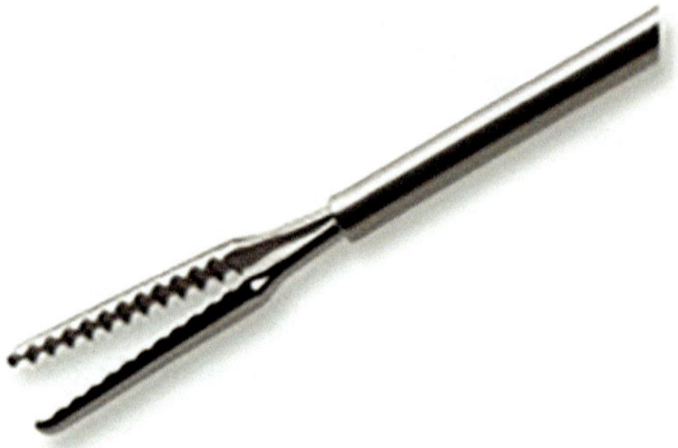

Fig. 4.12 Serrated jaws forceps (23G and 25G)

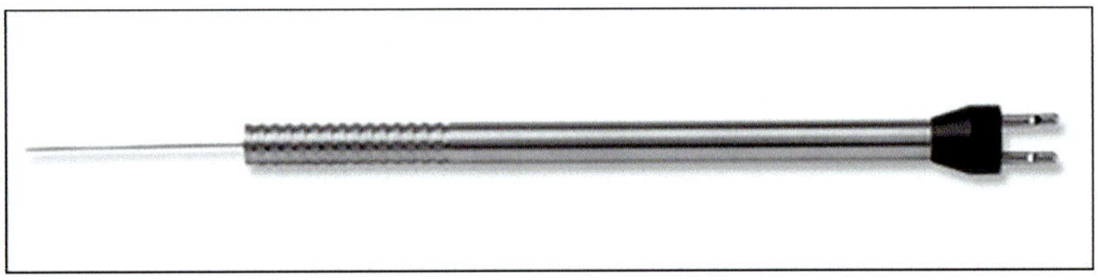

Fig. 4.13 Endodiathermy probe

Fig. 4.14 Vertical scissors (25G, DORC)

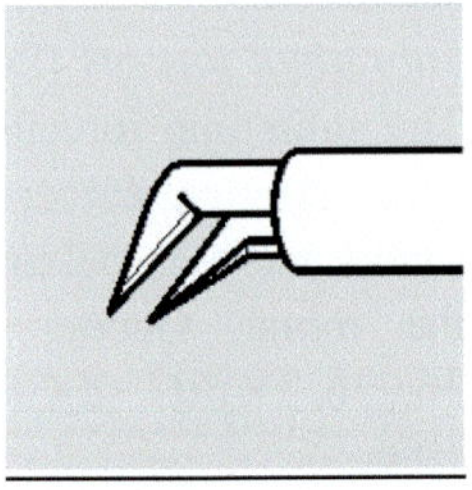

Fig. 4.15 Encircling bands (Labtician, Canada)

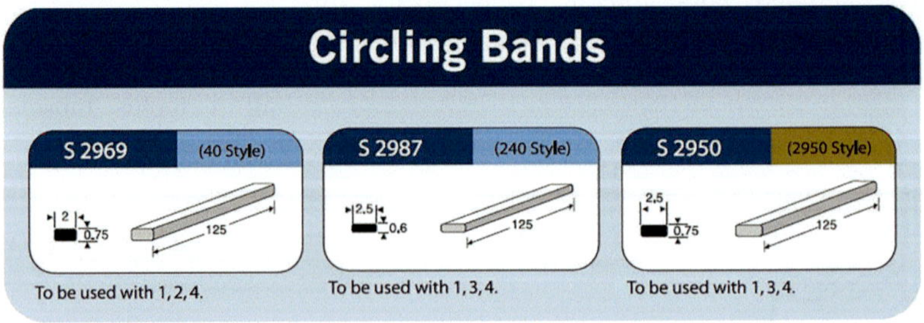

which connects both ends is located at the inferotemporal quadrant.

Segmental sponges

The buckle can cover the rupture in a radial or circumferential position.

(1) a normal sized (3.77 × 5 mm) silicone sponge. Our most commonly used silicone sponge. Indication: Ora dialysis, all breaks <= 3 mm in width for a radial buckle. This sponge requires a 7 mm marking (Fig. 4.17).

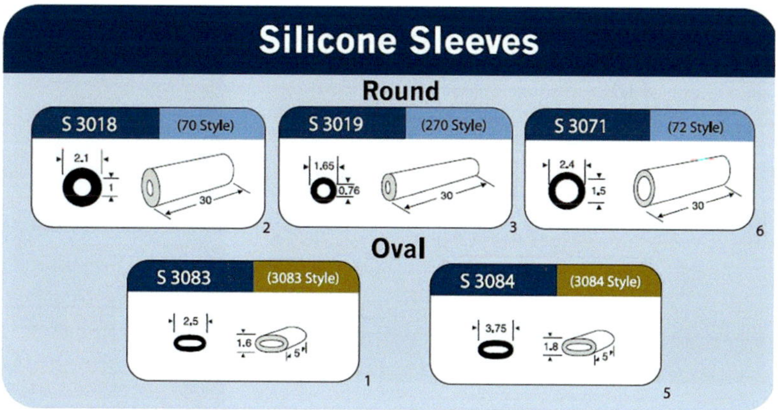

Fig. 4.16 Silicone sleeves (Labtician, Canada)

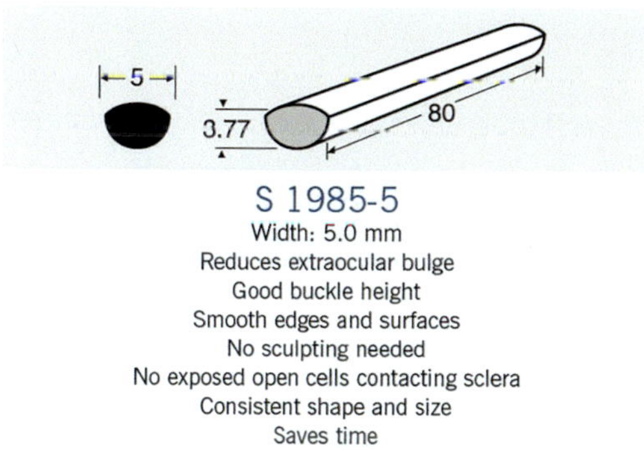

Fig. 4.17 Segmental sponge (Labtician, Canada)

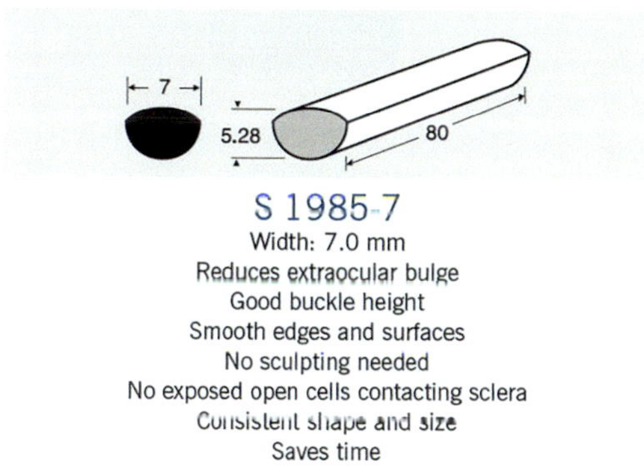

Fig. 4.18 Segmental sponge (Labtician, Canada)

(2) a large silicone sponge (5.28 × 7.5 mm). Less commonly used silicone sponge. Indication: Big breaks, i.e., <= 5 mm in width for a radial buckle. This sponge requires a 9.5 mm marking (Fig. 4.18).

4.8.1 Sutures for Episcleral Buckling

Mersilene 5–0 (Fig. 4.19)
Indication: Suturing of an encircling band (tyre). Ethicon.

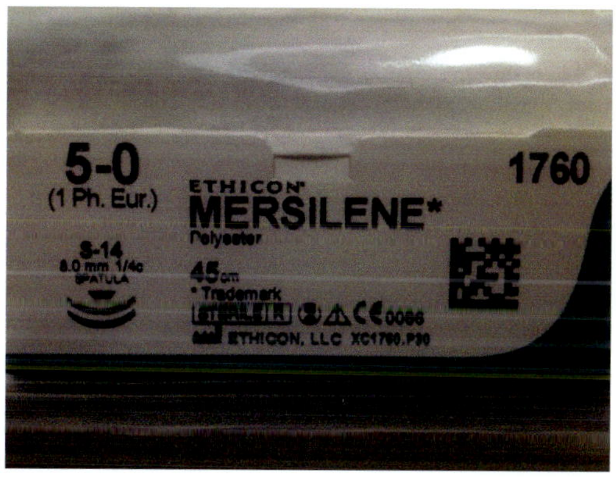

Fig. 4.19 Mersilene suture 5–0

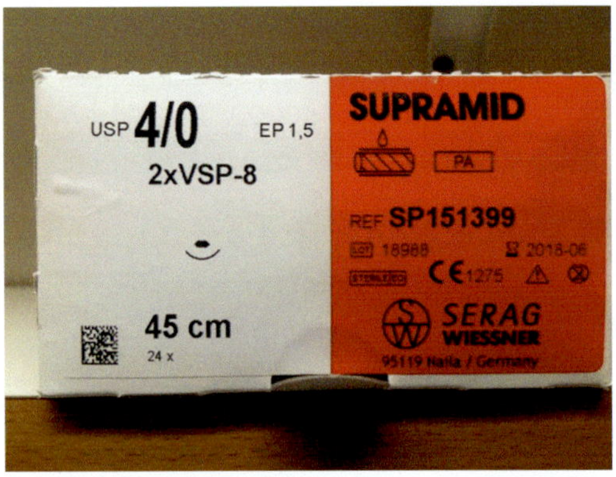

Fig. 4.20 Supramid suture 4–0

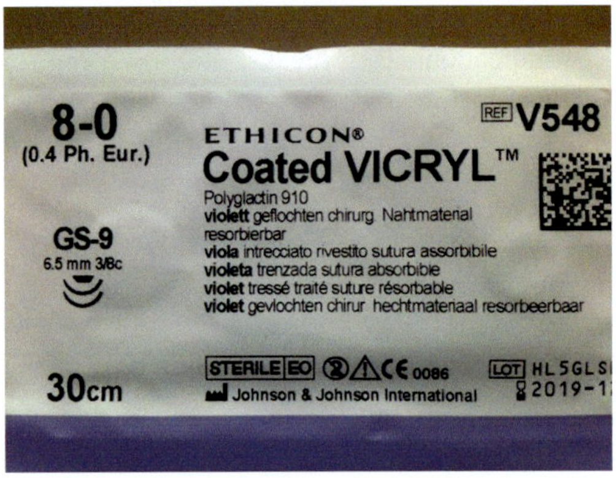

Fig. 4.21 Vicryl suture 8–0

Supramid 4–0 (Fig. 4.20)
Indication: Suturing of an episcleral sponge. Serag WIessner, Germany.

Vicryl 6–0 (Fig. 4.21)
Indication: Suture of conjunctiva. Ethicon.

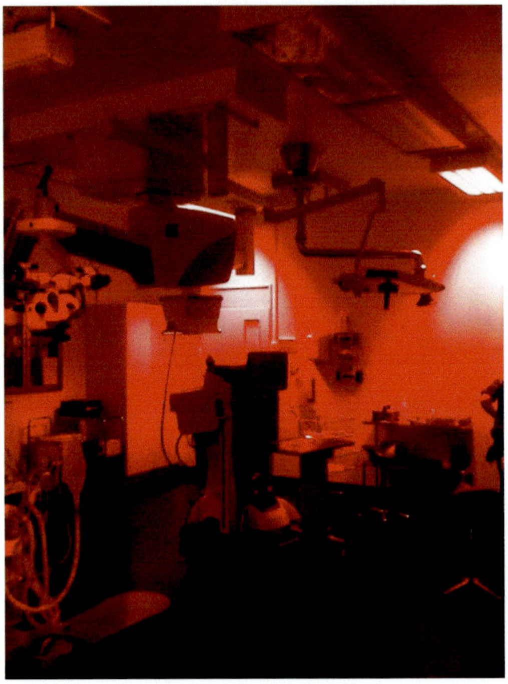

Fig. 4.22 Vitreoretinal OR with red neon light

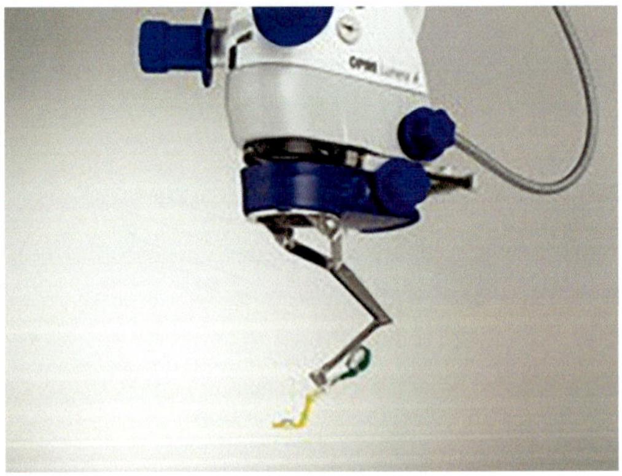

Fig. 4.23 Zeiss microscope with Resight viewing system

4.9 Surgical Setup

In our OR we use neon lights which we painted with red color in order to minimize bright white light on the OR field and in the microscope oculars. At the same time, it allows sufficient illumination for the staff (Fig. 4.22). We use a Zeiss Lumera microscope with Resight Biom viewing system (Fig. 4.23). The 120D, 90D, and 60D loupes can be changed as required during surgery. For positioning of the head, we use a pillow that stiffens around the patient's head with the use of a vacuum pump (Germa AB, Sweden) (Figs. 4.24 and 4.25).

The typical surgical setup in our OR is a 4-port vitrectomy with a chandelier light at the inferonasal position. Extra light fiber is fixated with a carbo band at the patient's forehead

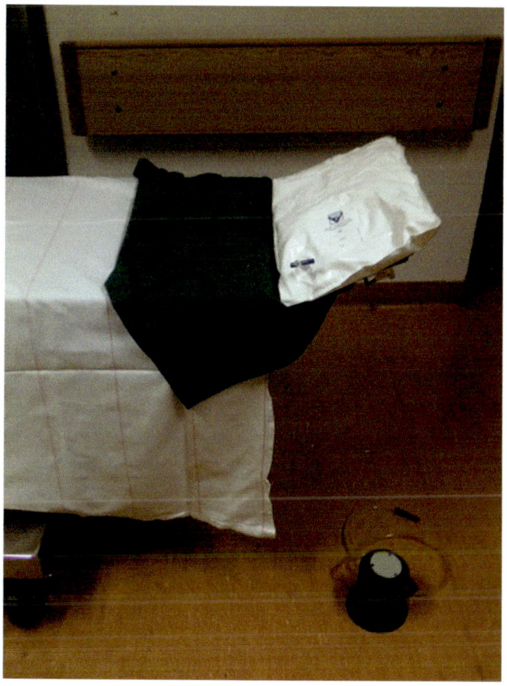

Fig. 4.24 We use a vaccum pillow which provides a customized positioning and fixation of the patients head

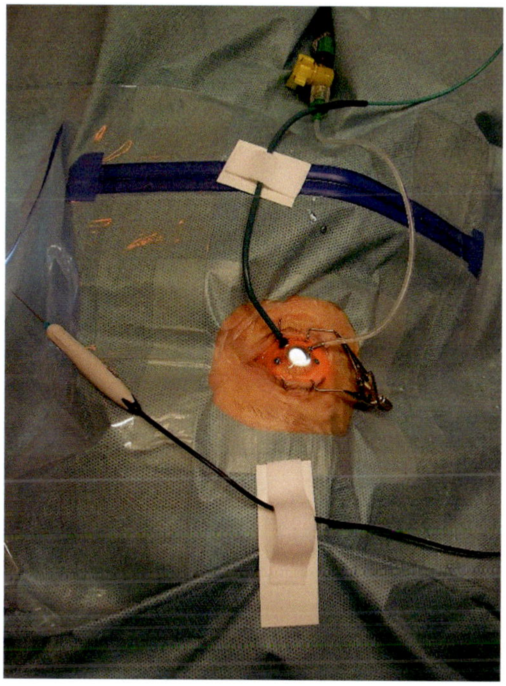

Fig. 4.26 Typical surgical setup with chandelier light fiber and handheld light fiber

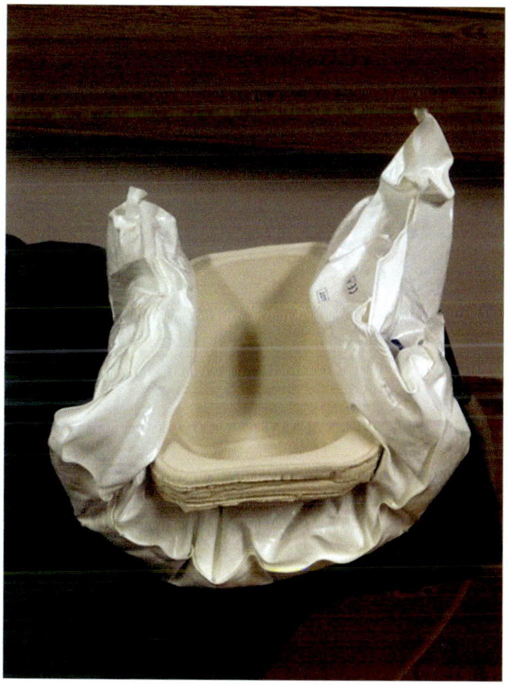

Fig. 4.25 A foot pump is required to pump up the pillow. The complete procedure takes a few seconds. (Germa, Sweden GE22393300000 55 × 30 cm)

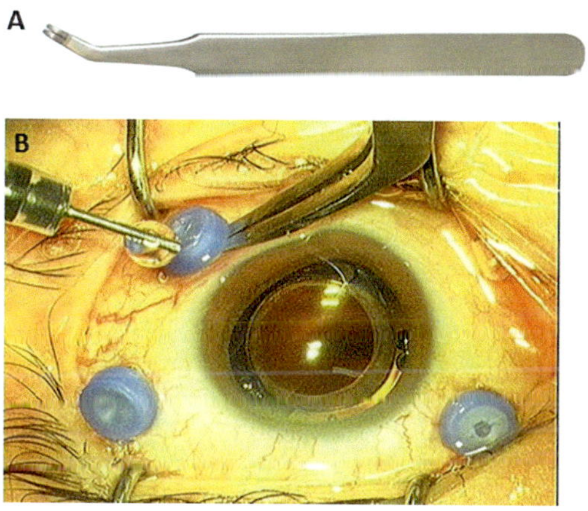

Fig. 4.27 **A, B**: We work with 25G and 27G vitrectomy **A**. The trocars forceps (DORC) is useful for manipulation of trocars **B**

(Fig. 4.26). A very practical instrument is the trocar forceps from DORC (Fig. 4.27A) to manipulate trocars during surgery (Fig. 4.27B). The standard instruments for a vitrectomy are depicted in Fig. 4.28.

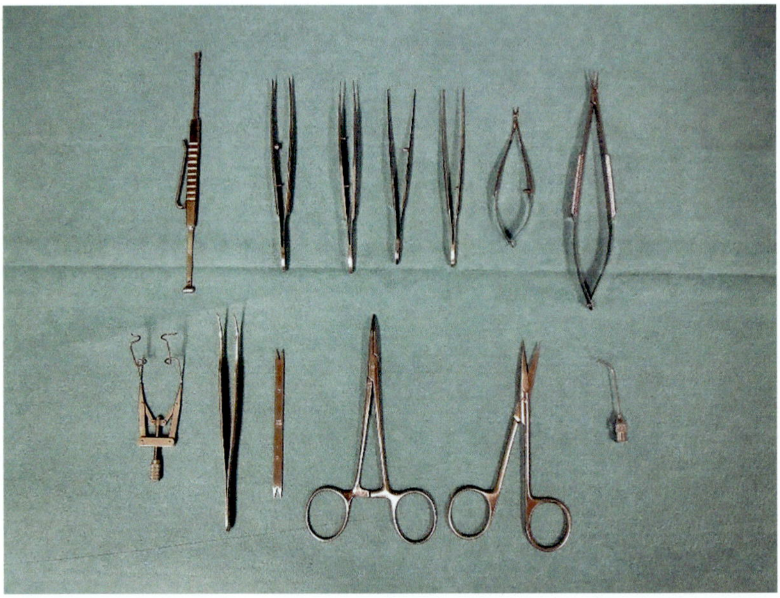

Fig. 4.28 The standard instruments for a vitrectomy

Gases and Liquids and Their Physiological Properties for Surgery

5

Ulrich Spandau, Zoran Tomic, and Diego Ruiz-Casas

In posterior segment surgery, various gases and liquids are used. It is, therefore, important to understand their characteristics and abilities. Four different intraocular gases are commonly used: air, sulphur hexafluoride (SF_6), perfluoroethane (C_2F_6) and perfluoropropane (C_3F_8). In the vitreous cavity, these gases are colourless, odourless and inert. When injected into the vitreous cavity, air does not expand, whereas pure SF_6, C_2F_6 and C_3F_8 gases do. All gases are, however, used in a non-expanding concentration (see Table 2.1).

Gases are temporary tamponades and are absorbed over several days (air) to months (C_3F_8). Air < SF_6 < C_2F_6 < C_3F_8; see Table 2.1. Silicone oil tamponades, however, are permanent tamponades and are usually removed between 4 weeks and 6 months after the initial surgery. Perfluorocarbon (PFCL) is a temporary, preoperative tamponade used especially for detachment surgery.

Remark If the term "water-filled eye" is used in this book, it means an eye filled with "balanced salt solution (BSS)". The BSS will be replaced postoperatively by aqueous humor.

In order to understand the function of the gases and liquids, one needs to know their physiologic abilities.

5.1 Physiologic Characteristics of Gases and Liquids: Specific Gravity

Substances with a specific gravity (SG) of 1 are neutrally buoyant, those with SG greater than one are denser than water, and will sink in it, and those with an SG of less than one are less dense than water, and so will float. The following diagram (see Table 5.1) gives the location of the fluids and gases depending on their relative weight within the vitreous cavity. Perfluorocarbon (PFCL) is the heaviest liquid and is always located on the bottom of the eye. Heavy silicone oils (Densiron Xtra®, Oxane Hd®) are heavier than water and tamponade, therefore, the inferior circumference. Conventional silicone oils are lighter than water and tamponade the superior circumference. The lightest tamponades used are gases; they are always located anteriorly.

In the eye, several gases or liquids may be present at the same time. In this context, the term phase is important. Phase is with regards to the physical properties of a spatially homogeneous field. One uses the term, for example, of a

U. Spandau (✉)
University of Stockholm, Stockholm, Sweden
e-mail: ulrich_spandau@yahoo.de

Z. Tomic
Milos Klinika, Belgrade, Serbia
e-mail: zorannos@yahoo.se

D. Ruiz-Casas
Hospital Ramón y Cajal, Madrid, Spain

U. Spandau et al. (eds.), *Retinal Detachment Surgery and Proliferative Vitreoretinopathy*,
https://doi.org/10.1007/978-3-031-11946-0_5

Table 5.1 Relative location of liquids, oils and gases in the vitreous cavity

Air/gas; SG = 0.0012	Vitreous space; SG = 1
Conventional silicone oils; SG = 0.97	
Water; SG = 1	
Heavy silicone oils; SG = 1.06	
Perfluorocarbon; SG = 1.75	

gaseous phase or liquid phase. A gas or liquid "bubble" refers to a spherical shape. Another important term is the meniscus: It refers to the curved surface of a liquid.

5.2 Physiologic Characteristics of Gases and Liquids: Surface Tension Pressure

The high surface tension between gas and fluid enables the formation of an effective seal around a retinal break, thus allowing the Retinal Pigment Epithelium (RPE) to absorb any remaining subretinal fluid to facilitate reattachment of the retina. The surface tension pressure of the gas/water interface is the greatest, and therefore, is the most effective in closing retinal breaks (70 mN/N). Because the specific gravity of any gas is lower than that of water, the intraocular gas bubble has a buoyancy that presses the retina against the RPE, and this effect is greatest at the apex of the bubble. Buoyancy forces can be directed by careful positioning of the patient's head so that a retinal break is placed at the apex of the bubble until chorioretinal adhesions are created by laser photocoagulation or cryotherapy can be established. Less effective are silicone oils because the surface tension pressure of silicone oil/water is only 50 mN/N.

5.3 All Gases and Liquids in Detail

5.3.1 Air

Room air can also be used as a tamponade. A focal detachment with a detached break between 11 and 1 o'clock can be tamponaded with room air. The air is resorbed after 1 week.

5.3.2 Expanding Gases

SF_6, C_2F_6 and C_3F_8 are expanding gases as dissolved nitrogen diffuses along the concentration gradient from the blood into the gas bubble and accumulates here. The postoperative extension may lead to strong increases in intraocular pressure when the gases are injected undiluted into the eye. To avoid this intraocular pressure rise, expanding gases are used in a concentration in which they do not expand. The non-expanding concentration of SF_6 is 20%, of C_2F_6 15% and of C_3F_8 14% (see Table 2.1). Patients with a gas-filled eye should not undergo anaesthesia with nitrous oxide, as it diffuses into gas-filled cavities and leads to an increase in volume. In addition, any air travel or trips to locations at greater heights (for example, patients living in mountainous areas) are strictly prohibited. This should be part of any routine consent procedure before vitreoretinal surgery. We also advise giving patients information leaflets with detailed instructions for themselves and referring physicians regarding these precautions.

Important: Air expands not at sea level. But patients with an air tamponade are not allowed to fly because air expands with increasing altitude. A plane flying at a height of 10.000 m above sea level has an air cabin pressure of 2400 m. The same also applies to a stay in the mountains.

5.3.2.1 *SF_6 (Sulphur Hexafluoride)*

The commonly used concentration of sulphur hexafluoride (SF_6) is 20%. It tamponades the eye for approximately 3–4 weeks. Indication: macular holes, diabetic retinopathy and retinal detachment surgery with superior breaks. SF_6 is not suitable for inferior breaks unless a specific posture can be maintained for prolonged periods of time (for example, supine position or on one side opposite to the break).

5.3.2.2 C_2F_6 *(Perfluoroethane)*

The usual concentration of C_2F_6 is 15%. It tamponades the eye for approximately 4–6 weeks. Indication: Difficult detachments with multiple breaks, inferior tears or PVR detachment.

5.3.2.3 C_3F_8 *(Perfluoropropane)*

The usual concentration of C_3F_8 is 12 to 14%. It tamponades the eye for approximately 8 weeks. It causes more ocular irritation than C_2F_6. The indications are similar to C_2F_6.

Remark: Short-acting gases such as room air and SF6 cause less virtual traction. There should therefore be preferred over C_2F_6 and C_3F_8. If possible choose a short-acting gas.

Surgical pearls no. 2

Injection of gas:

(1) Errors in preparing the correct concentration of the air–gas mixture are potential sources of disasters if different gases with varying concentrations are used regularly in one theatre. Concentration levels, which are too high, can lead to a massive rise in the intraocular pressure, whereas lower concentrations may result in a shorter tamponade than desired. In every theatre, a strict protocol for preparing the air–gas mixture must be followed. We recommend that every surgeon supervises the preparation of the mixture and checks on the gas used.

(2) Gases are in 100% concentration in gas containers. They must be diluted with air before injection into the eye. Example: 20% of SF_6 and a 50 ml syringe: draw 10 ml 100% SF_6 in the syringe and dilute to 50 ml with room air.

(3) If you intend to inject a gas into the eye, first perform a fluid–air exchange. The gas-filled syringe is then connected to the three-way tap. The scrub nurse can inject the gas. At the same time, you hold a flute needle behind the lens to release pressure, so that the globe remains normotensive (Fig 5.1). Always leave some 5–10 cc in the syringe. This gives you some extra volume to inject should the globe be hypotensive after removing the trocars.

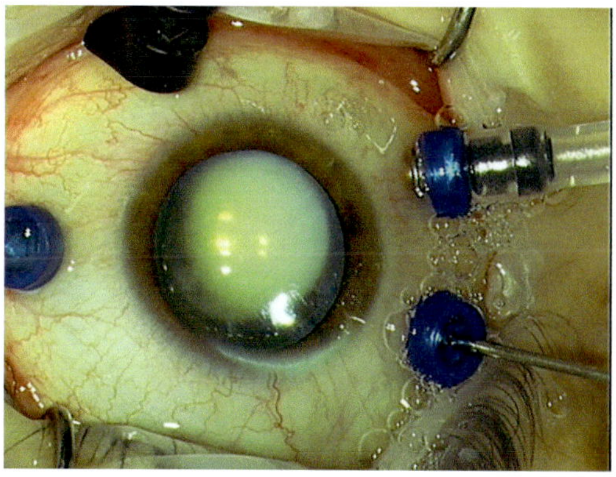

Fig. 5.1 An expanding gas is injected through the IV line to the top right into the eye. To the bottom right, a flute needle is held in a cannula to relieve intraocular pressure

5.3.3 Liquids

5.3.3.1 Perfluorocarbon

Perfluorocarbon (PFCL, "heavy water") has the highest density of all intraocular used liquids, see Table 5.1; the eye is filled up from the posterior pole to the ora serrata. In the supine position, PFCL exerts the most pressure on the posterior pole and less pressure anteriorly (Fig 5.2); it flattens the retina from the posterior pole to the ora serrata. A big advantage is a good visibility under PFCL. One disadvantage is that it always needs to be completely removed, as it is retinotoxic if left within the eye for weeks to months, especially if it is dislocated into the subretinal space. PFCL is now an essential tool in retinal detachment surgery. It is used to flatten the detached retina and push subretinal fluid through the breaks into the vitreous. Additional advantages are an instant apposition of photoreceptors and retinal pigment epithelial cells in order to promote reattachment and facilitate laser treatment around the breaks. It also stabilizes the detached retina, thereby facilitating trimming of the vitreous base and decreasing the risk of

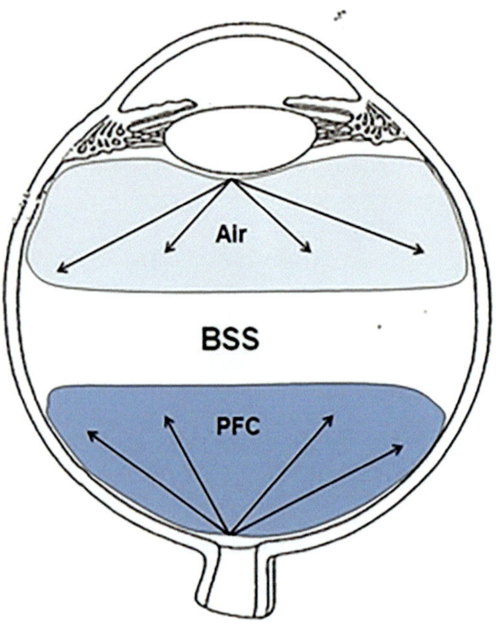

Fig. 5.2 Opposite effects of air and PFCL in the vitreous cavity. Air exerts pressure onto the retina from anterior to posterior whereas PFCL exerts pressure from posterior to anterior

iatrogenic breaks during surgery. Because it does not mix with vitreous, it clearly delineates vitreous remnants in the anterior periphery. One can fill PFCL without problems over the break itself; it will not spill through the break in the subretinal space due to its high surface tension. Finally, it can be used as a protectant of the posterior pole in cases of dislocated IOL or lens matter. Inject a small bubble of PFCL on the posterior pole in order to perform any necessary manipulations in these cases at some distance from the macula.

In the supine position, air exerts the most pressure on the anterior retina (ora serrata) and less on the posterior retina (Fig 5.2). Because air is lighter than water or PFCL, the eye will be filled with air from the ora serrata and then down to the optic disc.

Dislocation of PFCL into the subretinal space can occur in two situations: If there is a large retinal break with significant residual traction on the retina or if one injects PFCL too briskly, thus splitting the PFCL stream into multiple small bubbles that can then be "blown" through the break into the subretinal space. Silicone oil tamponades are permanent tamponades and are usually removed between 4 weeks and 6 months after the initial surgery. Silicone oils with a lower viscosity (1000 csts conventional oil or heavy oils, which are a mixture of 1300 csts conventional oil and a heavy liquid) tend to emulsify earlier and are usually removed within 3 months. An advantage of these lower viscosity silicone oils is that they can easily be injected and removed with 25- and 23-gauge ports. The higher viscosity of 5000 csts silicone oils tend to emulsify later and can usually be left within the vitreous cavity for longer periods of time.

5.3.3.2 Light Silicone Oils

Conventional silicone oil is lighter than water and floats in the vitreous and in the anterior chamber. Indications for silicone oil tamponade are retinal detachments with multiple (superior and inferior) breaks, a giant tear, advanced proliferative diabetic retinopathy, PVR detachment and a macular hole (if a prone position is not possible).

Light silicone oils are available with different viscosities of 1000 csts (centistokes), 1300 csts, 2000 csts and 5000 csts. 1300 csts silicone oil is more and more replaced by 1000 csts silicone oil. 1000 csts silicone oil emulsifies more rapidly and is suitable for a tamponade of about three months. Occasionally, 5000 csts silicone oil should be left intraocularly as a permanent tamponade in cases with multiple redetachments after previously attempted oil removal or severe hypotony. All oils can easily be injected and withdrawn through 25- and 23-gauge trocars.

5.3.3.3 Heavy Silicone Oils (Densiron Xtra® and Oxane Hd®)

Densiron Xtra® and Oxane Hd® are a mixture of silicone oil and perfluorohexyloctane (F_6H_8) and are known as heavy silicone oils (Fig. 3a and b).

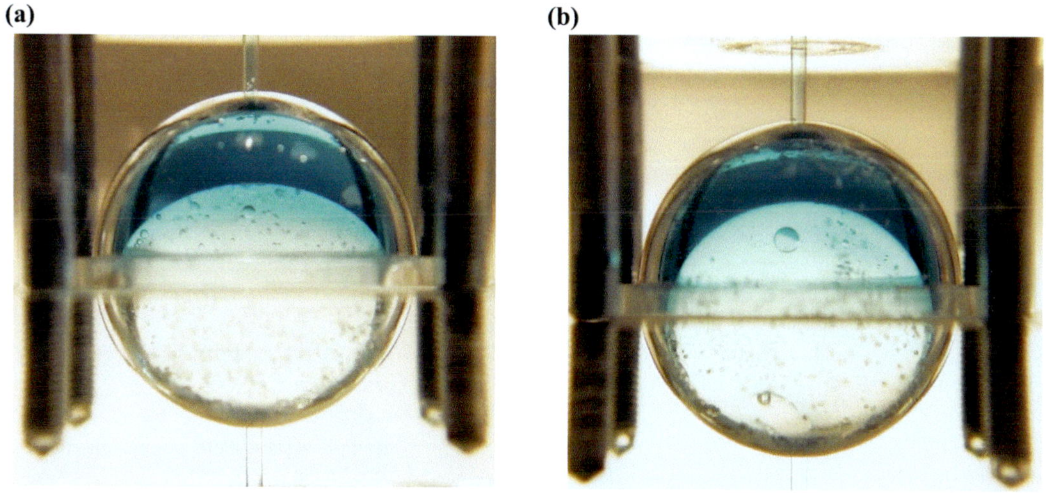

Fig. 5.3 **a** Tamponade with Densiron Xtra® in an eye model. The blue fluid is aqueous. Densiron Xtra® is less convex than Oxane Hd® and therefore tamponades the inferior retina better. Densiron Xtra® is widely accepted by vitreoretinal surgeons. With friendly permission of Dr. David Wong. **b** Tamponade with Oxane Hd® in an eye model. Oxane Hd® is much lighter than Densiron Xtra®. It is much more convex and tamponades the inferior retina less effectively than Densiron Xtra®. With friendly permission of Dr. David Wong

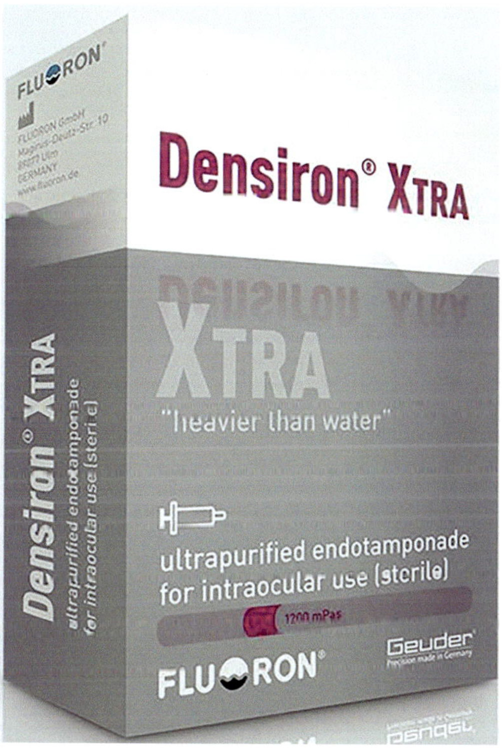

Fig. 5.4 Densiron Xtra from Fluoron, Germany

They are heavier than water, and therefore, support the inferior periphery. Indications are Inferior detachment.

Oxane Hd® and Densiron Xtra® (Fig. 5.4) should not come in contact with pure PFCL for longer periods of time because they would mix. However, a short contact (for example, during direct PFCL-heavy silicone oil exchange) is possible. Oxane Hd® should be removed after two months and Densiron Xtra® after about 3–4 months as their tendency to emulsify is comparable to 1300 csts conventional silicone oil. The features of these tamponades are summarized in Table 5.2.

IMPORTANT: There is no 100% tamponade, neither for gases nor for oils. This is because any tamponade will form the smallest possible surface, thereby forming a sphere within the eye that will never be able to cover all areas of the inner surface of the eye. This is also true for the so-called "double tamponades" of silicone oil and PFCL. These two substances will mix well but then they will form an hourglass-shaped tamponade within the eye with one part trying to

Table 5.2 Properties of gases and liquids for a tamponade. (Densiron Xtra® is heavier than Oxane Hd® (see density) but almost as viscous as 1300 csts silicone oil (see viscosity), and therefore, almost as easy to remove)

Gas	Tamponade duration (days)	Concentration in %	Indication
Air	7		Superior break between 11 and 1 o'clock
SF_6	14–21	20	Superior breaks from 9 to 3 o'clock
C_2F_6	30	15	Superior breaks from 8 to 4 o'clock
C_3F_8	60	14	Superior breaks from 7 to 5 o'clock
Silicone oils (viscosity)	Tamponade duration (Months)	Density (g/cm^3)	
Silicone oil (1000 and 1300 csts)	appr. 3–6	0.97	Multiple breaks, PVR, trauma, choroidal detachment
Silicone oil (5000 csts)	>= 12	0.97	Multiple breaks, PVR, trauma, choroidal detachment
Densiron Xtra® (1400 csts)	2–3	1.06	Inferior RD

folate upwards and one part sinking down. Thus, a belt of fluid surrounds the tamponade in the middle of the eye. Finally, a "complete" vitrectomy is not possible. Remnant vitreous will always lead to an incomplete tamponade.

Hot Topics Within Retinal Detachment Surgery

6

Ulrich Spandau, Zoran Tomic, and Diego Ruiz-Casas

6.1 Timing for Macula off Detachments

The right timing for macula on and off detachments is always a big discussion topic among VR surgeons and with the patients. The main notion nowadays is that immediate surgery is warranted as long as the macula is attached and that surgery can be delayed if the macula is detached. But new studies give a new picture.

*Is there an association between macula off detachments and visual acuity within the **first two weeks**?* Yes, there is. The visual acuity of a macula off retinal detachment that has persisted less than 1 week is significantly better than after 1–2 weeks [1].

*Is there an association between macula off detachments and visual acuity within the **first week**?* Yes, there is. The best mean postoperative vision was seen in patients with a detachment of <1 week duration [2].

*Is there an association between macula off detachments and visual acuity within the **first three days**?* Yes, there is. Recent macula off retinal detachments should be repaired within 72 h of the loss of central vision [3]. See Figs. 6.1 and 6.2.

*Is there an association between macula off detachments and visual acuity within **one day**?* Yes, there is. Duration of macular detachment affects the final VA even among patients whose duration of macular detachment is <3 days. Post-hoc analysis showed significant differences in final VA between detachments of 1 day versus 3 days [4].

*Is there a **maximal** time limit for macula off detachments?* Yes, there is. After a duration of 6 weeks, a macula off detachment has a significantly poor postoperative visual prognosis [2]. See Figs. 6.3 and 6.4.

*Is there an association between the **age of the patient** and final visual acuity?* Yes, there is. Patients younger than 60 years are more likely to achieve visual improvement despite the duration of the detachment.

*How long does **visual acuity** improve **after** a retinal detachment?* The postoperative recovery takes up to 1 year. A visual acuity improvement is observed up to 1 year postoperative [1].

*Is there an association between visual acuity recovery and **myopia**?* Yes, in myopia recovery of visual acuity is poorest in patients with myopia of −6D and more [1].

Is there an association between morphology of macula and visual acuity? Yes, the bullous macula off detachments have a worse prognosis than flat macula off detachments [1].

U. Spandau (✉)
University of Stockholm, Stockholm, Sweden
e-mail: ulrich_spandau@yahoo.de

Z. Tomic
Milos Klinika, Belgrade, Serbia
e-mail: zorannos@yahoo.se

D. Ruiz-Casas
Hospital Ramón Y Cajal, Madrid, Spain

U. Spandau et al. (eds.), *Retinal Detachment Surgery and Proliferative Vitreoretinopathy*,
https://doi.org/10.1007/978-3-031-11946-0_6

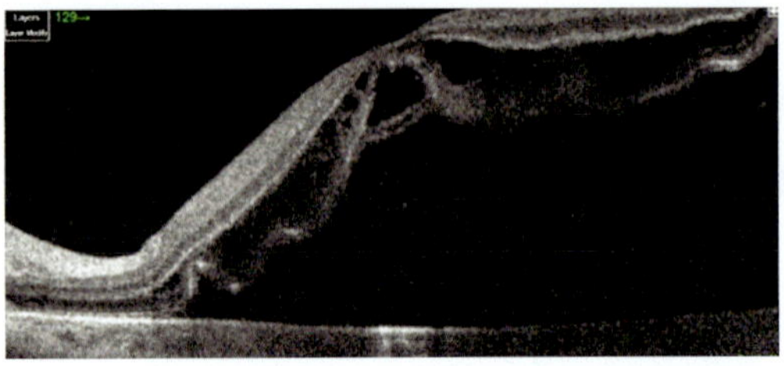

Fig. 6.1 An OCT of a detached macula secondary to retinal detachment. The macula is detached since two days

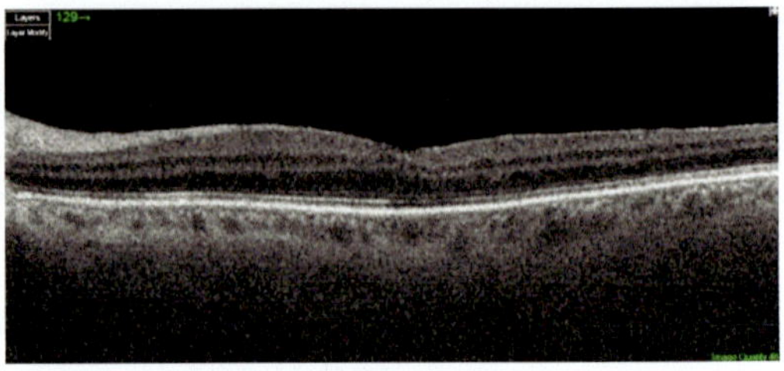

Fig. 6.2 The same eye as in Fig. 6.1. An OCT of an attached macula after successful vitrectomy

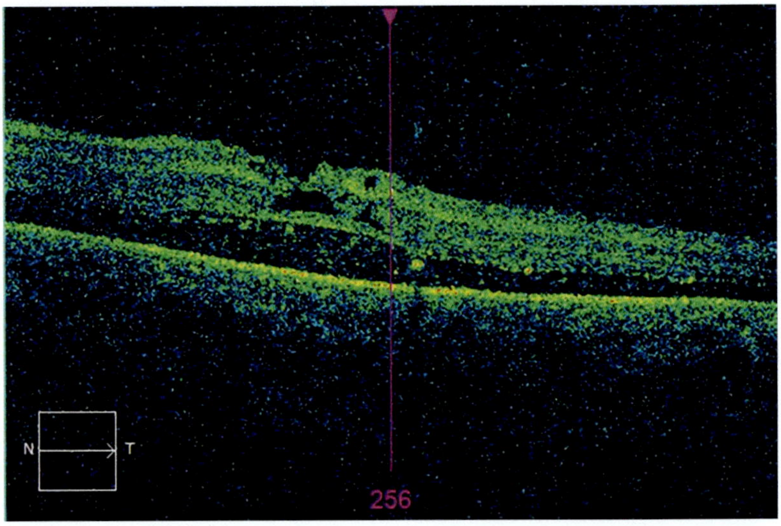

Fig. 6.3 A 12-year-old retinal detachment. 2 weeks postoperative OCT

Does a macula off detachment cause other symptoms aside VA decrease? Many patients following retinal detachment surgery complain of distortion and aniseikonia. There are several studies looking at the frequency of these symptoms. Most studies suggest in the 30–40% range that the vision is better but the image is pinched in and smaller. These symptoms are interestingly more pronounced after vitrectomy than after pneumatic retinopexy [5, 6].

Conclusion: A macula on detachment versus a 1-day old macula off detachment, who do we prioritize? According to these studies, the macula off patient has more to lose than the macula on patient. Within the first three days, we should ideally prioritize macula off patients toward macula on patients.

6.2 Cerclage or No Cerclage, That is the Question

The usage of an encircling band has decreased dramatically in the last decennium. 10–20 years ago, an encircling band was a standard procedure for a retinal detachment procedure (Fig. 6.3). Nowadays an encircling band is a rare procedure. So why do we use an encircling band?

The aim and effect of a segmental buckle is the sealing of retinal rupture. The aim and effect of an encircling band is primary the relief of the vitreous base and secondary the closure of a retinal rupture. This sealing of ruptures is restricted to the location of the band. You can reduce this problem by choosing a wider band.

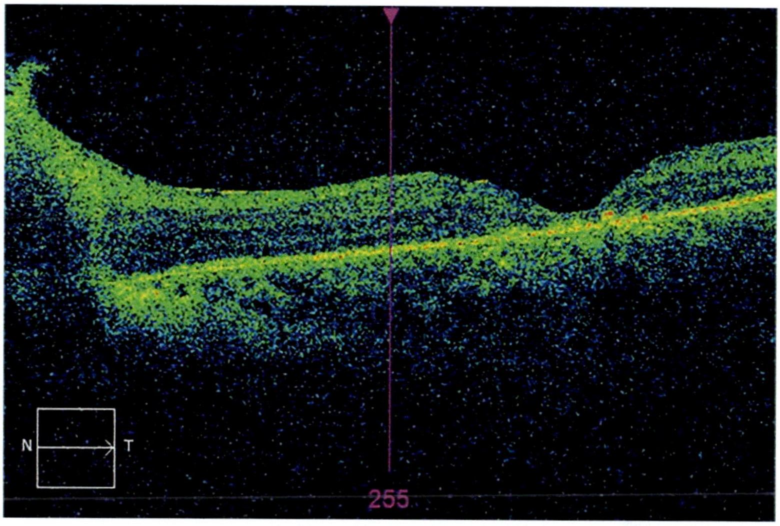

Fig. 6.4 The same eye as in Fig. 6.3. 1-year postoperative follow-up. The submacular fluid resorbed, and vision did not improve

We use a 3.5 mm band. Alternatively, a segmental strip can be placed under the band increasing the width of the band.

What are the disadvantages of an encircling band? An encircling band causes myopia of approximately 2–3 diopters and anisometropia. Remark: An encircling band in a newborn causes myopia of approximately −10 diopters. In addition, an encircling band constricts the sclera resulting in a decrease in ocular blood flow (Ingrid Kreissig). A too tight encircling band may cause Anterior Segment Ischemia caused by disruption of ciliary artery circulation. The typical signs are corneal edema, anterior chamber flare, ocular hypotension and in severe cases iris neovascularization. Cutting off the encircling band restores the ocular circulation and symptoms. Removal of the band is not necessary.

Although it is obvious that not all patients with a retinal detachment require an encircling band, the question remains which patient needs one and for which patient a band is an overtreatment (Fig. 6.5)

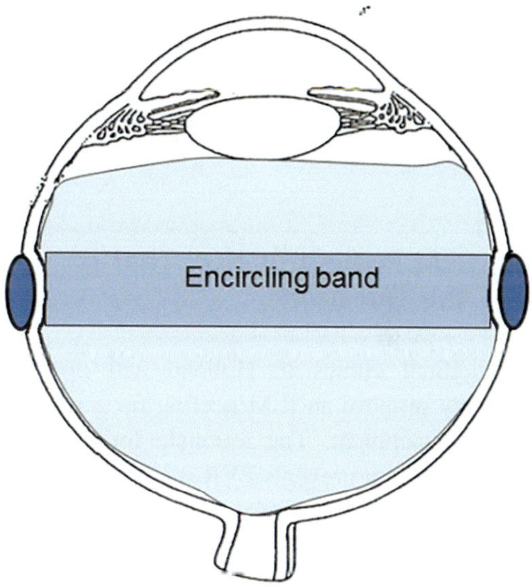

Fig. 6.5 An encircling buckle creates a scleral impression and relieves the vitreous base

The randomized VIPER study shows that in pseudophakic eyes a vitrectomy with the encircling band has no advantage over a vitrectomy alone [7]. This applies to non-complicated detachments. In the case of an inferior detachment, an encircling band with vitrectomy is superior to a vitrectomy alone [6].

Which eyes are highly recommended for a cerclage?

(1) Grave myopia
(2) Children
(3) PVR detachment

Which eyes should be considered for a cerclage?

(1) (Not grave) Myopia with lattice
(2) Recurrent detachment
(3) Inferior detachment (alternative Densiron Xtra)

The strongest indication is for high myopia, children and PVR detachment. A lower indication is for myopia with lattice and for recurrent detachment. In myopia with lattice, many surgeons prefer an episcleral buckling (without vitrectomy) or a vitrectomy with long-acting gas. In recurrent detachments, there are a few aspects to consider. The first aspect is the presence of PVR. In this case, we recommend an encircling band. If, however, a redetachment with a new break is present, then there is no need for a cerclage. We would repeat vitrectomy and laser treat the new break. If, however, the same detachment (as the primary) detachment is present and *no new* breaks are found then we would also recommend an encircling band.

6.3 ILM Peeling or Not, That is the Question

Vitreoretinal clinics in Holland and northern Germany propose an ILM peeling for a primary retinal detachment. The rationale for the ILM peeling is that it prevents PVR membranes in the central pole in case of a redetachment. The question, however, is which eye develops a PVR detachment and which eye does not. Most eyes reattach after a primary surgery without PVR development so that an ILM peeling in the majority of eyes is not necessary.

We recommend and perform an ILM peeling in eyes with a primary PVR detachment and in eyes with a recurrent detachment.

6.4 Gas or Silicone Oil, That is the Question

Gas has two great advantages over silicone oil. The surface tension pressure of a gas is much higher than for silicone oil which enables a more effective sealing of retinal holes. Secondly, the gas is a temporary tamponade. Long-term damages of gas are, therefore, not existent compared to silicone oil.

According to the silicone oil study, C_3F_8 is superior (higher reattachment rate and better visual outcome) to SF_6 in complicated detachments. The silicone oil study does not compare C_3F_8 with silicone oil (Silicone oil study, 1992). The advantages and disadvantages of C_3F_8 and silicone oil are listed in Tables 6.1 and 6.2. For complicated retinal detachments, we prefer silicone oil. The main reason is that the recurrent detachment risk in complicated RD's is higher than in easy detachments. And a recurrent detachment under silicone oil is better than a recurrent detachment under gas. Why? A recurrent detachment under gas develops fast into a PVR detachment. A recurrent detachment under silicone oil may also occur but only little PVR develops. Under gas an immediate surgery is required under silicone oil you can postpone for 1 week.

Remark: Sf_6, C_2F_6 and C_3F_8 are due to the fluorine atoms being heavier than air. The gases sink therefore to the ground whereas the lighter air stays above. Shake, therefore, the gas syringe

Table 6.1 The pros and cons of C_3F_8

Advantages of C_3F_8	Disadvantages of C_3F_8
Disappears spontaneously	Only temporary tamponade
	Specific head positioning (not for children, disabled)
	Air travel must be postponed (risk of expansion)
	Vision is restricted (not for monocular patients)
	Cataractogenic

Table 6.2 The pros and cons of silicone oil

Advantages of silicone oil	Disadvantages
"Non-temporary" longer tamponade	The need for the second operation
Does not require positioning	Scaffold for reproliferation (?)
Earlier visualization (option for monocular patients)	Cataractogenic
Air travel is possible	
Lower risk of hypotony	

before injection. Hold the Charles flute needle behind the lens to aspirate the air so that the gases can fill the vitreous cavity from posterior to anterior.

6.5 Sf_6 Versus C_2F_6 and C_3F_8

The short-lasting gas, Sf_6, causes less complications than the long-lasting gases C_2F_6 and C_3F_8. C_2F_6 and C_3F_8 have a higher detachment rate in VMTS treatment than Sf_6. C_2F_6 and C_3F_8 cause more ocular irritation, IOP spikes and PVR risk than Sf_6. Use only Sf_6 in pneumatic retinopexy and not C_2F_6 and C_3F_8. Use C_2F_6 and C_3F_8 only if the detached breaks are located below the 3–9 o′clock midline.

6.6 Summary

Prophylactic ILM peeling is only recommended in PVR detachments, SF_6 should be preferred over long-acting gases. And *indications* for combined encircling band/vitrectomy are:

(1) Pediatric detachment
(2) Grave myopia
(3) Recurrent detachment
(4) PVR detachment
(5) Myopic eyes with lattice
(6) Inferior detachment

References

1. Kreissig I. A practical guide to minimal surgery for retinal detachment. Thieme, Germany ISBN 9783131606914.
2. Mowatt L, Shun-Shin GA, Arora S, Price N. Macula off retinal detachments. How long can they wait before it is too late? Eur J Ophthalmol. 2005 Jan-Feb;15(1):109–17. PMID: 15751248.
3. Yorston D, Donachie PHJ, Laidlaw DA, Steel DH, Sparrow JM, Aylward GW, Williamson TH. Members of the BEAVRS retinal detachment outcomes group. Factors affecting visual recovery after successful repair of macula-off retinal detachments: findings from a large prospective UK cohort study. Eye (Lond). 2021; 35(5):1431–1439. https://doi.org/10.1038/s41433-020-1021-y. Epub 2020 Jun 24. PMID: 32581389; PMCID: PMC8182892.
4. Greven MA, Leng T, Silva RA, Leung LB, Karth PA, Moshfeghi DM, Sanislo SR, Schachar IH. Reductions in final visual acuity occur even within the first 3 days after a macula-off retinal detachment. Br J Ophthalmol. 2019;103(10):1503-1506. https://doi.org/10.1136/bjophthalmol-2018-313191. Epub 2018 Dec 1. PMID: 30504489.
5. Brosh K, Francisconi CLM, Qian J, Sabatino F, Juncal VR, Hillier RJ, Chaudhary V, Berger AR, Giavedoni LR, Wong DT, Altomare F, Kadhim MR, Newsom RB, Marafon SB, Muni RH. Retinal displacement following pneumatic Retinopexy vs pars plana vitrectomy for Rhegmatogenous retinal detachment. JAMA Ophthalmol. 2020 Jun 1;138(6):652–9. https://doi.org/10.1001/jamaophthalmol.2020.1046. PMID:32324204;PMCID:PMC7290408.
6. Francisconi CLM, Marafon SB, Figueiredo NA, Juncal VR, Shaikh S, Bhambra N, Ta Kim DT, Brosh K, Qian J, Chaudhary V, Berger AR, Giavedoni LR,

Wong DT, Altomare F, Chow DR, Di Simplicio S, Kadhim MR, Deonarain D, Hillier RJ, Muni RH. Retinal displacement after pneumatic Retinopexy versus vitrectomy for Rhegmatogenous retinal detachment (ALIGN). Ophthalmology. 2021;S0161–6420(21)00943-X. doi: https://doi.org/10.1016/j.ophtha.2021.12.007. Epub ahead of print. PMID: 34929256.

7. Walter P, Hellmich M, Baumgarten S, et al. Vitrectomy with and without encircling band for pseudophakic retinal detachment: VIPER study report No 2-main results. Br J Ophthalmol. 2017;101(6):712–8. https://doi.org/10.1136/bjophthalmol-2016-309240.
8. Baumgarten S, Schiller P, Hellmich M et al. Vitrectomy with and without encircling band for pseudophakic retinal detachment with inferior breaks: VIPER Study Report No. 3. Graefes Arch Clin Exp Ophthalmol. 2018;256(11):2069–2073. https://doi.org/10.1007/s00417-018-4106-6

7 Biometry and Anaesthesia

Ulrich Spandau and Zoran Tomic

7.1 Biometry

Biometry is challenging in eyes with a retinal detachment because the macula is detached and the Axial Length (AL) measurement is wrong. Start with an IOL Master of the healthy eye. Then measure the corneal power (K1 and K2) of the "detached" eye. Axial length measurement of the detached eye is not possible. Use the axial length measurement of the healthy eye for the "detached" eye.

An example is depicted in Fig. 7.1. The right eye has a retinal detachment and the left eye is normal. You can see that the Axial Length (AL) of the right is too short because the laser light measures from the cornea to the detached retina. If you would choose an IOL with these measurements, then you would require a 49D IOL (which does not exist). The solution is to use the axial length of the left eye as AL of the right eye. The result is depicted in Fig. 7.2. Important: Do NOT use the corneal measurements (K1 and K2) of the left eye for the right eye. In case of astigmatism, this may result in a high error in IOL measurement.

U. Spandau (✉)
University of Stockholm, Stockholm, Sweden
e-mail: ulrich_spandau@yahoo.de

Z. Tomic
Milos Klinika, Belgrade, Serbia
e-mail: zorannos@yahoo.se

BUT: This simple method does not function in case of anisometropia. It is, therefore, essential to check the glasses and to ask the patient if one eye was more near or far sighted than the other. If this is the case, then the following thumb rule will help us: 1 mm ≈ 2.5 to 3D. This means that 1 mm of AL correlates to 2.5–3D of corrected visual acuity. Example: The left eye has a retinal detachment and the IOL Master measures an AL of 23 mm in the right eye and 21 mm in the left eye. The glasses have refraction of −3D (right eye) and −6D (left eye). The AL of the right eye must be shorter than the AL of the left eye. The AL of 21 mm of the left eye is, therefore, wrong but using the AL of the right eye (23 mm) would also be wrong. Now we use the thumb rule: 6D–3D = 3D. 3D correlates to 1 mm. The AL of the left eye is, therefore, approximately 24 mm.

One more tip in case of a white nucleus. The IOL Master can often not measure the AL in case of a hard nucleus. In these cases, an A-scan is recommended. If it is not possible to measure the axial length with the A-scan, then change the settings in the A-scan from "Normal" to "Aphakic". In the "Aphakic" setting, the A-scan measures "over" the nucleus, he pretends that there is no nucleus and in this case, you will ALWAYS get a reliable AL measurement. If you succeeded with an AL measurement, then add 0.3 mm to the AL. The reason for this is that the A-scan machine measures too short in the aphakia setting. Example: The eye has a white

U. Spandau et al. (eds.), *Retinal Detachment Surgery and Proliferative Vitreoretinopathy*,
https://doi.org/10.1007/978-3-031-11946-0_7

Akademiska Sjukhuset

Namn:
Personnummer:
Födelsedatum:
Mätdatum: 2015-12-22
Ögonkirurg: **Akademiska Sjukhuset**

Formel: SRK®/T
Önskad ref.: -2 D
n: 1.3375

ZEISS

Mätvärdena AL ska kontrolleras på plausibilitet, patologiska förändringar kan föreligga!

OD höger	**OS** vänster
AL: 17.90 mm (*)	AL: 25.81 mm (*)
K1: 39.25 D / 8.60 mm (*)	K1: 41.50 D / 8.13 mm (*)
K2: 41.25 D / 8.18 mm (*)	K2: 43.00 D / 7.85 mm (*)
R / SE: 8.39 mm / 40.25 dpt(*)	R / SE: 7.99 mm / 42.25 dpt(*)
Cyl.: -2.00 D (*)	Cyl.: -1.50 D (*)
Status: Fakisk	Status: Fakisk

Hoya 251 (OD)		**Alcon SN60WF** (OD)		**Hoya 251** (OS)		**Alcon SN60WF** (OS)	
A konst:	118.5	A konst:	119	A konst:	118.5	A konst:	119
IOL (D)	REF (D)	IOL (D)	REF (D)	IOL (D)	REF (D)	IOL (D)	REF (D)
49.5	-3.48	51.0	-3.45	19.5	-3.16	20.0	-3.15
49.0	-3.03	50.5	-3.01	19.0	-2.79	19.5	-2.78
48.5	-2.59	50.0	-2.57	18.5	-2.41	19.0	-2.42
48.0	**-2.15**	**49.5**	**-2.15**	**18.0**	**-2.05**	**18.5**	**-2.06**
47.5	-1.72	49.0	-1.72	17.5	-1.68	18.0	-1.70
47.0	-1.29	48.5	-1.30	17.0	-1.32	17.5	-1.35
46.5	-0.87	48.0	-0.89	16.5	-0.97	17.0	-1.00
Emme. IOL:	45.45	Emme. IOL:	46.90	Emme. IOL:	15.11	Emme. IOL:	15.53

AMO Verisyse 50 retropup (OD)		**AMO Tecnis ZA9003** (OD)		**AMO Verisyse 50 retropup** (OS)		**AMO Tecnis ZA9003** (OS)	
A konst:	116.9	A konst:	118.9	A konst:	116.9	A konst:	118.9
IOL (D)	REF (D)	IOL (D)	REF (D)	IOL (D)	REF (D)	IOL (D)	REF (D)
45.0	-3.42	50.5	-3.28	18.0	-3.19	20.0	-3.23
44.5	-2.95	50.0	-2.84	17.5	-2.78	19.5	-2.86
44.0	-2.48	49.5	-2.41	17.0	-2.38	19.0	-2.49
43.5	**-2.02**	**49.0**	**-1.98**	**16.5**	**-1.99**	**18.5**	**-2.13**
43.0	-1.56	48.5	-1.56	16.0	-1.60	18.0	-1.77
42.5	-1.11	48.0	-1.14	15.5	-1.22	17.5	-1.41
42.0	-0.66	47.5	-0.73	15.0	-0.84	17.0	-1.06
Emme. IOL:	41.25	Emme. IOL:	46.60	Emme. IOL:	13.88	Emme. IOL:	15.44

(* = Ändra manuellt, ! =Värde osäkert)

Fig. 7.1 The biometry of a right eye (OD) with retinal detachment. The left eye (OS) is healthy. Observe the different Axial Lengths (AL)

cataract and you excluded a retinal detachment with the B-scan. Take your A-scan, change the settings to "Aphakia" and now you measure easily an AL of 22.5 mm. The final AL is 22.5 + 0.3 = 22.8 mm.

In conclusion: In case of retinal detachment, perform normal biometry of the healthy eye and measure the corneal power (K1 and K2) of the "detached" eye. Axial length measurement of the detached eye is not possible. Then use the axial length of the healthy eye for the detached eye. Finished.

Akademiska Sjukhuset

Namn: J
Personnummer: I
Födelsedatum: I
Mätdatum: 2015-12-22
Ögonkirurg: **Akademiska Sjukhuset**

Formel: SRK®/T
Önskad ref.: -2 D
n: 1.3375

ZEISS

Mätvärdena AL ska kontrolleras på plausibilitet, patologiska förändringar kan föreligga!

OD höger

AL: 25.81 mm (*)
K1: 39.25 D / 8.60 mm (*)
K2: 41.25 D / 8.18 mm (*)
R / SE: 8.39 mm / 40.25 dpt(*)
Cyl.: -2.00 D (*)

Status: Fakisk

OS vänster

AL: 25.81 mm (*)
K1: 41.50 D / 8.13 mm (*)
K2: 43.00 D / 7.85 mm (*)
R / SE: 7.99 mm / 42.25 dpt(*)
Cyl.: -1.50 D (*)

Status: Fakisk

OD:

Hoya 251		**Alcon SN60WF**	
A konst:	118.5	A konst:	119
IOL (D)	REF (D)	IOL (D)	REF (D)
21.5	-3.13	22.0	-3.09
21.0	-2.73	21.5	-2.70
20.5	-2.34	21.0	-2.32
20.0	**-1.96**	**20.5**	**-1.94**
19.5	-1.58	20.0	-1.57
19.0	-1.20	19.5	-1.20
18.5	-0.83	19.0	-0.84
Emme. IOL: 17.36		Emme. IOL: 17.82	

AMO Verisyse 50 retropup		**AMO Tecnis ZA9003**	
A konst:	116.9	A konst:	118.9
IOL (D)	REF (D)	IOL (D)	REF (D)
20.0	-3.23	22.0	-3.18
19.5	-2.81	21.5	-2.79
19.0	-2.39	21.0	-2.40
18.5	**-1.98**	**20.5**	**-2.02**
18.0	-1.57	20.0	-1.65
17.5	-1.17	19.5	-1.28
17.0	-0.77	19.0	-0.91
Emme. IOL: 16.01		Emme. IOL: 17.73	

OS:

Hoya 251		**Alcon SN60WF**	
A konst:	118.5	A konst:	119
IOL (D)	REF (D)	IOL (D)	REF (D)
19.5	-3.16	20.0	-3.15
19.0	-2.79	19.5	-2.78
18.5	-2.41	19.0	-2.42
18.0	**-2.05**	**18.5**	**-2.06**
17.5	-1.68	18.0	-1.70
17.0	-1.32	17.5	-1.35
16.5	-0.97	17.0	-1.00
Emme. IOL: 15.11		Emme. IOL: 15.53	

AMO Verisyse 50 retropup		**AMO Tecnis ZA9003**	
A konst:	116.9	A konst:	118.9
IOL (D)	REF (D)	IOL (D)	REF (D)
18.0	-3.19	20.0	-3.23
17.5	-2.78	19.5	-2.86
17.0	-2.38	19.0	-2.49
16.5	**-1.99**	**18.5**	**-2.13**
16.0	-1.60	18.0	-1.77
15.5	-1.22	17.5	-1.41
15.0	-0.84	17.0	-1.06
Emme. IOL: 13.88		Emme. IOL: 15.44	

(* = Ändra manuellt, ! = Värde osäkert)

Fig. 7.2 The corrected biometry. The AL of the left eye is used as AL for the right eye

7.2 Anaesthesia

We use **local** anaesthesia for (1) Pneumatic retinopexy, (2) Lenssparing vitrectomy with cryopexy and gas (Moorfield technique) and (3) Combined (25G, 27G) phaco + vitrectomy with chandelier light.

We use **general** anaesthesia for (4) Encircling band + vitrectomy + retinotomy + C3F8 (Stockholm technique), (5) Bimanual peeling + retinotomy for PVR detachment

And (6) Episcleral buckling (Segmental buckle with chandelier light and microscope) with chandelier light.

In the latter cases, peribulbar anaesthesia is sufficient. We use 50% Carbocain 20 mg/ml and 50% Marcain 5 mg/ml. We inject approximately 5–6 ml into the inferotemporal orbital region. In painful procedures such as episcleral buckling,

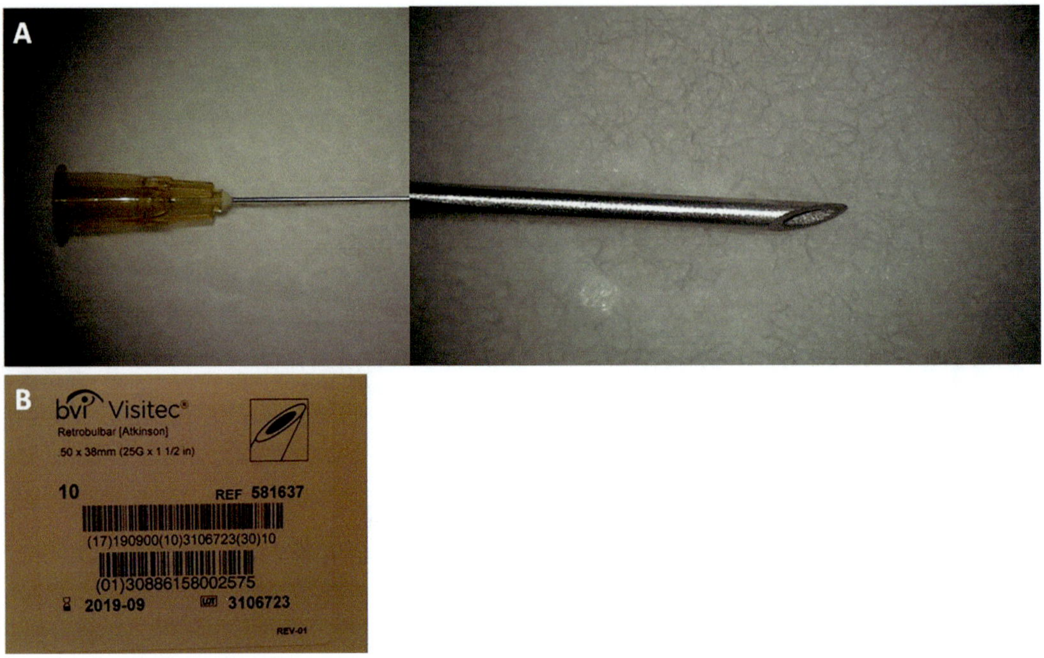

Fig. 7.3 A retrobulbar cannula rom Atkinson. The blunt tip prevents a scleral perforation

we add 3 ml into the superior orbital and 1–2 ml through the caruncle. If the patient complains during surgery about pain, we add only Carbocain and inject 2–3 ml into the caruncle. The anaesthetic effect comes after approximately 1 min.

Surgical pearls no. 111 (Fig 7.3)
Scleral perforation: If you use a 25G or 23G cannula, you may perforate the globe during retrobulbar anaesthesia. Use a blunt 25G retrobulbar cannula from Atkinson instead. The blunt tip prevents a scleral perforation.

Part II
Surgical Techniques for Retinal Detachment

All videos of this part are found in a playlist on my youTube channel:
https://youtube.com/playlist?list=PL0dKYclPD7yMn861X0g-aHCS6KZ5NcH1N
Chapter 8: No video
Chapter 9: No video
Chapter 10: **Pneumatic Retinopexy (Toronto Technique)**
Pneumatic retinopexy with Biom
Chapter 11: No video
Chapter 12: **Combined Phaco/Vitrectomy (Frankfurt Technique)**
Retinal detachment for dummies
27G-retinal detachment without PFCL
Retinal detachment high myopia with PFCL
Chapter 13: No video
Chapter 14: No video
Chapter 15: **Episcleral Buckling for Detachment Surgery with BIOM**
Episcleral buckling with BIOM 1
Episcleral buckling with BIOM 2
Complication during episcleral buckling
27G vitrectomy and episcleral buckling. How would you operate this case?
Scleral buckling for PVR C2.

8 What is the Best Surgical Technique?

Ulrich Spandau, Zoran Tomic,
and Diego Ruiz-Casas

The following surgical techniques are employed at the University of Stockholm for the surgical repair of a retinal detachment:

(1) Pneumatic retinopexy
(2) Lenssparing vitrectomy with cryopexy and gas (Moorfield technique)
(3) Combined phaco + vitrectomy with chandelier light (Frankfurt technique)
(4) Encircling band + vitrectomy + retinotomy + C3F8 (Stockholm technique)
(5) Bimanual peeling + retinotomy for PVR detachment
(6) Episcleral buckling (Segmental buckle with chandelier light and microscope)

Pneumatic retinopexy is very popular in California and Canada. Detachments with ruptures from 8 o'clock over 12 o'clock to 4 o'clock and macula off are treated with gas injection. A few days later the break is sealed with laser photocoagulation. This technique can also be used for pediatric detachments. The break is treated with cryopexy and the retina is reattached with gas injection. The risk for a recurrent RD is increased but without loss of visual outcome. The final reattachment rate is similar to phaco/vitrectomy. We use this technique with a small indication spectrum: Focal detachments with ruptures between 10 and 2 o'clock. Chandelier light is introduced. The rupture is treated with cryopexy under the view of BIOM and a gas bubble is injected.

The *Moorfield technique* is the most common technique for RD at Moorfield Hospital, London. This technique is used for all types of RDs except inferior RDs. Even macula off detachments are operated with this technique. A lens sparing vitrectomy is performed, the retinal ruptures are treated with cryopexy and gas is injected. The surgical time is short and the surgical material is small. The rate of primary attachment is 94%. The risk for macular folds is increased.

The *combined phaco/vitrectomy* was developed by Prof. Eckardt in Frankfurt, and is nowadays the gold standard technique for RD. In patients with an age over 50 years, phacoemulsification is performed and a chandelier light is inserted. A complete vitrectomy with vitreous base shaving is performed. The anterior vitreous can be removed completely reducing the risk for a PVR redetachment. In case of an inferior detachment, a Densiron Xtra tamponade can be used.

The *Stockholm technique* is the standard technique for retinal detachments at St Eriks University hospital in Stockholm. This technique

U. Spandau (✉)
St Eriks hospital, University of Stockholm, Stockholm, Sweden
e-mail: ulrich_spandau@yahoo.de

Z. Tomic
Milos Klinika, Belgrade, Serbia
e-mail: zorannos@yahoo.se

D. Ruiz-Casas
Retina Department, Hospital Ramón y Cajal, Madrid, Spain

U. Spandau et al. (eds.), *Retinal Detachment Surgery and Proliferative Vitreoretinopathy*,
https://doi.org/10.1007/978-3-031-11946-0_8

is especially advisable for myopic patients and inferior detachments but can be employed for all types of detachments. The surgery is usually performed without phacoemulsification. An encircling band is placed, a central and peripheral vitrectomy is performed, the subretinal fluid is removed through a posterior retinotomy and C_3F_8 is injected.

For *PVR detachments* we place an encircling band, insert a chandelier light and remove all membranes with bimanual peeling. In recurrent cases, a retinotomy is preferred. This technique is surgically very demanding and requires several intravitreal instruments.

Episcleral buckling is less and less common but this technique is still state of art for ora dialysis, young myopes and old detachments without PVR. We will demonstrate a simple surgical technique. Indirect binocular ophthalmoscopy is not necessary. For visualization of the fundus, a chandelier light is inserted and a microscope with a viewing system is employed. Cryopexy and suturing of the segmental buckle are done under the microscope.

8.1 What Surgical Technique Do We Use in Daily Practice?

For small focal detachments, we use pneumatic retinopexy. In macula-on detachments, we use mostly the Moorfield technique. In macula off detachments, we use the phaco/vitrectomy technique. In myopic patients, we use the Stockholm technique. In inferior detachments, we use the phaco/vitrectomy technique with Densiron Xtra.

8.2 Best Surgical Technique

The best surgical technique depends on the viewpoint. The best surgical technique is different if you take the reattachment rate as the primary outcome parameter or if you take visual acuity as the primary outcome parameter. We all know what a good visual acuity is but what is a good attachment rate?

8.2.1 Best Reattachment Rate

A primary reattachment rate of 100% is not achievable. The best primary attachment rate you can achieve is 94%. Your rate should be between 90 and 94%. A final reattachment rate of 100% is also difficult to achieve and depends if you include silicone oil-filled eyes or not.

8.2.2 Primary Outcome Parameter: Reattachment Rate

For phakic eyes, the best reattachment rate is achieved with scleral buckling (94%) and cerclage/vitrectomy (91%). The attachment rate is significantly worse for vitrectomy alone (83%) [1]. These numbers relate to a single surgery. In pseudophakic eyes, the primary reattachment rate is 92% for cerclage/vitrectomy and 83% for vitrectomy alone [2]. Pneumatic retinopexy has a low primary reattachment rate of 65–88% [3].

8.2.3 Primary Outcome Parameter: Visual Acuity

If you choose visual acuity as the primary outcome parameter, then you will be really surprised because pneumatic retinopexy is in this case the best technique. We recommend reading the randomized study from Hillier and colleagues from Toronto, Canada [4]. A primary detachment was randomized for pneumatic retinopexy or vitrectomy. The best visual acuity results were achieved with pneumatic retinopexy irrespectively for phakic or pseudophakic eyes. The VA outcome was significantly worse in the vitrectomy group. The primary attachment rate, however, was only 88% in the pneumatic group versus 92% in the vitrectomy group but the final attachment results were equal.

In a big retrospective study from Ryan and colleagues, phakic detachments were operated on with the techniques such as scleral buckling, vitrectomy and combined cerclage/vitrectomy. Scleral buckling had the best visual outcome [1].

In a big retrospective study by Joseph and colleagues, pseudophakic detachments were operated on with vitrectomy and combined cerclage/vitrectomy. Both techniques had similar visual outcomes [2].

8.3 Friday 4 o'clock Detachment and Binocular Occlusion

In California, pneumatic retinopexy is very popular and so popular that a Friday afternoon detachment is called a friday retinopexy. Why? Because pneumatic retinopexy is a fast procedure and stabilizes the eye until Monday. Are there other options?

In the old times of buckling surgery, a technique was used which is practically unknown today to young surgeons: Binocular occlusion. Both eyes are occluded with an eye patch, the patient shall rest and only take off the eye patches for toilet and eating. The result of binocular occlusion is that macula endangering retinal detachments will not progress and the macula will not detach until Monday. In case of acute vitreous hemorrhage, 50% of eyes will settle overnight and 89% will settle enough by 4 days to make the retina visible and available for laser or cryopexy to close a tear [5].

Conclusion: In case of a retinal detachment endangering the macula and arriving at your clinic at Friday 4 o'clock: Prescribe binocular occlusion, the macula will not be detached on Monday morning.

8.4 Summary

A good primary reattachment rate lies between 90 and 94%. The *best primary reattachment* rate can be achieved in phakic eyes with scleral buckling and in pseudophakic eyes with combined cerclage/vitrectomy. The *best visual acuity* can be achieved with scleral buckling and pneumatic retinopexy. Choose the technique which functions best with your hands. But try to think outside the box and try other techniques. All techniques are summarized in the following figures (Figs. 8.1, 8.2, 8.3 and 8.4).

Pneumatic retinopexy:

Pros:

Visual function recovery: High

Material: Very low

Surgical time: Short (10 min)

Anaesthesia: Local

Cons:

Attachment rate: 65-88%

OPD visits: High

Type of detachment: All RD´s except inferior and PVR

Fig. 8.1 Pros and Cons of pneumatic retinopexy

Vitrectomy, cryopexy, gas:

Pros:

Material: Mediocre

Surgical time: Short (20 min)

Attachment rate: 85%-92%

Visual function recovery: Good

Anaesthesia: Local

Cons:

Type of detachment: All RD´s except inferior and PVR

Fig. 8.2 Pros and Cons of vitrectomy, cryopexy and gas (Moorfield technique)

Combined phaco/vitrectomy:

Pros:

Attachment rate: 85%-92%

Type of detachment: All RD´s except PVR

Visual function recovery: Good

Anaesthesia: Local

Cons:

Material: High

Surgical time: Mediocre (45 min)

Fig. 8.3 Pros and Cons of phaco/vitrectomy, laser and gas (Frankfurt technique)

Encircling band, vitrectomy, gas:
Pros:
Attachment rate: 92%
Type of detachment: All
Cons:
Visual function recovery: Mediocre
Material: High
Surgical time: High (75 min)
Anaesthesia: General anaesthesia

Fig. 8.4 Pros and Cons of combined encircling band and vitrectomy (Stockholm technique)

References

1. Ryan EH, Ryan CM, Forbes NJ, Yonekawa Y, Wagley S, Mittra RA, Parke DW, Joseph DP, Emerson GG, Shah GK, Blinder KJ, Capone A, Williams GA, Eliott D, Gupta OP, Hsu J, Regillo CD. Primary retinal detachment outcomes study report number 2: Phakic retinal detachment outcomes. Ophthalmol. 2020;127(8):1077-1085. https://doi.org/10.1016/j.ophtha.2020.03.007. Epub 2020 Mar 9. PMID: 32312634
2. Joseph DP, Ryan EH, Ryan CM, Forbes NJK, Wagley S, Yonekawa Y, Mittra RA, Parke DW, Emerson GG, Shah GK, Blinder KJ, Capone A, Williams GA, Eliott D, Gupta OP, Hsu J, Regillo CD. Primary retinal detachment outcomes study: Pseudophakic retinal detachment outcomes: primary retinal detachment outcomes study report number 3. Ophthalmol. 2020;127(11):1507-1514. https://doi.org/10.1016/j.ophtha.2020.05.005. Epub 2020 May 8. PMID: 32437865
3. Chan CK, Lin SG, Nuthi AS, Salib DM. Pneumatic retinopexy for the repair of retinal detachments: a comprehensive review (1986–2007). Surv Ophthalmol. 2008;53(5):443–78. https://doi.org/10.1016/j.survophthal.2008.06.008. PMID: 18929759.
4. Hillier RJ, Felfeli T, Berger AR, Wong DT, Altomare F, Dai D, Giavedoni LR, Kertes PJ, Kohly RP, Muni RH. The Pneumatic Retinopexy versus Vitrectomy for the Management of Primary Rhegmatogenous Retinal Detachment Outcomes Randomized Trial (PIVOT). Ophthalmol. 2019;126(4):531-539. https://doi.org/10.1016/j.ophtha.2018.11.014. Epub 2018 Nov 22. PMID: 30468761.
5. Lincoff H, Stopa M, Kreissig I. Ambulatory binocular occlusion. Retina. 2004;24:246–53.

9 Special Surgical Techniques for Vitrectomy of Retinal Detachment

Ulrich Spandau, Zoran Tomic, and Diego Ruiz-Casas

9.1 Surgery of an Encircling Band

Instruments

Mersilene 5–0

Silk 3–0

Encircling band (S2987, Labtician, Canada) (Fig. 9.1) and sleeve (S3083, Labtician, Canada) (Fig. 9.1)

Strabismus hook (of Gass)

Orbita spatula.

The surgery of an encircling band step-by-step:

1. **Limbal peritomy 360°**
2. **Dissect Tenon from the sclera**
3. **Place 4 holding sutures (Silk 3–0) on the straight muscles**
4. **Place the encircling band under all 4 straight muscles**
5. **Check that the band is not twisted**
6. **Insert both ends of the band into the sleeve at the inferotemporal quadrant**
7. **Mark the sclera with a caliper at Axial Length/2 mm behind the limbus**
8. **Place the first stitch (Mersilene 5–0) posterior to the scleral marking and hold the band at the same time anterior to the marking**
9. **Place the second stitch anterior to the scleral marking and hold the band at the same time posterior to the marking**
10. **Tie the suture and continue with the next three quadrants**
11. **Tighten the band.**

The surgery in detail:

1. **Limbal peritomy 360°**
2. **Dissect Tenon from the sclera**
3. **Place 4 holding sutures (silk 3–0) on the straight muscles**
   Open the conjunctiva 360° at the limbus with a Westcott scissors and anatomic forceps. Then dissect the tenon capsule from the sclera using a strabismus forceps. Dissect to the equator. Then place a strabismus hook with a hole under the rectus muscle and insert a silk 3–0 suture. Pull back the hook with a suture and place a knot on the suture. Repeat this step with all 4 rectus muscles.
4. **Place the encircling band under all 4 straight muscles**
5. **Check that the band is not twisted**
   Start at the inferotemporal position. Pull the holding sutures of the inferior and temporal rectus, insert the orbital spatula and insert the silicone band behind the temporal rectus.

U. Spandau (✉)
University of Stockholm, Stockholm, Sweden
e-mail: ulrich_spandau@yahoo.de

Z. Tomic
Milos Klinika, Belgrade, Serbia
e-mail: zorannos@yahoo.se

D. Ruiz-Casas
Hospital Ramón y Cajal, Madrid, Spain

U. Spandau et al. (eds.), *Retinal Detachment Surgery and Proliferative Vitreoretinopathy*,
https://doi.org/10.1007/978-3-031-11946-0_9

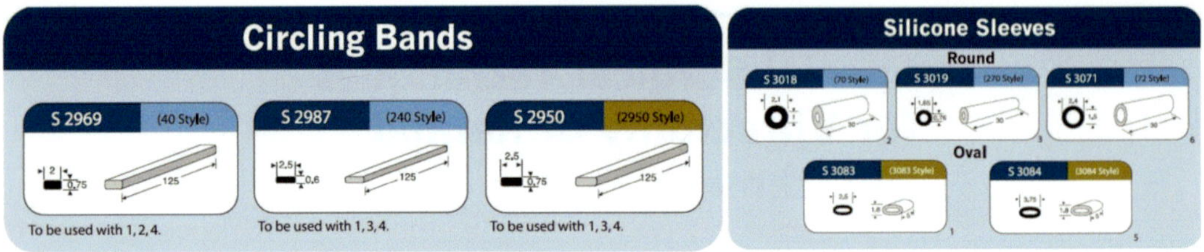

Fig. 9.1 Circling bands and silicone sleeves (Labtician, Canada)

Double check that the encircling band is located behind the complete muscle. Then pull the sutures of the temporal and superior rectus, insert the orbital spatula and place the band behind the superior rectus (Fig. 9.2); and so on until you are back to the inferotemporal position with both ends. Then check all 4 quadrants that the band is not twisted.

6. **Insert both ends of the band into the sleeve at the inferotemporal quadrant**
   Now comes the most difficult step for this surgery: Place the sleeve on the special forceps (Labtician, Canada) and insert the first end (this is easy) and then the second end (this is very tricky). If you succeed, then tighten the band a little bit.
7. **Mark the sclera with a caliper at Axial Length/2 mm behind the limbus**
8. **Place the first stitch (Mersilene 5–0) posterior to the scleral marking and hold the band at the same time anterior to the marking**

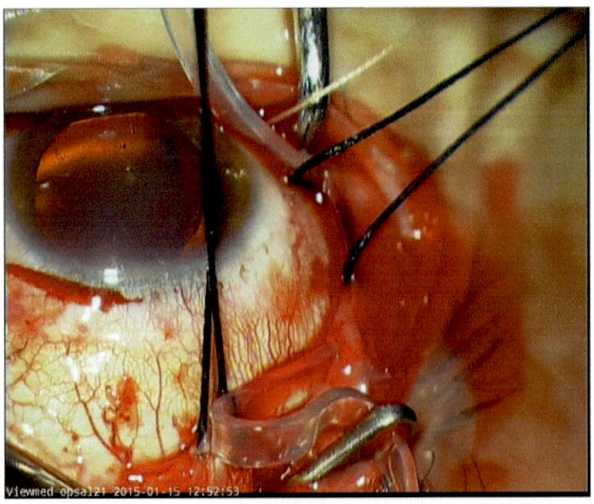

Fig. 9.2 With a strabismus hook with hole the encircling band can be placed under all rectus muscles

9. **Place the second stitch anterior to the scleral marking and hold the band at the same time posterior to the marking**
10. **Tie the suture and continue with the next three quadrants.**
    We continue now at the superotemporal quadrant. Pull the sutures and insert the orbital spatula. Then mark the sclera at AXL/2, i.e., the eye has an AXL = 23 mm, then mark the sclera at 11.5 mm. The marking is located in the middle of the band. Fixate then the band with a forceps anterior to the marking and place the first stitch (Mersilene 5–0) 1.5 mm posterior to the marking. Then fixate the band posterior to the first stitch and place a second stitch with the same suture 1.5 mm anterior to the marking. Then tie the suture and continue with the next three quadrants. The final suture is located at the sleeve.
11. **Tighten the band**
    Now tighten the band. The globe should be a little bit hypotensive, approximately 8 mmHg, to achieve a good impression. You can either tighten the band until the band lies tense on the sclera or tighten the band maximally 8 mm.

Surgical pearls no. 93
Anterior segment ischemia is caused by disruption of ciliary artery circulation secondary to the encircling band. The ocular blood flow and pulse are reduced (**2**). The typical signs are corneal edema, anterior chamber flare, ocular hypotension, and in severe cases iris neovascularization. Cutting off the encircling band restores the ocular circulation and symptoms. Removal of the band is not necessary.

9.2 Usage of a Chandelier Light

Surgery for retinal detachment means bimanual vitrectomy and the usage of a chandelier light. Bimanual vitrectomy is an essential part of modern Minimal Incision Vitreoretinal Surgery (MIVS). By inserting a stationary chandelier light in the sclera (4-port vitrectomy, Fig. 9.3), the surgeon has two active hands. To operate with two active hands is a new and exciting method of surgery. For example, in retinal detachment surgery, you can indent the sclera with one hand and vitrectomize the vitreous base with the other hand. In diabetic retinopathy, you can apply laser photocoagulation up to the ora serrata with the help of a scleral depressor. You can remove membranes with two different instruments and also apply counteraction and so on.

For optimal use of a chandelier light three requirements have to be met:

(1) Inferonasal insertion enabling a good rotation of the globe.
(2) A rigid cable allowing aiming the light source in all directions in the vitreous cavity.
(3) Strong light source for optimal illumination.

The chandelier light is best positioned inferonasally, because here its location does not affect the rotation of the eye. The 12 o'clock or 6 o'clock insertion sites disturb the rotation of the globe and the light fiber is easily dislocated when the globe is rotated upwards or downwards. The rigid cable allows bending of the light fiber and henceforth the ability to maneuver the light to different directions in the vitreous cavity. The light source of modern vitrectomy machines (Constellation, Stellaris, Eva) is sufficient for optimal illumination of chandelier light. The light source of old vitrectomy machines (Accurus) is *not* sufficient for optimal illumination of chandelier light. In the latter case, an external light source (Photon or Xenon) is required for a sufficient illumination of the vitreous cavity.

Practical tips for insertion of chandelier light

If you have never used a chandelier light before, then start with one which can be easily inserted. The 25-gauge chandelier light from ALCON and the 23-gauge chandelier light from DORC are simple to use (see Table 9.1) as the light fiber can be placed inside a normal one-step trocar (Figs. 9.4 and 9.5).

The chandelier light from Synergetics is trickier to put in place, but on the other hand, it provides excellent panoramic illumination of the vitreous cavity. Rotate the globe with a swab in a superotemporal direction so that there is space for the insertion of the chandelier light inferonasally. With the sclerotomy needle supplied by the manufacturer, one first performs a transconjunctival sclerotomy 3.5 mm posterior to the limbus with a perpendicular (not lamellar) path.

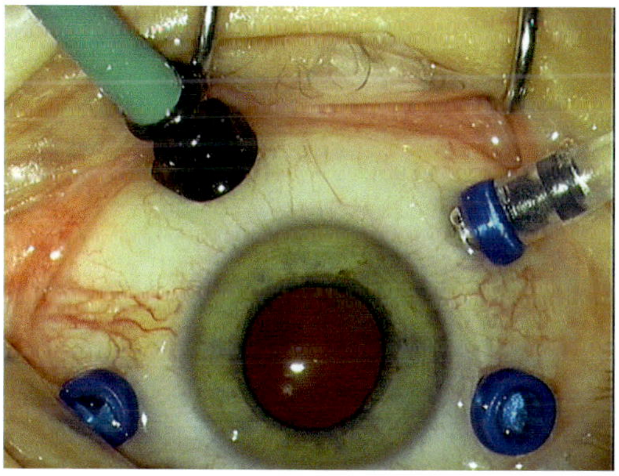

Fig. 9.3 An eye with 4-port vitrectomy. In addition to the known three-port system, a chandelier-light fibre was firmly inserted into the sclera (top left)

Table 9.1 Features of different types of chandelier lights

Chandelier light	ALCON[a]	DORC[b]	Synergetics[c]
Light source	Photon	Xenon	Photon
Illumination	Good	Good	Very good
Rigid cable	Yes	No	Yes
Maneuverability	Average	Reduced	Good
Method of insertion	Trocar	Trocar	Sclera
Difficulty of insertion	Simple	Simple	Average

ALCON[a]: Chandelier Accurus 8,065,751,574; DORC[b]: 23-gauge Chandelier light 3269.EB06; Synergetics[c]: 25-Gauge Awh Chandelier 56.20.25

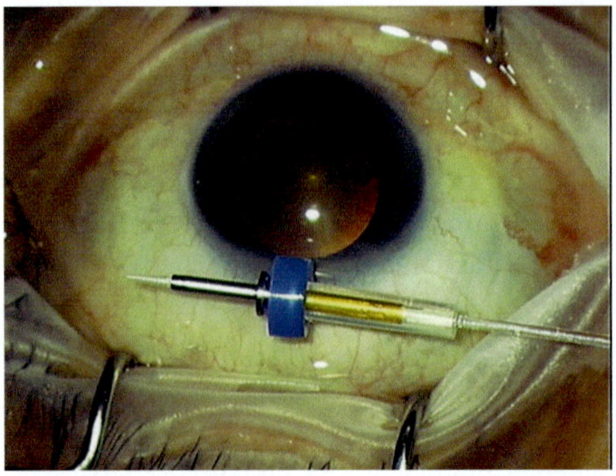

Fig. 9.4 A 23-gauge chandelier light from DORC, which is very easy to insert because it is placed in a trocar. Similar chandelier lights are available from Alcon and Synergetics

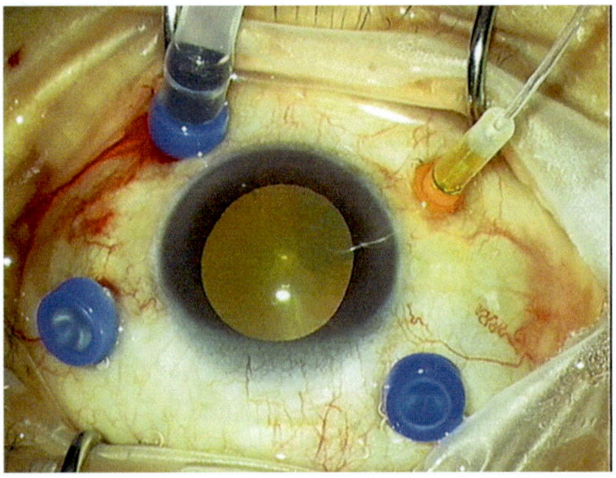

Fig. 9.5 Same 23-gauge chandelier light. Place inferonasally a 23-gauge trocar. Then insert the light fiber into an ALCON or DORC trocar (with or without valve). DORC: 23-gauge Chandelier light 3269.EB06

The chandelier light is then inserted into the sclerotomy. This procedure requires some practice. The Synergetics chandelier light requires an external Photon light source. By bending the rigid cable of the chandelier light, you can manipulate the light source. Sometimes you need to tape the cable to the drape.

Surgical pearls no. 65

Chandelier light:

(1) The insertion of the chandelier light is rather difficult in avitreal eyes because the globe is soft. Use a 25G trocar stiletto for the sclerotomy.

(2) Conjunctival chemosis or hemorrhage may make it difficult to identify the sclerotomy. In such cases, open the conjunctiva focally with scissors and forceps in order to visualize the sclerotomy.

9.3 Use of Heavy Liquid or Posterior Retinotomy

Subretinal fluid can be removed in two ways:

(1) With the use of heavy liquid from peripheral break. The subretinal fluid is pushed from posterior to anterior (Fig. 9.6).

(2) Posterior retinotomy. The subretinal fluid is pushed from anterior to posterior (Fig. 9.6).

(1) *With the use of heavy liquid from peripheral break*: Heavy liquid (PFCL) attaches to the retina and presses the subretinal fluid through a peripheral break.

(2) *Posterior retinotomy*: The central retinal rupture is iatrogenic and called posterior retinotomy (Fig. 9.7). The retinotomy is

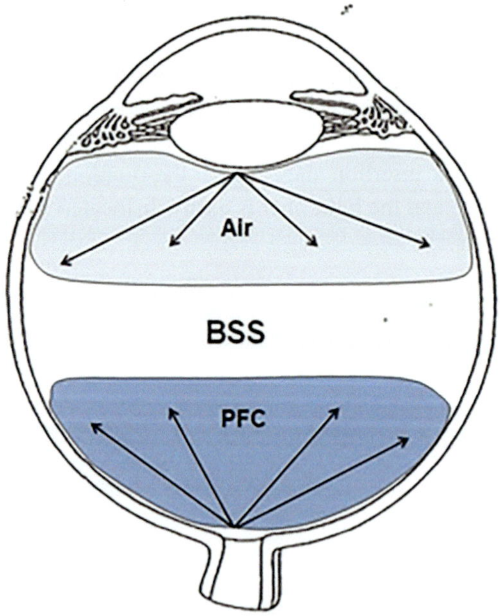

Fig. 9.6 Opposite effects of air and PFCL in the vitreous cavity. Air exerts pressure onto the retina from anterior to posterior, whereas PFCL exerts pressure from posterior to anterior

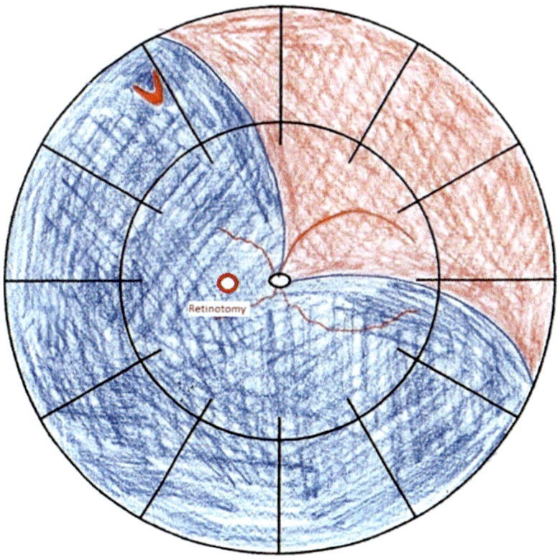

Fig. 9.7 A central retinotomy is created to remove the subretinal fluid. It is located outside the temporal arcade

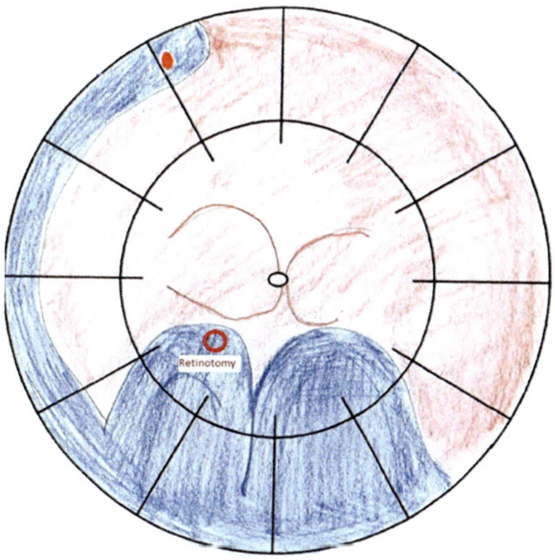

Fig. 9.8 The posterior retinotomy is placed at the site of maximal subretinal fluid

located outside the temporal arcade at the site of the maximal amount of subretinal fluid (Figs. 9.7 and 9.8). The disadvantage of a central retinotomy is focal destruction of the nerve fiber layer resulting in a nerve fiber layer defect. Another disadvantage of a central retinotomy is an additional rupture in the central pole which has to be laser treated and tamponaded.

Bibliography

1. Vitrectomy with silicone oil or sulfur hexafluoride gas in eyes with severe proliferative vitreoretinopathy: results of a randomized clinical trial. Silicone Study Report 1. Arch Ophthalmol 1992;110(6):770–9.
2. Kreissig I. Minimal surgery for retinal detachment. Thieme. ISBN 3131110619.
3. Heimann H, Bartz-Schmidt KU, et al. Scleral buckling versus primary vitrectomy in rhegmatogenous retinal detachment: a prospective randomized multicenter clinical study. Ophthalmol. 2007; 114(12):2142–54.

10 Pneumatic Retinopexy (Toronto Technique)

Ulrich Spandau

10.1 Introduction

Pneumatic retinopexy is very popular in California and Canada, but elsewhere it is rarely used. According to a randomized study (PIVOT study) from the University of Toronto, pneumatic retinopexy is superior to vitrectomy for RD repair (Hillier RJ, Ophthalmology. 2019). In this study, a primary detachment was randomized in pneumatic retinopexy or vitrectomy. The best visual acuity results were achieved with pneumatic retinopexy. The VA outcome was significantly worse in the vitrectomy group. The primary detachment rate, however, was only 88% in the pneumatic group versus 92% in the vitrectomy group, but the final attachment results were equal. At the University from Toronto study all RD´s with breaks from 7 over 12 to 5 o'clock are included, irrespectively if the macula is on or off and irrespectively if the eye is phakic or pseudophakic. The surgery is performed without microscope and BIOM. This means that the search for the break is done at the slitlamp and with binocular indirect ophthalmoscopy on the surgical table. This technique is less trained nowadays. The retinal break can be sealed on the surgical table with cryopexy or a few days later with laser photocoagulation. The latter method is better because laser effects seal the break faster than cryopexy.

This educative video illustrates this surgical technique: https://www.aao.org/clinical-video/pneumatic-retinopexy-laser-cryo-retinopexy.

There are two possible techniques for pneumatic retinopexy: (1) Binocular ophthalmoscopy with helmet or (2) the microscope with BIOM and insertion of a chandelier light. Here we describe the second method. We employ a microscope with BIOM for the search of the retinal break. We use cryopexy and not laser. In addition, we limit the indication to a focal detachment with a retinal break between 10 o'clock and 2 o'clock and attached superior arcade (Fig. 10.1).

Remark: It is important only to use a short-lasting gas for this technique such as air or SF_6. A long lasting gas may induce breaks.

Anaesthesia: We use always subtenonal or peribulbar anaesthesia. General anaesthesia is not necessary.

10.2 The surgery

Figures 10.2, 10.3, 10.4, 10.5 and 10.6

1. Insertion of a chandelier light (Figs. 10.2 and 10.3)
2. Flick in the BIOM (Fig. 10.4)
3. Cryopexy of the break (Fig. 10.5)

U. Spandau (✉)
St. Eriks Hospital, University of Stockholm, Stockholm, Sweden
e-mail: ulrich_spandau@yahoo.de

U. Spandau et al. (eds.), *Retinal Detachment Surgery and Proliferative Vitreoretinopathy*,
https://doi.org/10.1007/978-3-031-11946-0_10

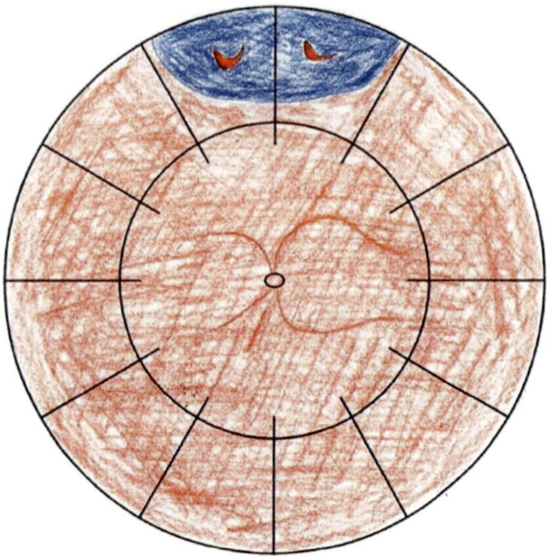

Fig. 10.1 A focal retinal detachment from 11:00 to 1:00 and two retinal breaks at 12 o'clock

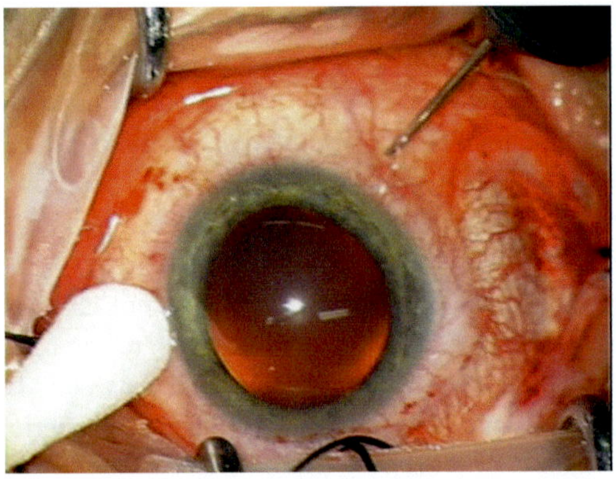

Fig. 10.2 Insertion of chandelier light

Insert the chandelier light on the opposite side of the break. If the break is localized at 12 o'clock then insert the chandelier light at 6 o'clock. Flick in the BIOM, localize the break, and freeze the break edges with cryopexy.

4. Removal of the chandelier light
5. AC tap
6. Injection of air or gas (Fig. 10.6)

Remove the chandelier light, suture the sclerotomy with a Vicryl 8–0 suture and remove a possible vitreous prolapse with a Vannas

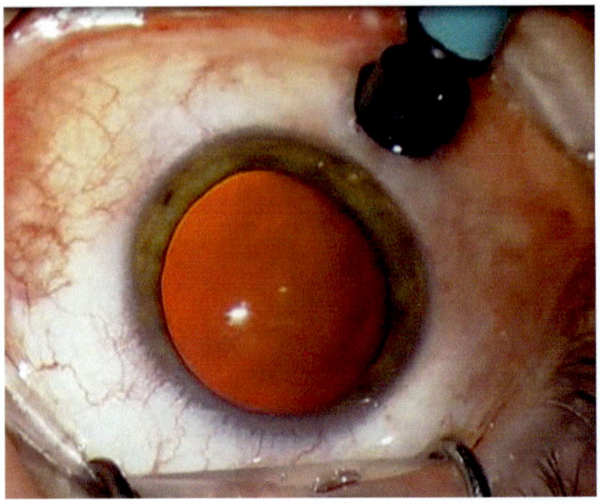

Fig. 10.3 Insertion of chandelier light (Synergetics, USA)

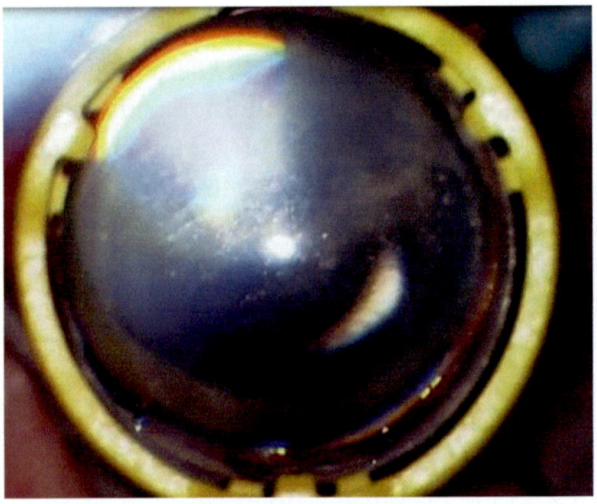

Fig. 10.4 Flick in the BIOM

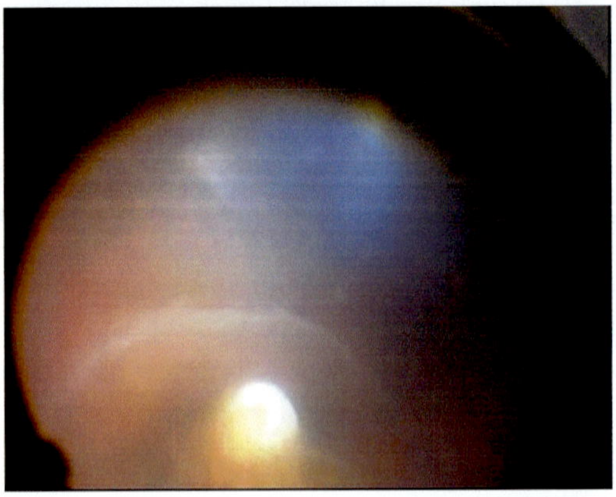

Fig. 10.5 Cryopexy of the retinal break

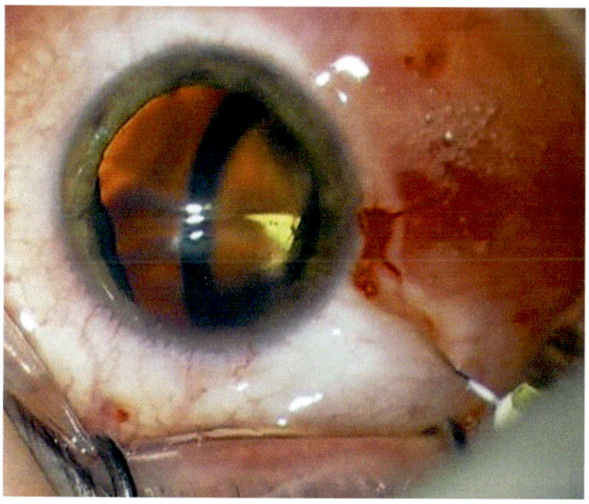

Fig. 10.6 Injection of 0.5 ml 100% SF_6

scissors. With a 30G needle cannula on a 3 cc syringe you can aspirate 0.3–0.4 ml aqueous from the anterior chamber. Then inject 0.5 ml 100% SF_6 into the vitreous cavity. Check the IOP with your index finger.

Tipps & tricks

Air as tamponade: Air is an excellent alternative to SF_6. The duration of an air tamponade is maximal 1 week. A shorter tamponade duration reduces the risk for complications such as a tractive detachment. Use air for a hole between 11 and 1 o'clock.

10.3 Postoperative Posture

The patient has to perform a so-called steamroller maneuver to expedite retinal reattachment by pushing the *subretinal fluid* through the retinal break (Fig. 10.7). After the gas is injected, the maneuver starts with immediate face down positioning for 4–6 h, 4 h in case of macula-on RD and 6 h in case of macula off RD. This is followed by gradual elevation of the head, 30°/h, until the head is upright. Then, the patient is allowed to position so that the apex of the bubble covers the retinal breaks.

Postoperative follow-up

Patients treated with pneumatic retinopexy need more postoperative visits and surgeries than patients with a vitrectomy and gas surgery. A 1-day and 1-week follow-up is recommended. If displaced fluid is observed on day one then a daily follow-up is recommended until it is clear that the displaced fluid does not increase.

The rate for a redetachment is higher with this technique. A reinjection of gas is also common for this technique. It is important to underline that the increased redetachment risk does not influence the visual acuity in a negative way. For example, in a patient with a superotemporal break in the detached retina and an inferotemporal break in the attached retina. It is possible that on day 1 or 2 after surgery, the superotemporal break is secure with retinopexy in situ, but the inferotemporal break may have become lifted by the displaced fluid. If a second bubble of SF_6 is injected and the patient is positioned flat on the side then the inferotemporal break will reattach.

Case report

A superotemporal retinal detachment is present Fig. 10.8. First all pathology in attached retina is lasered. After a 0,3 cc ac tap, 0,6 cc Sf6 is injected into the vitreous cavity. As postoperative posture the face is positioned down for 6 h. Then the face is positioned on the right side with head elevated. On the next day the retina is attached. The retinal break is lasered with indirect ophthalmoscopy. Positioning is continued for 1 week (Fig. 10.9).

10.4 Complications

Sometimes an inferior detachment occurs. The cause is displaced fluid (Fig. 10.10). Observe if a break is present. The key point is that displaced fluid should be unassociated with any open break and reduce over time. It is important not to operate these cases prematurely but to wait. Schedule daily controls. In the most cases the subretinal fluid decreases within one week. In rare cases it may take several weeks. If a new

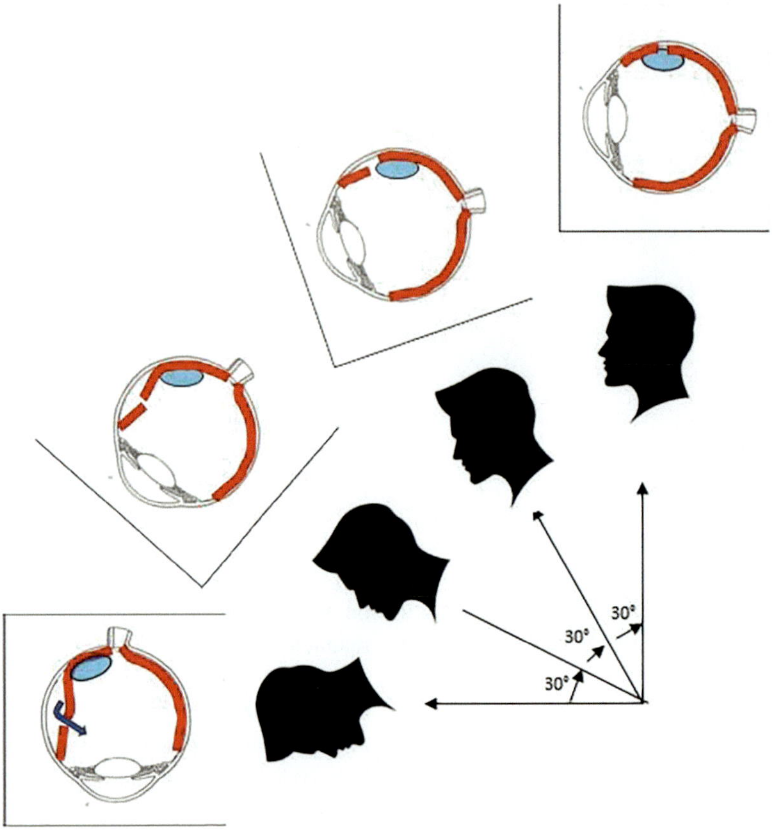

Fig. 10.7 Steam roller maneuver

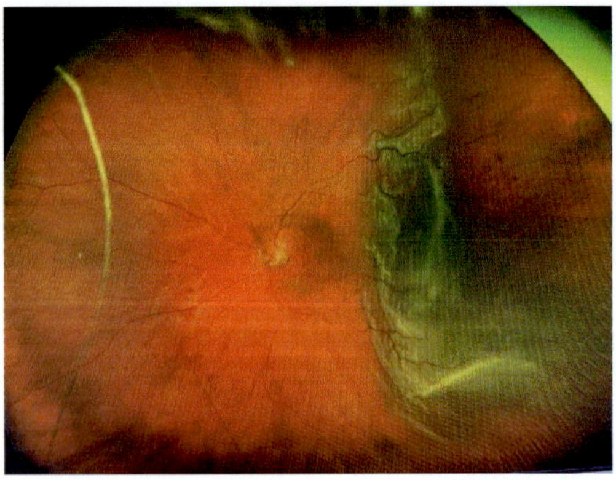

Fig. 10.8 A superotemporal detachment. Photocourtesy RH Muni

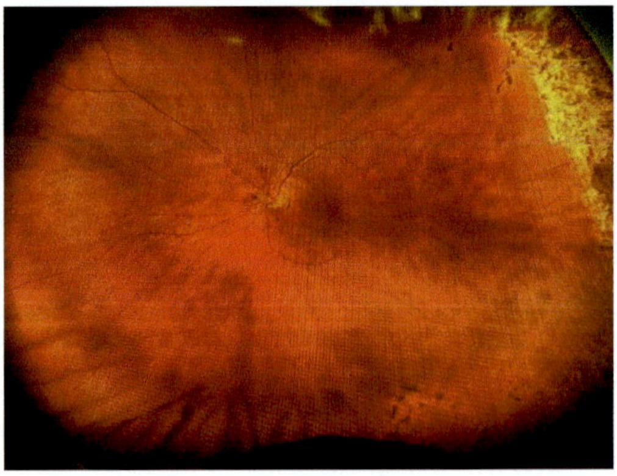

Fig. 10.9 4 weeks postop. Photocourtesy RH Muni

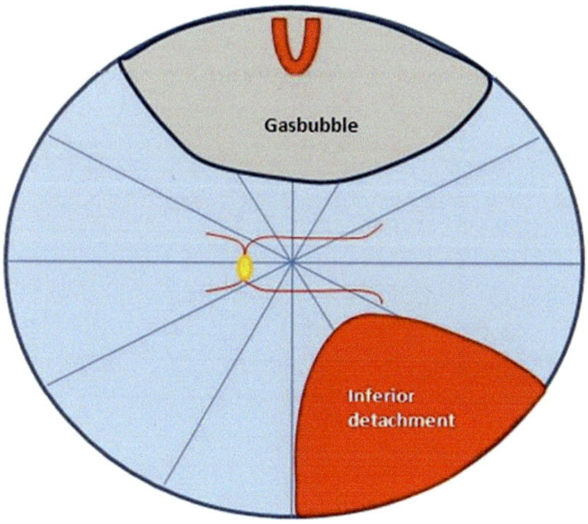

Fig. 10.10 A typical postoperative phenomenon. The inferior detachment is in the most cases only displaced fluid and disappears with time. Exclude a retinal rupture within the focal detachment and observe

break is present, you can either inject again Sf6 (PIVOT study) or alternatively perform a 25G or even better 27G vitrectomy + laser + C_2F_6 tamponade.

10.5 FAQ

Q: How high is your success rate?
A: 90%, but remember: We use a very restricted indication with breaks only from 10 o'clock to 2 o'clock.

Q: Can I perform pneumatic retinopexy with laser instead of cryo?
A: Yes, you can. Perform a paracentesis and drain anterior chamber fluid. Then inject 0.5 ml 100% SF_6 into the vitreous cavity. One or two days later, when the retinal break is attached you can perform a laser coagulation.

Q: How high is the percentage of RD's you perform with this technique?
A: Approximately 20%. But the VR colleagues from the University from Toronto use this technique in 80% of all cases (macula on and off, phakic and pseudophakic, RD from 8 over 12 to 4 o'clock.)

Q: Do you see additional advantages of this technique?
A: The material and costs for this surgical technique is minimal.

11 Vitrectomy with Cryopexy and Gas (Moorfield Technique)

Ulrich Spandau

11.1 Introduction

This surgical method is the most common employed technique for retinal detachments at Moorfield eye hospital in London. This technique is a fusion of pneumatic retinopexy and phaco/vitrectomy. In this technique the vitreous is removed so that the gas tamponade cannot cause a vitreous traction. At Moorfield's hospital this technique is used for all types of retinal detachment, even for macula-off detachments. The technique in short: A core and peripheral vitrectomy is performed. The vitreous base is not shaved. Then a retinal cryopexy is performed and gas is injected. A phacoemulsification is *not* performed. An advantage of this technique is that it requires very little material and instruments: Endodiathermy, laser, PFCL and a chandelier light are not needed. At our hospital we limit the indication for this technique to all detachments with ruptures from 8 over 12 to 4 o'clock. We do *not* operate macula-off detachments with this technique in order to prevent a macular fold (Figs. 11.1, 11.2 and 11.3). Another advantage is that cryopexy can be performed on a detached break whereas laser requires an attached break.

Remark: We switched from pneumatic retinopexy to the Moorfield technique because this technique is easy and fast. We use this technique in approximately 30% of retinal detachments.

Anaesthesia: We use subtenonal or peribulbar anaesthesia. General anaesthesia is not necessary.

11.2 Surgery

Instruments

1. 25/27-Gauge 3-port trocar system
2. Cryopexy

Tamponade

Postoperative: 20% SF_6.

The main surgical steps:

1. 25G/27G 3-port system
2. Core and peripheral vitrectomy
3. Cryopexy of retinal ruptures
4. Aspiration of subretinal fluid
5. Fluid/air exchange
6. Gas tamponade
7. Removal of trocars

The surgery step-by-step:

1. 25G/27G 3-port system
2. Core and peripheral vitrectomy
3. Aspiration of subretinal fluid

Insert three 25G or 27G trocar cannulas. Then start with a core vitrectomy and continue with a

U. Spandau (✉)
St. Eriks Hospital, University of Stockholm, Stockholm, Sweden
e-mail: ulrich_spandau@yahoo.de

U. Spandau et al. (eds.), *Retinal Detachment Surgery and Proliferative Vitreoretinopathy*,
https://doi.org/10.1007/978-3-031-11946-0_11

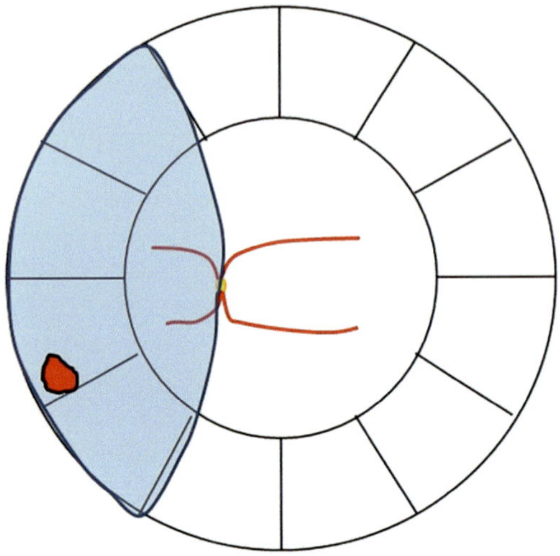

Fig. 11.1 A nasal retinal detachment with attached macula and one retinal break at 8 o'clock

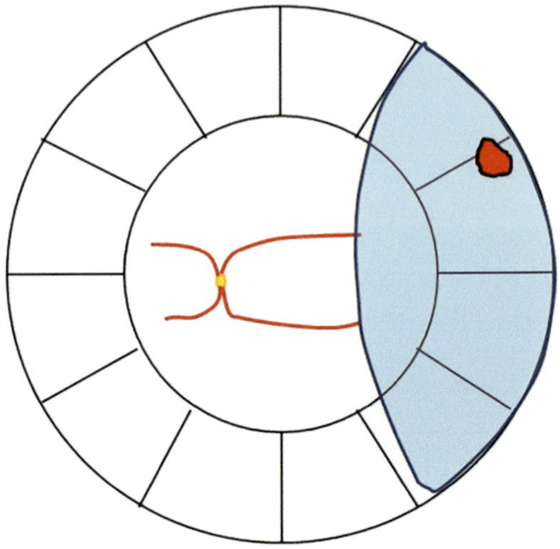

Fig. 11.3 A temporal retinal detachment with attached macula and one retinal break at 2 o'clock

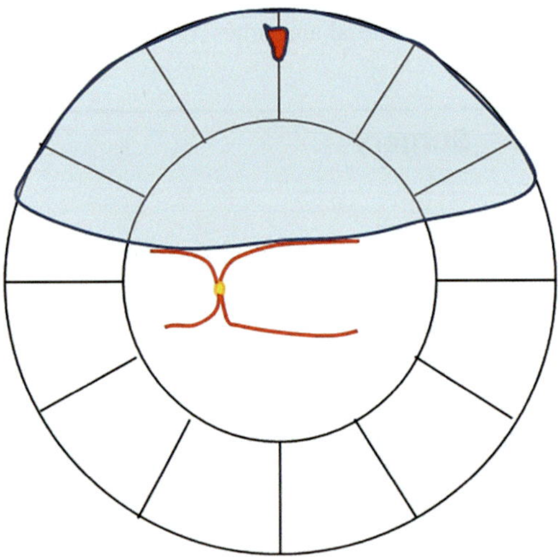

Fig. 11.2 A superior retinal detachment with attached macula and one retinal break at 12 o'clock

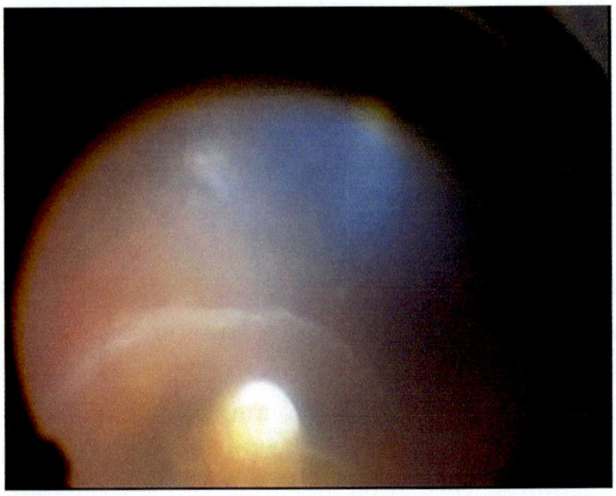

Fig. 11.4 Cryopexy of the retinal break. Note the retinal bleaching

peripheral vitrectomy. A vitreous base shaving is not required. Aspirate then as much subretinal fluid as possible with the vitreous cutter.

4. Cryopexy of retinal ruptures
5. Fluid/air exchange
6. Gas tamponade
7. Removal of trocars.

Treat now the retinal ruptures with cryopexy (Fig. 11.4). The cryopexy is performed on a detached retina. Continue with a fluid against air exchange. Try to remove some subretinal fluid. Stop the fluid against air exchange as soon as the subretinal fluid reaches the temporal arcade, an approximately 70–80% fluid air fill is sufficient. Then continue with a 20% SF_6 tamponade. Remove finally all trocar cannulas.

11.3 Postoperative Posture

Macula-on detachments: The head is positioned so that the apex of the gas bubble is located against the break.

Macula-off detachments: After the gas is injected, postoperative posture starts with immediate face down positioning for approximately 4 h. Then the steam roller maneuver is employed to push the subretinal fluid towards the break. The steam roller maneuver is a sequence of head positions utilized in order to reduce the time required to achieve retinal reattachment, followed by gradual elevation of the head (30 degrees per hour) until the head is upright. Then, the patient is positioned so that the apex of the bubble covers the retinal breaks.

11.4 Helpful Tips

In case of a bullous detachment we insert a chandelier light, indent the sclera, remove the vitreous traction at the break and aspirate some subretinal fluid. Then we proceed with cryopexy and fluid x air exchange. The advantage is that very little subretinal fluid is pushed towards the central pole.

Caution: You can use this technique also for **macula off** detachments but the risk for macular fold is increased because a complete removal of subretinal fluid is not performed.

To avoid this complication, we comply with the following precautions:

1. We operate only macula-on detachments, the superior arcade should be attached.
2. We aspirate as much subretinal fluid with the vitreous cutter as possible.
3. We perform a fluid against air exchange only until the subretinal fluid reaches the superior arcade.

11.5 Questions and Answers

Q: Do you perform this technique in eyes with PVR?

A: No, I use this technique only for fresh detachments.

Q: Do you perform routinely a PVD?

A: No, not routinely. If you induce PVD, you have less ERM induction.

Q: What is the pathophysiological advantage of this technique compared to pneumatic retinopexy?

A: In the Moorfield technique the vitreous traction at the retinal rupture is removed.

Q: Why do you perform cryopexy in a fluid filled eye? Cryopexy is easier in an air filled eye because the tear is attached.

A: I prefer cryopexy in a fluid filled eye because the view to fundus and to the break is better. If the tear is very detached and I am not able to apply cryopexy then I remove partially the subretinal fluid.

Q: Do you operate macula off detachments with this technique?

A: No. But Moorfield hospital does so. They recommend a postoperative steam roller maneuver or alternatively a strict head down posture for approximately 4 h.

12 Combined Phaco/Vitrectomy (Frankfurt Technique)

Ulrich Spandau

A rhegmatogenous retinal detachment (RRD) with multiple breaks is a surgery for experienced surgeons, as there is a significant complication profile. The beginner should start with a localized detachment (one to two quadrant detachments and a single break), as this is usually easier to manage.

Regarding surgery, we recommend two things, which simplify vitrectomy very much: Phacoemulsification and usage of a chandelier light. We recommend performing phacoemulsification in all patients older than 50 years because the anterior vitreous and the vitreous base can be removed completely. See our treatment algorithm (Fig. 12.1). Secondly, we recommend the usage of a chandelier light because it facilitates every step of the vitrectomy. Complete removal of the anterior vitreous is only possible after the removal of the natural lens. Visualization and removal of the vitreous base are easier with chandelier light. The retinal breaks are located in the periphery and need to be indented with the scleral depressor: Nobody indents as well as your second hand.

U. Spandau (✉)
St. Eriks Hospital, University of Stockholm, Stockholm, Sweden
e-mail: ulrich_spandau@yahoo.de

12.1 PFCL or no PFCL?

Some vitreoretinal clinics use PFCL as a routine, others don't. PFCL is an excellent tool for vitreoretinal surgery and we recommend using it, if necessary. We use PFCL in large, macula-off detachments and we work without PFCL in focal, macula-on detachments. In giant tears, we always use PFCL due to the risk of slippage.

12.2 25G or 27G?

27G is superior to 25G in myopic eyes. 27G sclerotomies require no suture. Myopic eyes tend to leak and 27G sclerotomies have only minimal leakage. Minimal leakage results also in improved gas tamponade. The disadvantages of 27G are the soft instruments. In normal eyes, a 25G cutter is, therefore, recommended. In addition, passive aspiration with a 25G fluid needle is more efficient than with 27G.

Anaesthesia:
We use always peribulbar anaesthesia. General anaesthesia is not necessary.

The surgery
Instruments

1. 25/27-Gauge 3-port trocar system
2. Chandelier light
3. 120D lens
4. Endodiathermy
5. Endolaser

U. Spandau et al. (eds.), *Retinal Detachment Surgery and Proliferative Vitreoretinopathy*,
https://doi.org/10.1007/978-3-031-11946-0_12

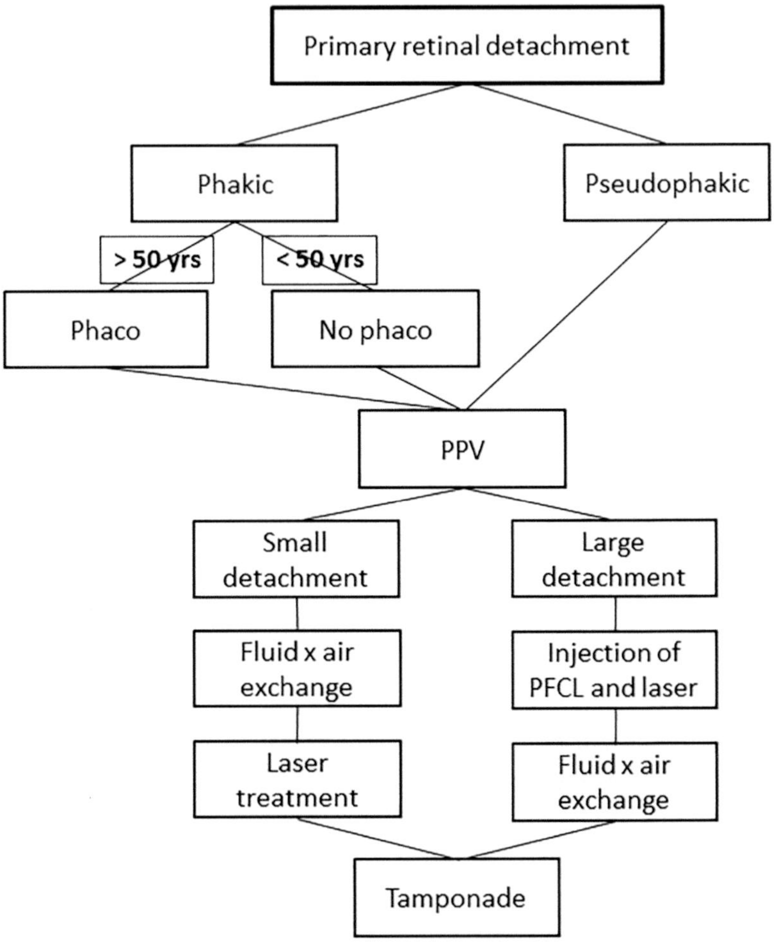

Fig. 12.1 Our treatment algorithm for retinal detachment surgery

6. Backflush instrument
7. Scleral depressor.

Dye
Possibly: Triamcinolone to stain the vitreous
Tamponade
Intraoperative: PFCL
Postoperative: 20% SF_6, 15% C_2F_6.

Main surgical steps:

1. **25G/27G 3-port system with chandelier light**
2. **Phacoemulsification with IOL**
3. **Core vitrectomy and posterior vitreous detachment**
4. **Marking of breaks with endodiathermy**
5. **Injection of PFCL up to the posterior edge of the break and drainage of subretinal fluid**
6. **Vitrectomy of tear flap and peripheral vitreous**
7. **PFCL injection up to ora serrata**
8. **Laser photocoagulation around breaks**
9. **Trimming of the vitreous base (Shaving)**
10. **Fluid/air exchange**
11. **Drainage of subretinal fluid**
12. **Complete laser coagulation**
13. **Gas tamponade**
14. **Removal of trocars**.

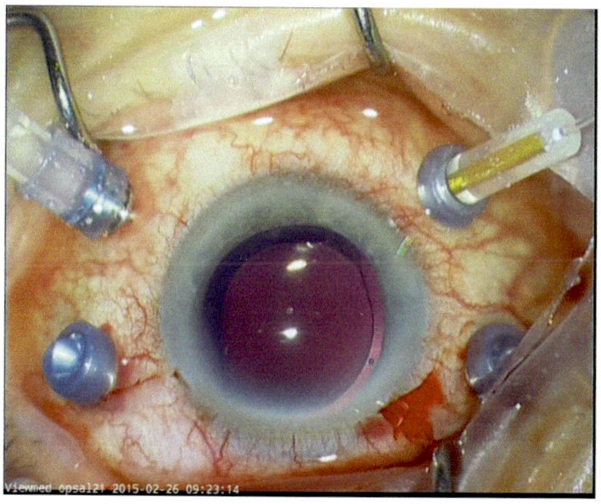

Fig. 12.2 Our regular setup for retinal detachment. 3-port vitrectomy and one chandelier light at the inferotemporal position

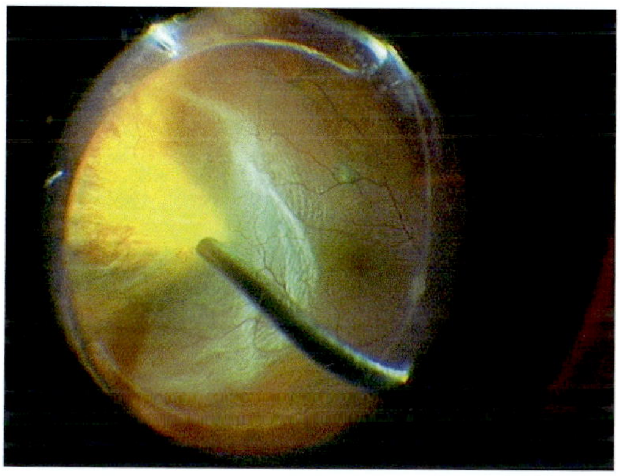

Fig. 12.3 The retinal break is hard to visualize

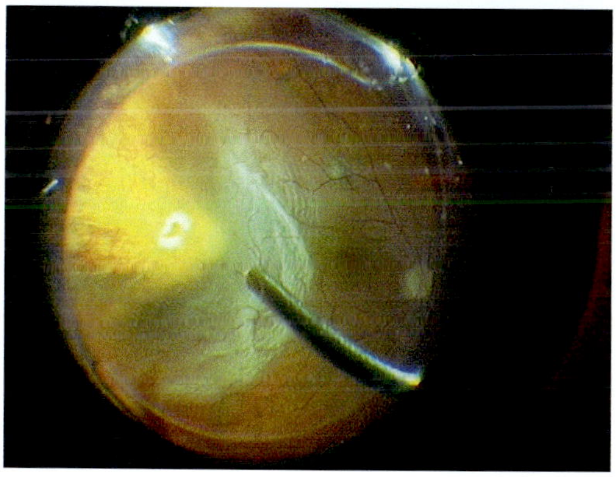

Fig. 12.4 After diathermy of the retinal edges the retinal break is easy to visualize

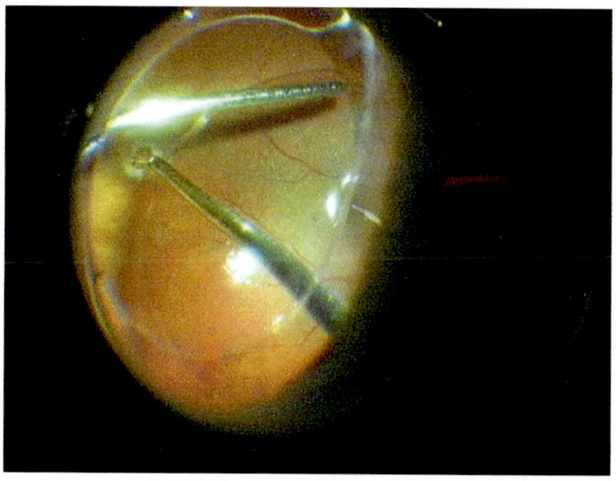

Fig. 12.5 Injection of PFCL and at the same time aspiration of subretinal fluid from the retinal break

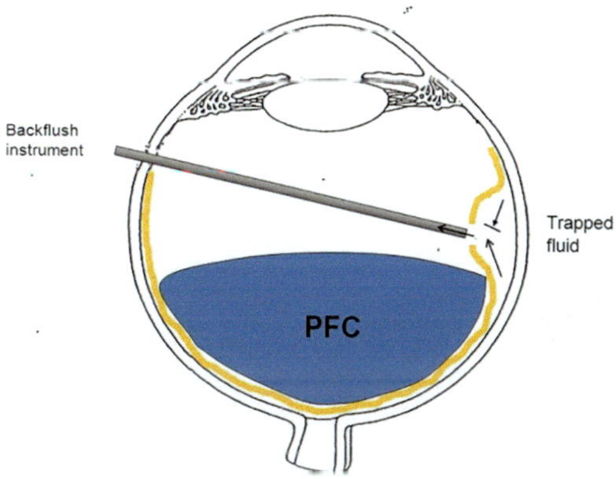

Fig. 12.6 Aspiration of subretinal fluid from retinal break. Note that only the posterior subretinal fluid can be removed and not the anterior located fluid. The latter will bre removed later

12.3 The Surgery Step-by-Step (Figs. 12.2, 12.3, 12.4, 12.5, 12.6, 12.7, 12.8, 12.9, 12.10, 12.11, 12.12, 12.13, 12.14, 12.15 and 12.16)

1. **25G/27G 3-port system with chandelier light (Fig.** 12.2)

Insert the trocars at the usual locations 3.5 mm behind the limbus. Visualize the location of the infusion cannula in order to avoid a choroidal

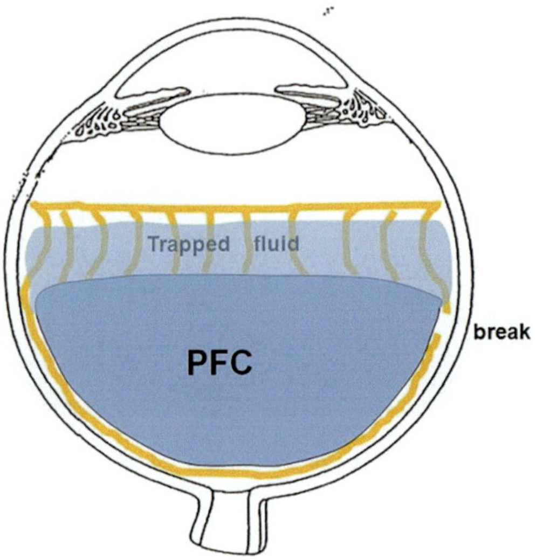

Fig. 12.7 Inject PFCL to the ora serrata. Note the trapped fluid anterior to the break

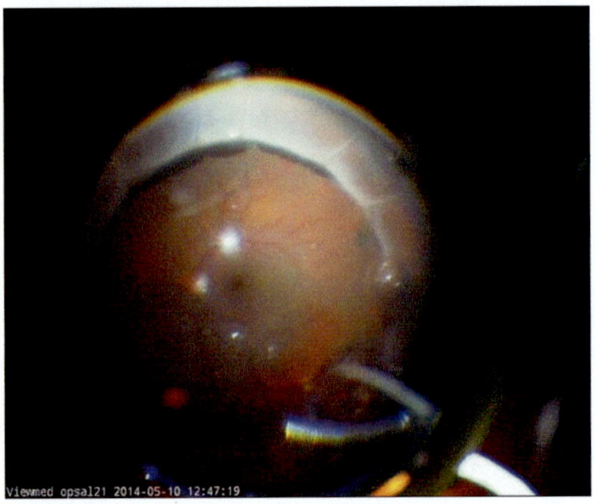

Fig. 12.8 Much trapped fluid anterior to the retinal break is visible

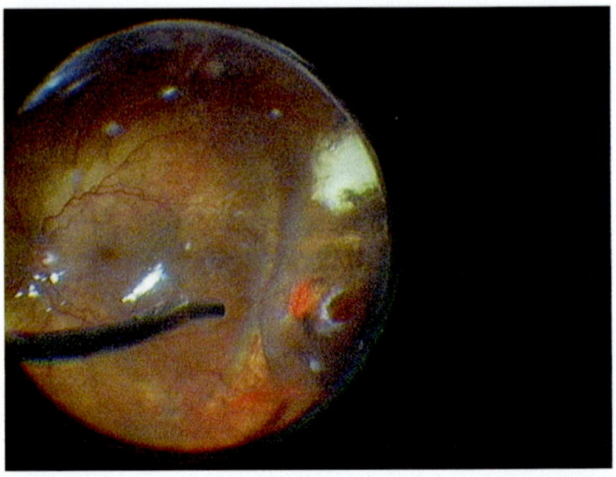

Fig. 12.9 Laser treat the complete break after removal of subretinal fluid

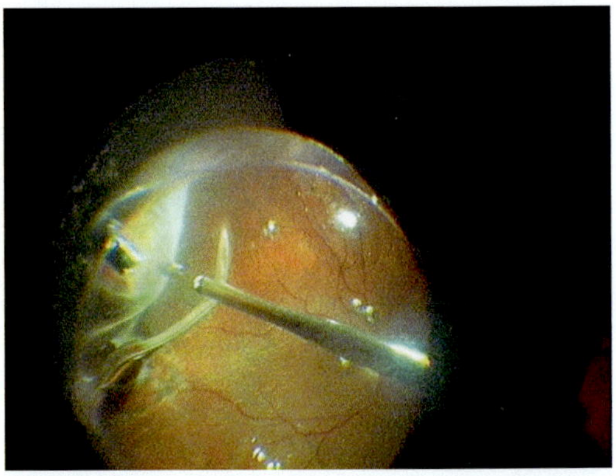

Fig. 12.10 Observe the "empty space" between retina and PFCL. The empty space is vitreous

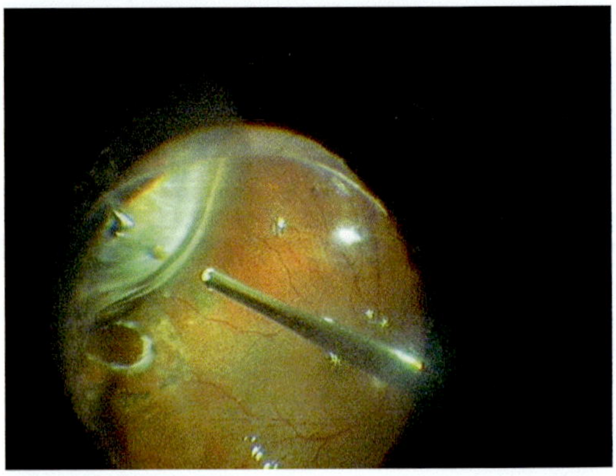

Fig. 12.11 Remove the peripheral vitreous and the PFCL will attach onto the retina

detachment. Then insert the chandelier light inferonasally 3.5 mm behind the limbus.

2. **Phacoemulsification**

The IOL can be implanted in this step or later when all the breaks are treated (step 10). The advantage of early IOL implantation is that one works with a stable anterior segment and the IOL implantation is usually easier at this stage compared to the end of the surgery. The disadvantage

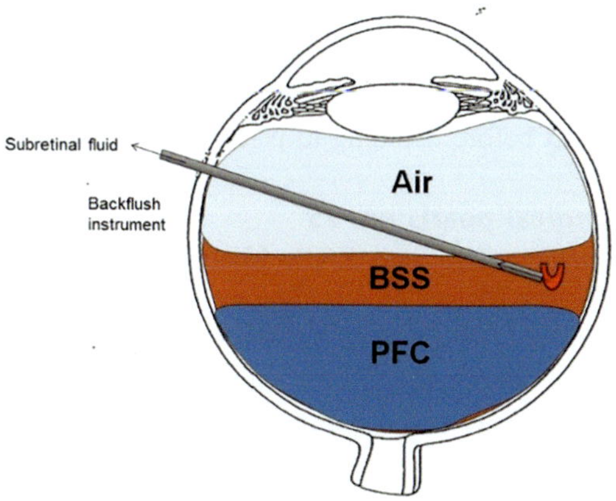

Fig. 12.12 Sandwich tamponade with air and PFCL. Aspirate first BSS and then PFCL until the PFCL meniscus reaches the posterior edge of the hole

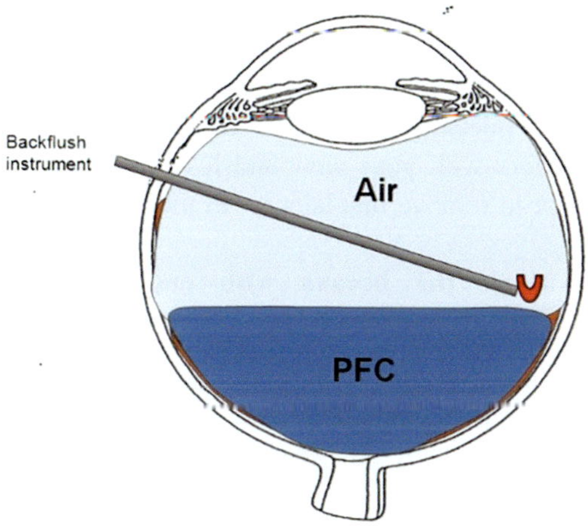

Fig. 12.13 If the PFCL has reached the inferior edge of the retinal break then aspirate the subretinal fluid anterior to the retinal break. Then you can continue to remove the residual PFCL

is that the edge of the IOL may interfere with the view of the retinal periphery and the vitreous base.

Surgical pearls no. 71

Phaco or no phaco: If a cataract is present, remove it during the same surgery. Why? The vitrectomy and the gas tamponade lead to an opacification of the lens resulting in a bad view to retina. The risk that you miss a recurrent detachment is high especially if it is inferior.

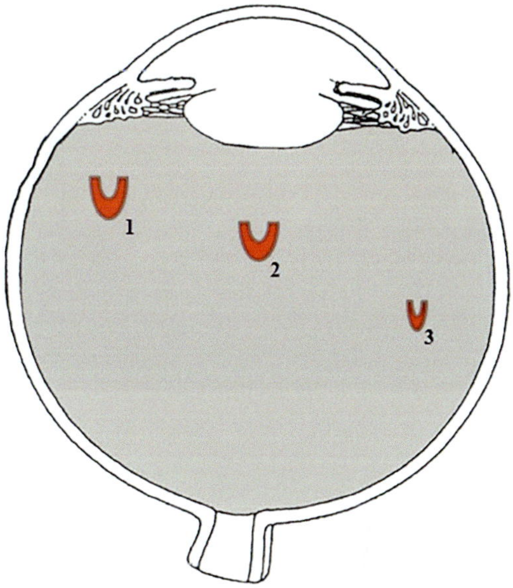

Fig. 12.14 If several holes are present then start to remove subretinal fluid from hole 1 and continue with hole 2 and then 3

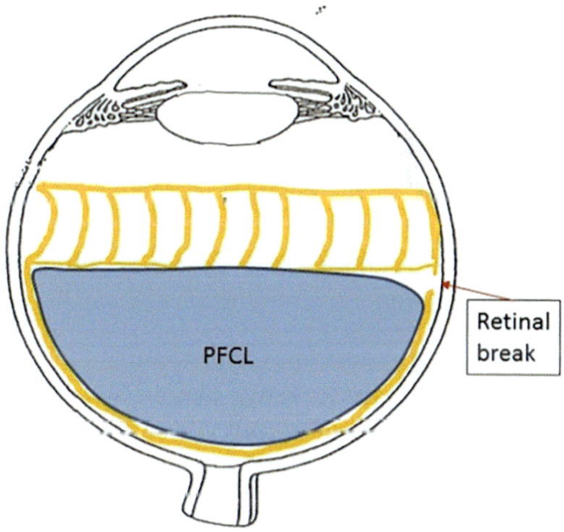

Fig. 12.15 Only if the complete trapped fluid is removed you can continue with removal of PFCL. Otherwise the trapped fluid will flow towards the posterior pole and detach the macula

Surgical pearls no. 72

Corneal suture: In case of an unstable anterior chamber, place a single 10–0 nylon suture at the end of the phaco and IOL. This avoids accidental opening of the corneal wound during indentation,

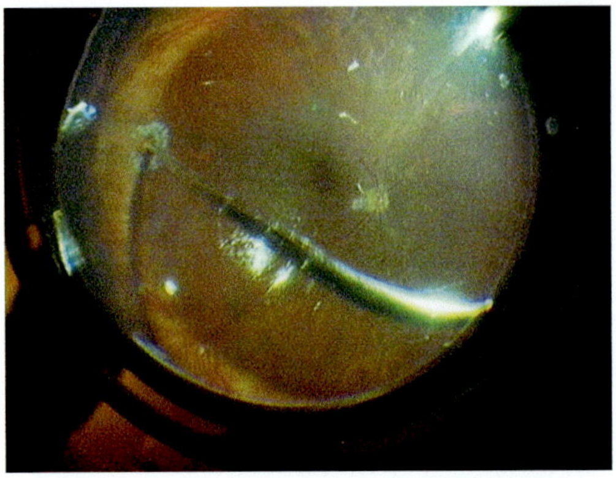

Fig. 12.16 Complete laser photo coagulation if necessary

which may lead to flattening of the anterior chamber and even dislocation of the IOL. The suture can be removed once the vitrectomy has been completed.

Surgical pearls no. 73
Corneal lubrication: A major problem during vitrectomy, especially in combined surgeries with a duration of over 1 h, is corneal epithelial oedema. With a generous application of methylcellulose (Celoftal, Alcon), the cornea remains clear for the complete surgery.

3. **Core Vitrectomy and posterior vitreous detachment**

Perform a core vitrectomy and identify the posterior vitreous face to verify that a PVD is present. If the vitreous is still attached, perform induction of a PVD. Then continue with vitrectomy, and search for retinal breaks. Carefully remove the vitreous close to the retina in the area of a detached, fluttering retina.

Surgical pearls no. 74
PVD in RRD: In about 15% of patients with RRD, the vitreous is still attached at the posterior pole. One group at risk is myopic patients below the age of 50 years with multiple small round breaks. The vitreous may be very adherent to the retina in such cases and trying to induce a PVD can lead to multiple iatrogenic breaks. These cases usually do very well with scleral buckling surgery. If in doubt, check the status of vitreous attachment/detachment with preoperative ultrasound before deciding to perform a vitrectomy.

Surgical pearls no. 75
Triamcinolone and RRD: Many cases of RRD are caused by strong vitreoretinal adhesion. It may not be possible to separate vitreous and retina simply by engaging the vitreous with the vitreous cutter and pulling it off the retina—you may enlarge pre-existing breaks or induce iatrogenic breaks in some cases. If you find very strong vitreoretinal adhesions, it is advisable to "stop pulling" and start "shaving" the vitreous of the retina. This is facilitated by staining the adherent vitreous with triamcinolone. When staining the vitreous with triamcinolone, use minimal amounts and direct the injection to the area of interest. We dilute triamcinolone 1:4 with BSS. Injecting too much triamcinolone may interfere with your view and it can be cumbersome to remove this later on in the procedure.

4. **Mark the breaks with endodiathermy (Figs.** 12.3 **and** 12.4)

The key concept of all retinal detachment surgeries is to identify and treat all retinal breaks. Perform a thorough internal search for breaks following Lincoff's rules that point to the most likely areas of retinal breaks. If you fail to identify and treat a retinal break in the detached retina, failure and retinal redetachment following vitrectomy are guaranteed. Mark the edges of the break with endodiathermy. A break, which is not marked, is hard to identify when it is attached to the underlying retinal pigment epithelium.

Surgical pearls no. 76
Unseen breaks and Schlieren phenomenon: Inject PFCL slowly and watch for the "Schlieren phenomenon". In particular, in long-standing RRD, the subretinal fluid appears like a muddy stream when entering the vitreous cavity. This "Schlieren phenomenon" may point to the location of the retinal break at the entry site of the Schlieren in cases of "unseen breaks".

5. **Injection of PFCL to the posterior edge of break and drainage of subretinal fluid**

The PFCL has three tasks in detachment surgery:

1. Stabilization of the mobile retina
2. Removal of the subretinal fluid
3. Elevation of the peripheral vitreous.

The PFCL pushes the subretinal fluid from the central pole towards the periphery and presses it through the retinal break into the vitreous cavity. First, the PFCL is injected up to the posterior edge of the most central break while we observe how the subretinal fluid is forced through the break into the vitreous cavity. You can accelerate this step by aspirating subretinal fluid actively with the Charles flute needle (Figs. 12.5 and 12.6). The PFCL also has the effect that the mobile retina is attached, and a vitrectomy in the vicinity of the detached retina is less dangerous (Fig. 12.7).

Surgical pearls no. 77

PFCL is quite expensive. In more complicated cases, it may be necessary to perform multiple manipulations under PFCL, occasionally removing and then again adding PFCL at a later stage. If PFCL needs to be removed, you can easily aspirate it back into the injection syringe for re-injection at a later stage of the procedure.

6. **Vitrectomy of the tear flap and the peripheral vitreous**

After ensuring the presence and completion of a PVD, the next step is to perform trimming of the vitreous base. Start within the area of the break(s) and also remove the flap, as the vitreous traction on the flap caused the detachment. The scleral depressor in the second hand is a great help when indenting the retina.

7. **PFCL injection up to ora serrata**

Depending on the anterior/posterior location of the break, there is more or less subretinal fluid anterior to the break (trapped fluid) (Figs. 12.7 and 12.8). If a break is located at the ora serrata you can drain the residual subretinal fluid with a complete PFCL fill. However, if the break is located between the equator and ora serrata, then complete drainage of subretinal fluid is not possible. The subretinal fluid is trapped between the break and the ora serrata (Figs. 12.7 and 12.8). In the first case, you can proceed with laser photocoagulation. In the latter case, a complete laser coagulation is not possible because the retinal break is partially detached. You can perform partial laser photocoagulation and complete the laser after the fluid/air exchange in step 10.

Surgical pearls no. 78

Iatrogenic break: If the retinal break and the bullous detachment are far apart from each other, it is difficult to drain the subretinal fluid from the break. In the first case, one can try to massage the subretinal fluid with a scleral depressor to the break. Or perform an iatrogenic break in the area of trapped fluid. Mark the inferior retina close to the ora serrata with endodiathermy. Then cut a hole with the vitreous cutter (setting: approx. 300 cuts/min) by suctioning the retina and then cutting it cautiously. Drain the subretinal fluid from this break. Another alternative is the aspiration of the subretinal fluid with a 41G cannula.

8. **Lasertherapy of breaks (Fig. 12.9)**

Apply three rows of laser burns around the breaks. The settings depend on the laser device.

It is possible that subretinal fluid has accumulated anterior to the break (so-called “trapped fluid”) which makes it difficult to apply a laser onto the anterior part of the break. Try to indent the break with the scleral depressor, so that the subretinal fluid is pushed away. Apply white laser burns. A good alternative is to freeze the break with a cryoprobe. If you do not succeed due to excess trapped fluid, then complete the laser treatment in a later step.

Surgical pearls no. 79

Laser necrosis: Be careful with your laser energy. Only a mild whitening of the RPE is necessary; 200 ms duration is sufficient; 300 ms is too much, otherwise you may create laser necrosis. Burns which are too strong will weaken the retina and are a predilection site for the formation of new retinal breaks. They may also cause contraction of the choroid or even choroidal haemorrhages. A typical beginner's mistake is to perform too much laser or cryotherapy as an extra safety measure that then may turn out to have exactly the opposite effect.

Surgical pearls no. 80

Lasercerclage: A circumferential 360° laser is not recommended. It is essential to identify and treat all retinal breaks. A circumferential laser has the big disadvantage that, in case of a redetachment, the breaks are difficult to find within the patches of chorioretinal atrophy.

Surgical pearls no. 81

Difficult to find holes: In case of a recurrent detachment, extensive laser treatment from the primary surgery makes it difficult-to-find holes. If you do not find the hole then laser treat according to the Lincoff rules.

9. **Trimming of vitreous base (Shaving) (Figs.** 12.10 **and** 12.11)

If it has not been performed before, a thorough vitrectomy of the vitreous base has to be performed at this stage using the scleral depressor. This procedure is also called "shaving". PFCL lifts the vitreous up and enables a secure and thorough trimming of the vitreous base. In those areas, where PFCL does not rest on the retina, there is a vitreous which has to be removed. Indent the sclera and move the vitreous cutter along the meniscus of the PFCL. Hereby you can manoeuver the vitreous cutter very close to the retina because the heavy liquid presses against the retina.

Surgical pearls no. 82

Trimming of vitreous base: There are various ways to trim the vitreous base (a) Bimanual technique using a scleral indentor, (b) removal under coaxial light (only with microscope illumination) by using a cotton wool swab or a scleral depressor to indent the sclera or (c) using the light fibre as an external scleral depressor (this gives you a focused beam of transscleral light to illuminate the vitreous base).

10. **Fluid against air exchange**

If the shaving is finished, a PFCL x air exchange is performed. Before we perform this procedure, we have a look at Diagram 12.1 to get a better sense of the situation in the vitreous cavity. Before the PFCL x air exchange the vitreous cavity is filled with PFCL and on top of it is a layer of water. During the PFCL x air exchange, there is an anterior phase of air, a middle phase of water and a posterior phase of PFCL. After the PFCL x air exchange, only air is in the eye, which is then replaced by gas. Postoperatively, water will accumulate again under the gas phase. Consequently, the gas does not effectively tamponade the lower pole.

The PFCL x air exchange is certainly the most difficult and most important manoeuver in the whole detachment surgery, mainly because visibility under air is bad. Therefore, it is essential to understand the characteristics of PFCL and air. PFCL and air "work" as antagonists. Air exerts pressure in the eye from peripheral (anterior) to central (posterior), but vice versa in case of PFCL, i.e. from posterior to anterior.

PFCL presses most of the subretinal fluid from the central pole to the periphery through the retinal break into the vitreous cavity, but a part of

Diagram 12.1 Diagram of the location of fluids during the PFCL x air exchange

Intraoperatively			Postoperatively
PFCL x air exchange			
Before	During	After	
BSS	Air	Gas	Gas
	BSS		
PFCL	PFCL		Aqueous

it flows beyond the break up to the ora serrata, where it cannot be aspirated ("trapped fluid") (Figs. 12.7 and 12.8). This "trapped fluid" can, however, be removed with air: The air attaches the retina beginning in the periphery and ending at the central pole, and thereby pushes the "trapped fluid" in the direction of the break (Figs. 12.12 and 12.13).

11. **Drainage of subretinal fluid**

How do we proceed in practice? Before you switch to air, hold the flute tip in the middle of the break. If necessary, take the scleral depressor to help. If several breaks are present, start with the most peripherally located break and then move to the next more central break (Fig. 12.14). Now, the scrub nurse switches the three-way tap from BSS to air. In the beginning, disturbing air bubbles arise and the view deteriorates. Remain calm and turn the front lens with the BIOM-focus wheel up. The visibility will gradually improve.

In the beginning, the break is covered with PFCL. After a short time, the PFCL is suctioned to the posterior edge of the break. Now the air presses the subretinal fluid in the direction of the break. The subretinal fluid is trapped between anteriorly located air and posteriorly located PFCL, the so-called "sandwich tamponade". Now you aspirate the subretinal fluid through the break and at the same time the BSS phase between air and PFCL (Figs. 12.12, 12.13 and 12.15).

Only when the "trapped fluid" and the BSS in the vitreous cavity are completely aspirated, can you continue to aspirate PFCL beyond the posterior edge of the break. This is very important because the subretinal fluid, which you do not aspirate, will continue to flow beyond the break in the direction of the optic disc.

If the "trapped fluid" is completely removed, you switch with the flute needle alternately between the PFCL bubble in order to reduce it and the break in order to aspirate fluid here. Try to aspirate without indenting the break. But sometimes you can only reach the break with the flute needle if you indent it with the scleral depressor. But you should not indent the break itself, but the retina on either side of the break. By indenting the break, you close it and prevent the aspiration of subretinal fluid. This procedure is usually not easy and requires patience.

The remaining PFCL is aspirated by holding the flute tip directly in front of the optic disc. Make sure that the PFCL is completely removed and that neither the retina nor the optic disc are affected.

If after complete removal of PFCL, residual subretinal fluid remains in the central pole, then you may either inject PFCL again up to the break and aspirate the fluid or—if it is only a small amount—leave it. The subretinal fluid will be absorbed on the first postoperative day.

Surgical pearls no. 83

Air test for detachment: When the retina is completely attached under air, you have drained the subretinal fluid completely. Air presses the entire subretinal fluid from the periphery to the optic disc, where it is easy to spot. This is only partly true for PFCL because PFCL pushes the subretinal fluid from the posterior pole to the periphery, where the "trapped fluid"is hard to detect.

Surgical pearls no. 84

Active aspiration: In 25G/27G the aspiration of subretinal fluid is easier and more effective with active (than passive) aspiration. If you do not want to use PFCL, e.g. because only a focal retinal detachment is present, then you should absolutely aspirate subretinal fluid with active aspiration.

Surgical pearls no. 85

Removal of PFCL: Two pearls for PFCL removal: (1) When using a flute needle with a silicone tip, the risk of retinal or optic disc touch is much lower. (2) If you are not sure whether you aspirated the entire PFCL, Instil a little water into the air-filled vitreous cavity (with a brief water x air exchange) and then completely remove the residual PFCL/water puddle.

12. **Complete laser coagulation (Fig. 12.16)**

If necessary, complete now the laser therapy around the retinal break in the air-filled eye.

13. **Tamponade**

Concerning the use of tamponade, there are significant differences between vitreoretinal units at the national and international level. The trend nowadays is to use SF_6 in a primary detachment and longer-acting gases and silicone oils for re-detachments.

We differentiate between detached breaks and attached breaks. The choice of tamponade depends only on the detached breaks. If all detached breaks are located above the 3 o'clock–9 o'clock meridian, we use SF_6. If one detached hole is located below the 3 o'clock–9 o'clock meridian, we use C_2F_6. If the detached break is located at the 6 o'clock meridian, we would use Densiron 68 or perform episcleral buckling. An alternative is, of course, C_3F_8.

Surgical pearls no. 86

(1) 27G and air tamponade: 27G sclerotomies leak very little. In case of a superior detachment with a break between 11 o'clock and 1 o´clock, we use often only air as tamponade. There is an excellent tamponade present for 7–10 days and laser treatment is effective after 3–4 days.
Why does it matter? Especially professionally active patients will appreciate regaining their visual acuity after 1 week. In comparison, C_3F_8 makes an eye blind and the patient earthbound for 2 months.
(2) Gas tamponade: air against gas exchange
If the retina and the breaks are fully attached, you can flick the BIOM out and insufflate the diluted gas. The gas container is connected to the three-way tap, the scrub nurse injects the gas and the surgeon decompresses the globe with the use of a flute instrument. The globe should remain normotensive.

Surgical pearls no. 87

Gas versus silicone oil: If the retina is attached under air in detachment surgery, then it will also be attached under gas, but that's not necessarily the case for silicone oil. Why? The surface tension pressure of the gas/water interface is the greatest, and therefore, is the most effective in closing retinal breaks (70 mN/N). So, when the retina is attached under air, then it is also attached under gas. The same statement is not true for silicone oil. Why? Because the surface tension of silicone oil/water with 50 mN/N is less than that of air/water. So, when the retina is attached under air it might not be attached under silicone oil.

14. **Removal of the trocar cannulas**

Finally, the trocars are removed. Remove first the instrument trocars and at the end the infusion trocar. In case of a gas tamponade, add some gas until the globe is normotensive. No suture is needed neither for gas nor for silicone oil.

12.4 Postoperative Posture

In case of macula-off detachment, we recommend 4–6 h face-down positioning in order to push the subfoveal fluid away. Then the face is positioned in a way that the apex of the gas bubble is located on the break.

In case of a macula on detachment, the patient is positioned straight away with face down so that the apex of the gasbubble presses against the break.

12.5 Complications

(1) *Posterior capsular defect*:

This is a stupid complication during detachment surgery because the tamponade will press the IOL forwards and gas or silicone oil will flow into the anterior chamber. In case of a gas tamponade, we would inject air into the anterior chamber to counterpress, and in case of a silicone oil tamponade, we would perform an iridectomy and fill the anterior chamber with Healon GV.

(2) *Slippage*:

In cases of giant tears, the retina in the area of the break may slip/glide postoperatively towards the posterior pole (slippage). This is associated with the risk of developing retinal folds postoperatively which, in the worst of cases, may involve the macula. This phenomenon is caused by inadequate drainage of subretinal fluid during the fluid–air exchange. To avoid slippage, perform a direct PFCL x silicone oil exchange.

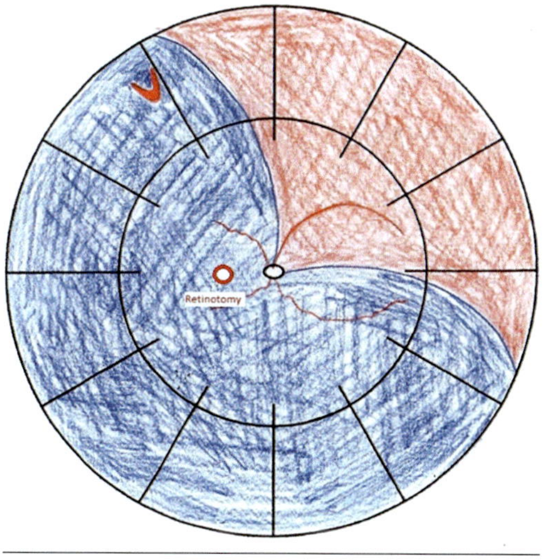

Fig. 12.17 A central retinotomy is created to remove the submacular fluid

12.6 How to Remove Submacular Fluid

An intravitreal gas tamponade in macula-off detachments requires the complete removal of subretinal fluid. Otherwise, a macular fold may develop.

A small amount of submacular fluid can be removed by postoperative face-down posture for 3–6 h. But big amounts of submacular fluid have an increased risk of macular folds.

Patients with silicone oil tamponade never had macular folds even in case of submacular fluid. A gas tamponade, however, may cause a macular fold because the gas has a high surface tension pressure and creates a retinal fold when pressing the submacular fold away. Why? The surface tension pressure of silicone oil is lower than that of gas.

What to do in case of much residual submacular fluid?

(1) Create a posterior retinotomy and aspirate the submacular fluid (Fig. 12.17).
(2) Use a silicone oil tamponade.

Summary: Residual submacular fluid is a common problem when performing vitrectomy for retinal detachment. There are several solutions to this problem. We recommend solutions 3 and 4: Posterior retinotomy or silicone oil tamponade.

12.7 Tips for PFCL Injections

We inject PFCL manually; one hand holds the PFCL syringe and the other hand holds the Charles flute needle. Hold the tip of the PFCL cannula in the middle of the vitreous cavity and inject a little bit. If air bubbles escape, then aspirate them at once with the flute needle. Then start to inject the PFCL at the posterior pole and keep the tip of the cannula always in the PFCL bubble in order to prevent small bubbles (Fig. 12.18). These small bubbles will fusion

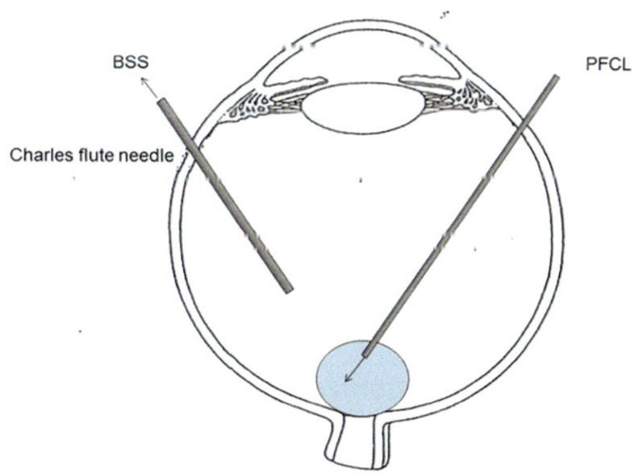

Fig. 12.18 Work bimanual. Start with a small PFCL bubble

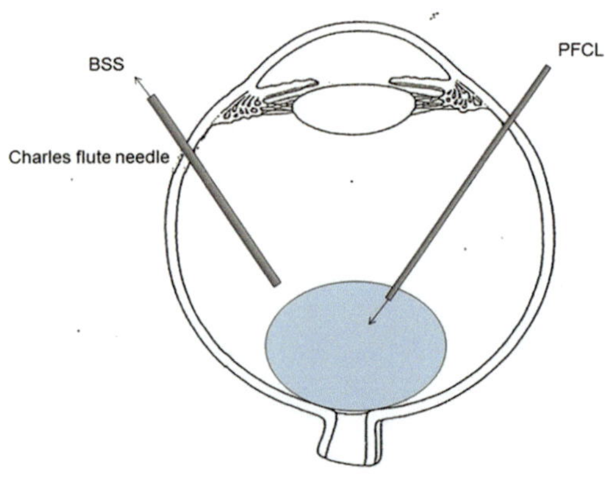

Fig. 12.19 Retract the injection needle slowly as the bubble is growing. But keep the tip constantly in the PFCL bubble to prevent emulsification

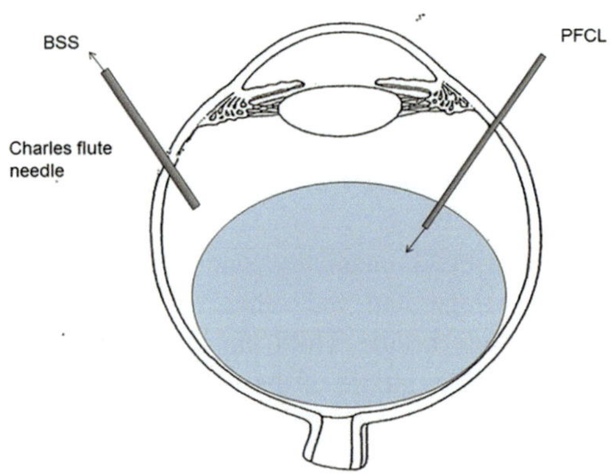

Fig. 12.20 Do not inject the PFCL towards the macula or a retinal break

after some time with the large bubble. Be cautious where the PFCL cannula is aiming. Aim never towards the macula or a retinal break (Fig. 12.19). The PFCL bubble becomes bigger and bigger, pull the PFCL cannula slowly backwards with the tip remaining constantly inside the bubble (Fig. 12.20).

12.8 Fractionized PFCL Injection

What does fractionized injection of PFCL mean?

The PFCL is not injected at once but in fractions (Fig. 12.21). First, inject the PFCL up to the posterior edge of the retinal break. Then remove the vitreous on height of the tear. Then inject PFCL up to the ora serrata. Remove now the vitreous base Fractionized PFCL injection helps to drain subretinal fluid, stabilize the retina and remove the vitreous base.

12.9 FAQ

How do you deal with what type of detachment?

The general recommendations are that in young phakic patients, one should perform a buckling surgery if possible. In old and pseudophakic patients, a PPV is recommended [1]. In pseudophakia with multiple breaks, we always perform a PPV; this is often named "primary vitrectomy for retinal detachment".

There is a strong tendency towards a combined phaco/vitrectomy for RRD in all phakic patients of 50 years or above. Phacoemulsification greatly facilitates the trimming of the vitreous base that is necessary for retinal detachment.

Must I change the position of the trocars according to the location of the detachment?

No. The trocars are always located at the same positions. You can, however, make small deviations according to the location of the break, i.e. to reach the break more easily. For example: If the retinal break is located at 12 o'clock, then place the trocars more towards 3 and 9 o'clock. This way you can reach the 12 o'clock break easier.

What do you do if a macular hole is present?

Always check for the presence of a macular hole. This is present in 0.5% of all retinal detachments and if you don't consider it, chances are that you will miss it. Check either during the preoperative examination or during the surgery. This is important for prognostication and your surgery, as you may be able to perform an ILM peeling during the vitrectomy in order to increase the chances of a postoperative hole closure. To correctly identify a macular hole in cases of macula-

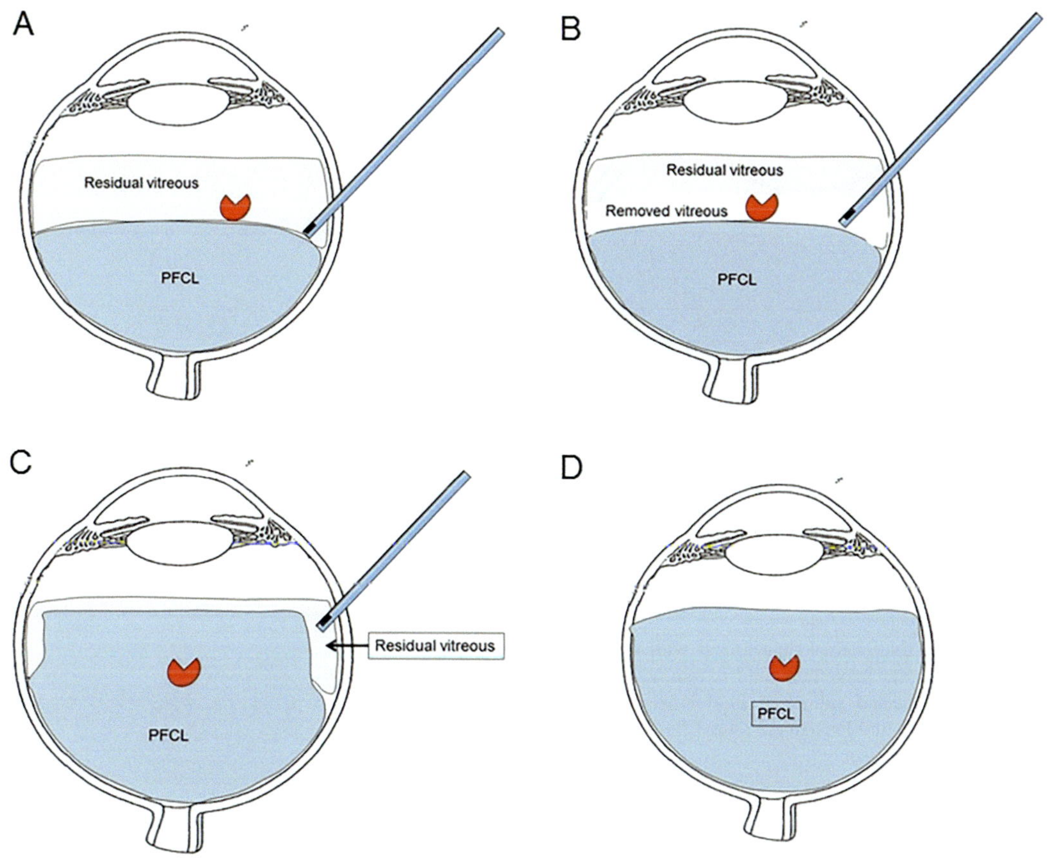

Fig. 12.21 **A** Inject PFCL to the inferior edge of the retinal break and remove the vitreous. **B** Remove the vitreous on height of the retinal break. **C** Now inject PFCL up to the ora serrata. **D** Remove the vitreous base (shaving)

off, RRD is difficult as the thinned retina at the fovea may be mistaken for a macular hole by the inexperienced examiner.

Should I perform an ILM peeling under PFCL?

If the macula is attached, then perform an ILM peeling in a water-filled eye. If the macula is detached, then ILM peeling is difficult. Stain first the ILM and create a small opening in the ILM. Then inject a small PFCL bubble, search for the small ILM opening and peel the ILM.

How do I remove the subretinal fluid in case of a big retinal detachment?

You remove the complete fluid with air, PFCL and a scleral depressor (Fig. 12.22). The anterior subretinal fluid is removed with air. The posterior

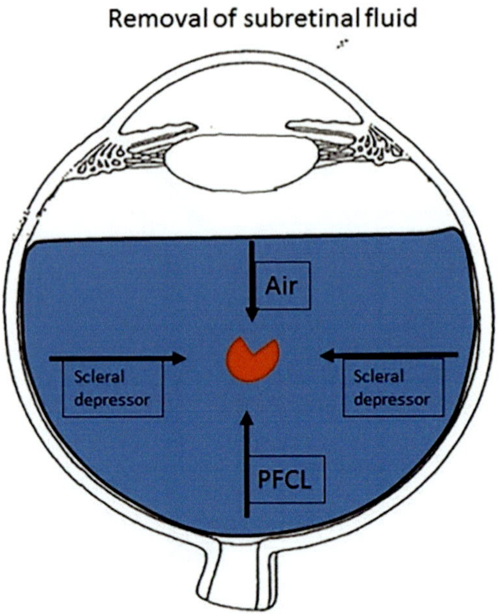

Fig. 12.22 A total retinal detachment with one retinal break. The anterior subretinal fluid is removed with air. The posterior located subretinal fluid is removed with PFCL. The horizontal located subretinal fluid is removed with a scleral depressor

located subretinal fluid is removed with PFCL. The horizontal located subretinal fluid is removed with a scleral depressor. Massage the fluid towards the retinal break.

References

1. Heimann H, Bartz-Schmidt KU et al. Scleral buckling versus primary vitrectomy in rhegmatogenous retinal detachment: a prospective randomized multicenter clinical study. Ophthalmology. 2007;114(12):2142–54.

Inferior Retinal Detachment with Densiron Xtra

13

Ulrich Spandau

In this chapter the surgical management of an inferior retinal is explained. A vitrectomy with a Dension Xtra temponade is described step-by-step. An inferior retinal detachment with a break at 4 o'clock (Fig. 13.1) can be operated with Sf_6 gas and postop positioning. An inferior detachment with a break at 4:30 (or 7:30) can be tamponaded with a long lasting gas such as C_2F_6 and C_3F_8. Inferior RDs with ruptures from 5:00 to 7:00, however, have an increased reattachment risk if you use long-lasting gases [1]. Especially, an inferior detachment with a break at 6 o'clock cannot be operated with a gas tamponade because no gas can tamponade a break at 6 o'clock (Fig. 13.2). An elegant choice for surgical management is a segmental buckle at the inferior pole. You can place an ora parallel buckle from 5 to 7 o'clock. An alternative is a vitrectomy with a Densiron Xtra tamponade. Densiron Xtra is heavier than water and tamponades therefore a break at 6 o'clock. Densiron Xtra has a viscosity comparable to 1300 cSt silicone oil.

Anaesthesia: We use always peribulbar anaesthesia. General anaesthesia is not necessary.

U. Spandau (✉)
St. Eriks Hospital, University of Stockholm, Stockholm, Sweden
e-mail: ulrich_spandau@yahoo.de

13.1 Surgery

Surgery

Instruments:

1. 25/27-Gauge 3-port trocar system
2. Chandelier light
3. Endodiathermy
4. Endolaser
5. Backflush instrument
6. Scleral depressor.

Tamponade

Intraoperative: PFCL

Postoperative: Densiron Xtra (Fluoron, Germany) (Fig. 13.3).

Individual steps:

1. **25G/27G 3-port system with chandelier light**
2. **Phacoemulsification with IOL**
3. **Core vitrectomy and posterior vitreous detachment**
4. **Marking of breaks with endodiathermy**
5. **Injection of PFCL up to the posterior edge of the break and drainage of subretinal fluid**
6. **Vitrectomy of the break flap and the peripheral vitreous**
7. **PFCL injection up to ora serrata**
8. **Laser photocoagulation around breaks**
9. **Trimming of the vitreous base (Shaving)**
10. **Fluid/air exchange**
11. **Drainage of subretinal fluid**

U. Spandau et al. (eds.), *Retinal Detachment Surgery and Proliferative Vitreoretinopathy*,
https://doi.org/10.1007/978-3-031-11946-0_13

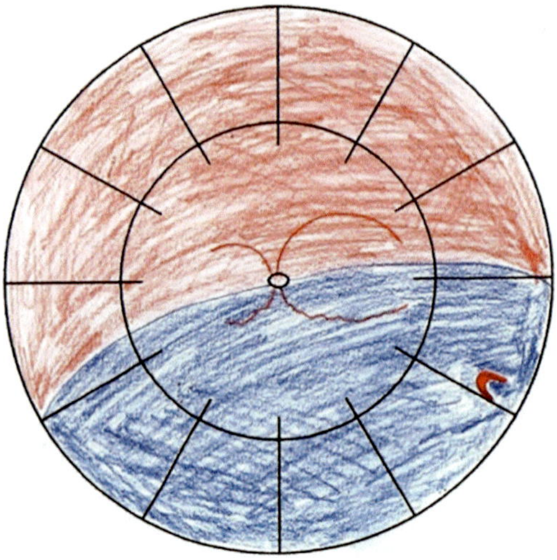

Fig. 13.1 An inferior detachment with a break at 4 o'clock

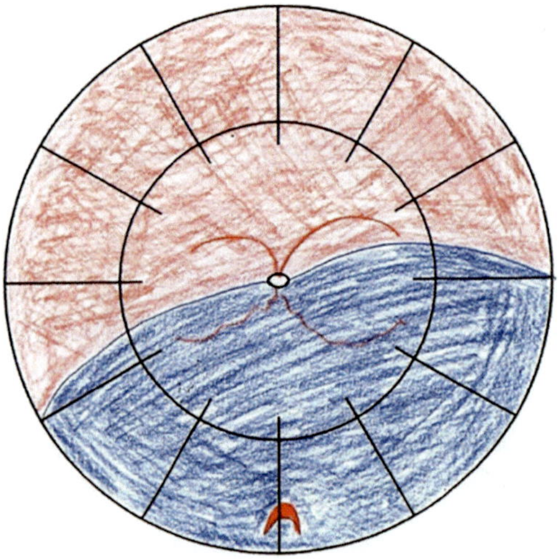

Fig. 13.2 An inferior detachment with a break at 6 o'clock

12. **Complete laser coagulation**
13. **Densiron Xtra tamponade**
14. **Removal of trocars**
15. **Suture of sclerotomies**
16. **Postoperative posture**.

The surgery step-by-step: **Figs.** 13.4, 13.5 **and** 13.6.

1. **25G/27G 3-port system with chandelier light (Fig.** 13.4)

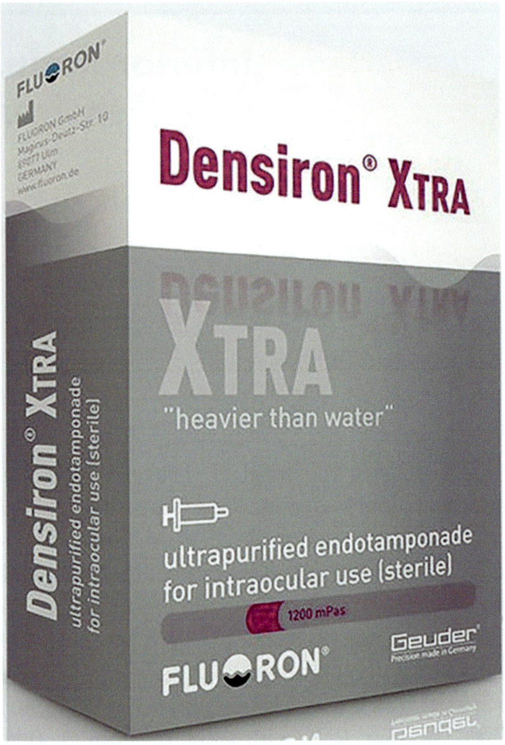

Fig. 13.3 Densiron Xtra (Fluoron, Germany)

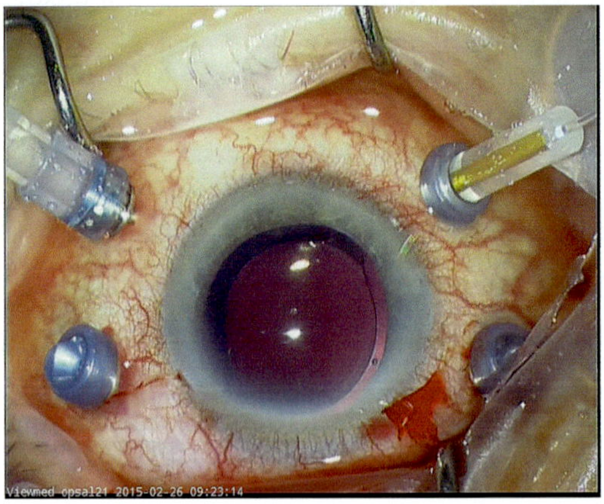

Fig. 13.4 Our regular setup for retinal detachment. 3-port vitrectomy and one chandelier light at the inferotemporal position

Insert the trocars at the usual locations 3.5 mm behind the limbus. Visualize the location of the infusion cannula in order to avoid a choroidal detachment. Then insert the chandelier light inferonasally 3.5 mm behind the limbus.

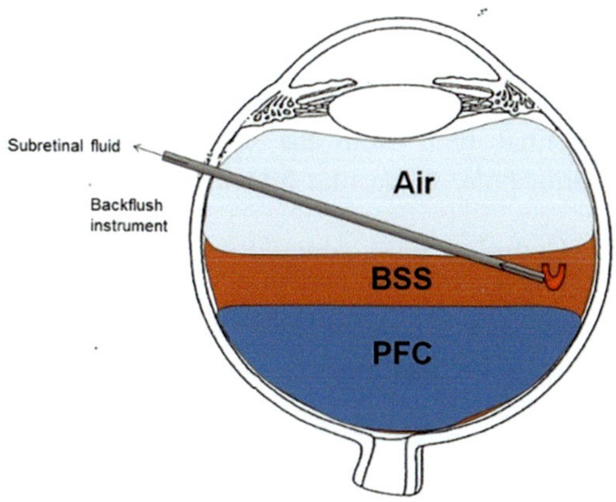

Fig. 13.5 Sandwich tamponade with air and PFCL. Aspirate first BSS and PFCL until the PFCL meniscus reaches the posterior edge of the hole

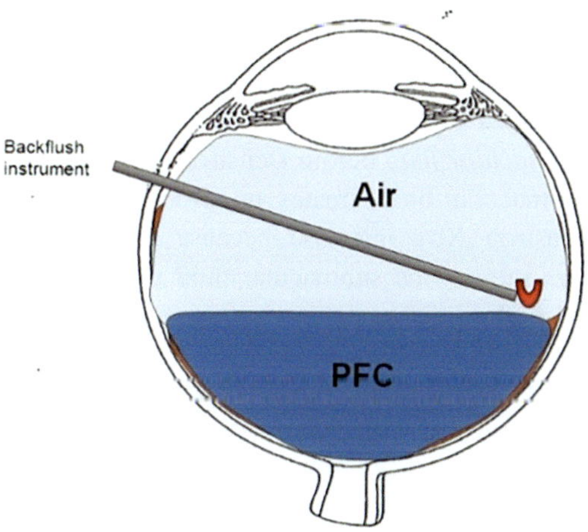

Fig. 13.6 If the PFCL has reached the inferior edge of the retinal break then aspirate the subretinal fluid. Then you can continue to remove the residual PFCL

2. **Phacoemulsification**

Continue with phacoemulsification and IOL implantation.

3. **Core vitrectomy and posterior vitreous detachment**

Perform a core vitrectomy and identify the posterior vitreous face to verify that a PVD is present. If the vitreous is still attached, induce a PVD. Then continue with vitrectomy, and search for retinal breaks. Carefully remove the vitreous close to the retina in the area of detached, fluttering retina.

4. **Mark the breaks with endodiathermy**

The key concept of all retinal detachment surgeries is to identify and treat all retinal breaks. Perform a thorough internal search for breaks following Lincoff´s rules that point to the most likely areas of retinal breaks. Mark the edges of the break with endodiathermy. A break, which is not marked, is hard to identify when it is attached to the underlying retinal pigment epithelium.

5. **Injection of PFCL to posterior edge of break and drainage of subretinal fluid**

The PFCL pushes the subretinal fluid from the central pole towards the periphery and presses it through the retinal break into the vitreous cavity. First, the PFCL is injected up to the posterior edge of the most central break, while we observe how the subretinal fluid is forced through the break into the vitreous cavity. The PFCL also has the effect that the mobile retina is attached, and a vitrectomy in the vicinity of the detached retina is less dangerous.

6. **Vitrectomy of the tear flap and the peripheral vitreous**

After ensuring the presence and completion of a PVD, the next step is to perform trimming of the vitreous base. Start within the area of the break(s) and also remove the flap, as the vitreous traction on the flap caused the detachment. The scleral depressor in the second hand is a great help when indenting the retina.

7. **PFCL injection up to ora serrata**
8. **Laser Therapy of breaks**

Inject PFCL up to the ora serrata. Continue with laser photocoagulation. Apply three rows of laser burns around the breaks. The settings depend on the laser device. It is possible that subretinal fluid has accumulated anterior to the break (so-called “trapped fluid”) which makes it difficult to apply a laser onto the anterior part of the break. Try to indent the break with the scleral depressor, so that the subretinal fluid is pushed away. Apply white laser burns. If a complete laser photocoagulation is not possible due to trapped fluid, then finalize laser photocoagulation after fluid x air exchange.

9. **Trimming of vitreous base (Shaving)**

If it has not been performed before, a thorough vitrectomy of the vitreous base has to be performed at this stage using the scleral depressor. This procedure is also called "shaving". PFCL lifts the vitreous up and enables a secure and thorough trimming of the vitreous base. In those areas, where PFCL does not rest on the retina, there is vitreous which has to be removed. Indent the sclera and move the vitreous cutter along the meniscus of the PFCL. Hereby you can manoeuvre the vitreous cutter very close to the retina because the heavy liquid presses against the retina.

10. **Fluid against air exchange**
11. **Drainage of subretinal fluid**

In the beginning, the break is covered with PFCL. After a short time, the PFCL is suctioned to the posterior edge of the break. Now the air presses the subretinal fluid in the direction of the break. The subretinal fluid is trapped between anterior located air and posterior located PFCL, so-called "sandwich tamponade". Now you aspirate the subretinal fluid through the break and at the same time the water phase between air and PFCL (Figs. 13.5 and 13.6).

If the "trapped fluid" is completely removed, you switch with the flute needle alternately between the PFCL bubble in order to reduce it and the break in order to aspirate fluid here. Try to aspirate without indenting the break.

The remaining PFCL is aspirated by holding the flute tip directly in front of the optic disc. Make sure that the PFCL is completely removed and that neither the retina nor the optic disc is affected.

Remark: Residual subretinal fluid in the central pole is no problem in case of a Densiron Xtra tamponade. Why? The Densiron Xtra pushes the subretinal fluid from the central pole to the inferior pole. A macular fold will not develop.

12. **Complete laser coagulation**

If necessary complete now the laser therapy around the retinal break in the air-filled eye.

13. **Densiron Xtra tamponade**

Densiron Xtra has a viscosity of 1300 csts. The injection time is therefore short. An oil injection is best performed bimanual. One hand holds the Charles flute needle to relieve air and the other hand holds the silicone oil syringe. Inject Densiron Xtra with a 25G silicone oil cannula (Alcon) and a 25G trocar cannula.

Tips and Tricks

Submacular fluid before Densiron Xtra injection. Submacular fluid creates no problem before a Densiron Xtra injection because the Densiron Xtra presses the submacular fluid from the central to the inferior pole.

14. **Removal of the trocar cannulas**
15. **Suture of sclerotomies**

Finally, the trocars are removed. Remove first the instrument trocars and at the end the infusion trocar. In case of a gas tamponade add some gas until the globe is normotensive. Suture the sclerotomies with Vicryl 8-0.

16. **Postoperative posture**

Densiron Xtra tamponades the inferior pole. A postoperative posture is not required.

13.2 Complications

In our experience, Densiron Xtra causes no complications. Some clinics report severe membrane formation under Densiron Xtra but we have never observed this phenomenon. An IOP increase can be controlled with antihypertensive eye drops. We remove Densiron Xtra after 6 weeks, but even a long-term tamponade causes no major problems. It may happen under the postoperative course that the retina is attached inferiorly but detaches superiorly. In this case, we perform a silicone oil exchange against 1300 or 5000 csts silicone oil. Densiron Xtra can be removed with a 25G metal cannula from Alcon. For a beginner it is however easier to remove it with a long 23G metal cannula from DORC.

Reference

1. Starr MR, Obeid A, Ryan EH, Ryan C, Ammar M, Patel LG, Forbes NJ, Capone A Jr, Emerson GG, Joseph DP, Eliott D, Gupta OP, Regillo CD, Hsu J, Yonekawa Y. Primary Retinal Detachment Outcomes (PRO) study group. Retinal detachment with inferior retinal breaks: primary vitrectomy versus vitrectomy with scleral buckle (PRO study report no. 9). Retina. 2021;41(3):525–30. https://doi.org/10.1097/IAE.0000000000002917 (PMID: 33600131).

14 Encircling Band, Vitrectomy, Retinotomy and C3F8 (Stockholm Technique)

Ulrich Spandau

This technique is the standard surgical technique for retinal detachments at the University hospital in Stockholm, Sweden. All types of detachments including an inferior detachment can be operated with this technique (Figs. 14.1 and 14.2). The typical patient has its natural lens and is myopic with lattice. The surgery is performed with encircling band, vitrectomy and C_3F_8 tamponade. The encircling band is 3.5 mm wide (Labtician, Canada). The advantage of this technique is that all types of detachments can be operated and that the redetachment rate is low. The disadvantage is that the encricling band creates myopia of 3dpt and that general anesthesia is required.

A second feature of this technique is that in the most cases a phacoemulsification is not performed. Only in case of a dense nucleus, a phacoemulsification is performed.

Another feature is that the subretinal fluid is removed with a posterior retinotomy. (Remark: The subretinal fluid can either be removed with PFCL from a peripheral rupture or with air from a central rupture. The central retinal rupture is iatrogenic and called posterior retinotomy.) But this technique is to the preference of the surgeon and a removal of subretinal fluid with PFCL is also possible.

U. Spandau (✉)
St. Eriks Hospital, University of Stockholm, Stockholm, Sweden
e-mail: ulrich_spandau@yahoo.de

Anaesthesia: We use always general anaesthesia because the placement of the encircling band causes pain.

14.1 Surgery

Instruments

(1) 25G or 27G 4 port vitrectomy with chandelier light
(2) Retinal detachment tray
(3) 3,5 mm encircling band (Labtician, Canada) (Fig. 14.3).

Main surgical steps

1. 4 holding sutures
2. Encircling band
3. Insertion of trocars and chandelier light
4. Maybe: Phaco + IOL
5. Core and peripheral vitrectomy
6. Marking of breaks with endodiathermy
7. Posterior retinotomy
8. BSS against air exchange
9. Laser treatment
10. C_3F_8 tamponade
11. Close the conjunctiva

Every step in detail

1. 4 holding sutures
2. Encircling band

Open the conjunctiva along the limbus 360 degrees with Westcott scissors, dissect the Tenon

U. Spandau et al. (eds.), *Retinal Detachment Surgery and Proliferative Vitreoretinopathy*,
https://doi.org/10.1007/978-3-031-11946-0_14

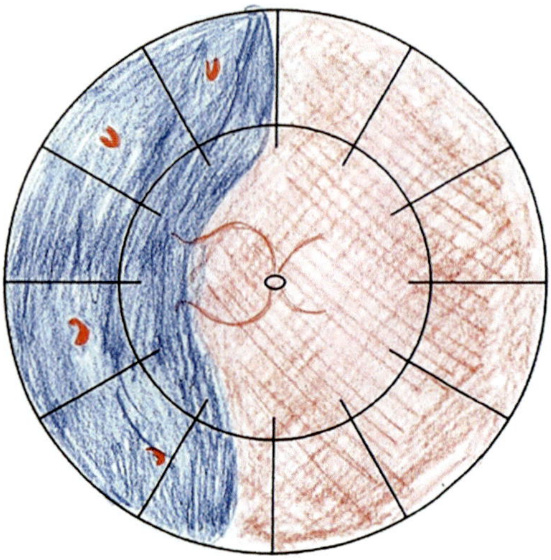

Fig. 14.1 All types of retinal detachments can be operated with this method

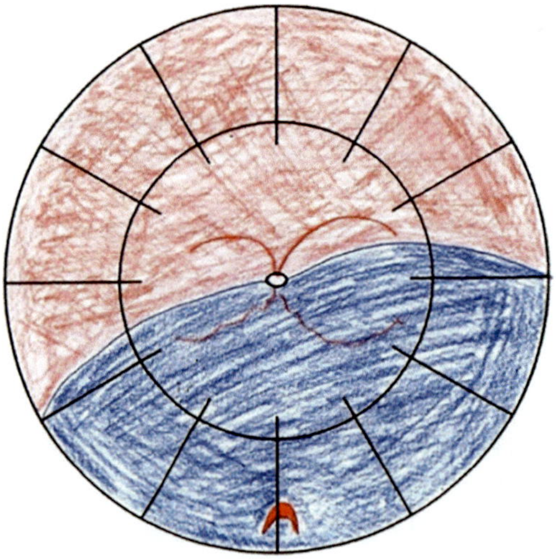

Fig. 14.2 Even an inferior detachment with a break at 6 o´clock can be operated with this technique. But the break must be located on the impression of the encircling band because the gas cannot tamponade this break

Fig. 14.3 3,5 mmencircling band from Labtician (S2970), Canada

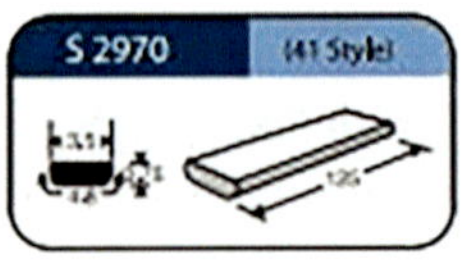

capsule from the sclera with a strabismus scissors and place four holding silk 3–0 sutures on all straight muscles. Place the encircling band under all 4 straight muscles and then fixate the band with a Mersilene 5–0 suture in each quadrant. The band should be located on the equator. You can measure this location, and it is the axial length divided by two (AXL/2).

3. Insertion of trocars and chandelier light
4. Maybe: Phaco + IOL
5. Core and peripheral vitrectomy

Insert then the trocars and a chandelier light. Start with a core vitrectomy. Be cautious with the natural lens. Then continue with a peripheral vitrectomy. Perform also a vitreous base shaving with scleral depression through vitreous base shaving; a thorough vitreous base shaving is not required.

6. Marking of breaks with endodiathermy
7. Posterior retinotomy

Mark the retinal breaks with an endodiathermy. Decide whether you want to continue with or without PFCL. If you choose to continue without PFCL need to remove the subretinal fluid with a central retinotomy. The retinotomy is

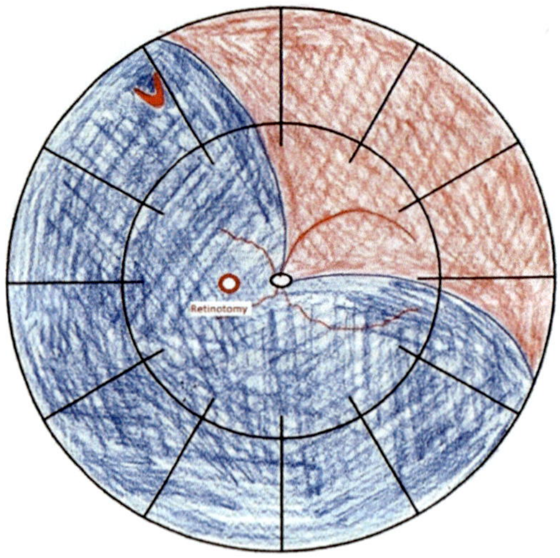

Fig. 14.4 Posterior retinotomy: Depending on the shape of the detachment you need to create a posterior retinotomy. The retinotomy is located outside the temporal arcade at the site of the maximal amount of subretinal fluid

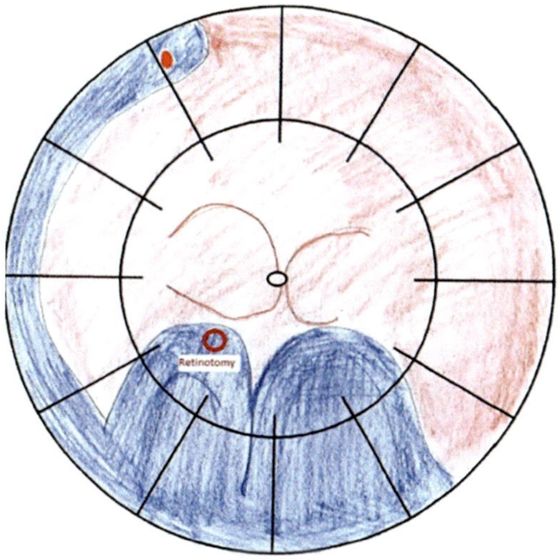

Fig. 14.5 Posterior retinotomy: Depending on the shape of the detachment you need to create a posterior retinotomy. The retinotomy is located outside the temporal arcade at the site of the maximal amount of subretinal fluid

located outside the temporal arcade at the site of the maximal amount of subretinal fluid (Figs. 14.4 and 14.5).

8. BSS against air exchange
9. Laser treatment
10. C_3F_8 tamponade
11. Close the conjunctiva

The next step is a BSS against air exchange. Remove the peripheral subretinal fluid first from the peripheral break and then from the posterior retinotomy. Continue with laser photocoagulation. Laser three rows of laser around the retinal ruptures. Then continue with the PFCL against air exchange. This is the most difficult step because visualization is poor. Remark: The best visualization system for an air-filled eye is the Resight system from Zeiss. We use a 14% C_3F_8 tamponade. Finalize surgery and close the conjunctiva with Vicryl 8–0.

14.2 FAQ

Q: **How is the risk for macular folds?**

A: The risk for slippage is small with this technique.

Q: **Choice of gas tamponade**

A: We recommend a long-lasting gas such as C_2F_6 or C_3F_8 for this technique because both gases cover the peripheral breaks as well the retinotomy well. Sf_6 may not be sufficient to cover the retinotomy.

Q: **What are the pros and cons of no phacoemulsification?**

A: Pros are reduced postoperative inflammation. Cons are that the anterior vitreous is not removed and that the visualization of the fundus is much reduced in the postoperative follow-up. This is especially true for the first postoperative week and improves at the second postoperative week.

15 Episcleral Buckling for Detachment Surgery with BIOM

Ulrich Spandau

15.1 Introduction

The principle of buckle surgery can be explained very easily when comparing it with a puncture in a bicycle tyre. The tyre is the sclera, and the tube is the retina. The first step in repairing a puncture is the search for a hole under water. Unfortunately, the same test is not available for the eye. Here, we use an indirect ophthalmoscope and Lincoff rules. When the puncture in the tube is found, we mark it and according to the size of the puncture we place a patch on it. In the eye, we mark the hole on the sclera and according to the size of the hole we suture a sponge on it. Then we pump the tyre up with air. If the tube remains filled, we solved the problem. If the tube gets soft again then either the old hole is not well patched or a second hole is present. This situation correlates completely to the eye. If the retina is attached the next day, then the problem is solved. If the retina remains detached, then either the first hole is not located on the buckle or a second break is present.

Minimal buckling versus maximal buckling technique

Episcleral buckling with encircling band or segmental sponges is possible in vitrectomized and not-vitrectomized eyes. Episcleral buckling is possible in eyes with PVD and without PVD. Nowadays two different episcleral buckling techniques are employed (Fig. 15.1): (1) Minimal buckling surgery with a segmental silicone sponge which seals only the hole. (2) Maximal buckling surgery with encircling band/tyre and a grooved strip which covers the hole.

Drainage versus no drainage

An external drainage is not necessary. Why? The RPE pumps nonstop subretinal fluid outside the eye. A bullous detachment is resorbed and attached after 1–2 days (Fig. 15.2). We recommend, however, an external drainage in a highly bullous detachment when the rupture is not attached on the buckle.

Radial buckle versus ora parallel buckle

The radial buckle is the most efficient buckle because it seals efficiently the complete horseshoe rupture. An ora parallel buckle seals often the horseshoe rupture only partially. So choose always a radial buckle if possible. If the rupture is located under a muscle then place the silicone sponge onto the muscle (radial) and place the suture in the sclera on each side of muscle.

Our surgical technique at the University of Uppsala for episcleral buckling is the following:

Minimal buckling surgery: The episcleral buckling technique we apply is the minimal buckling technique according to Kreissig/Lincoff (1).

U. Spandau (✉)
St. Eriks Hospital, University of Stockholm, Stockholm, Sweden
e-mail: ulrich_spandau@yahoo.de

U. Spandau et al. (eds.), *Retinal Detachment Surgery and Proliferative Vitreoretinopathy*,
https://doi.org/10.1007/978-3-031-11946-0_15

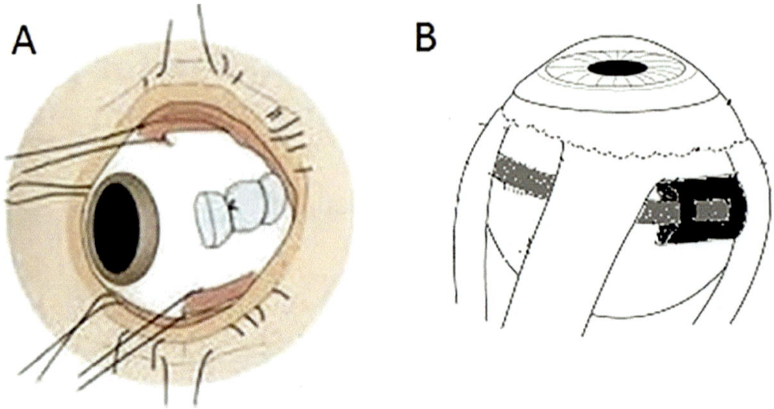

Fig. 15.1 Minimal buckling surgery with a radial sponge (**A**). Maximal buckling surgery with an encircling band and a grooved strip (**B**)

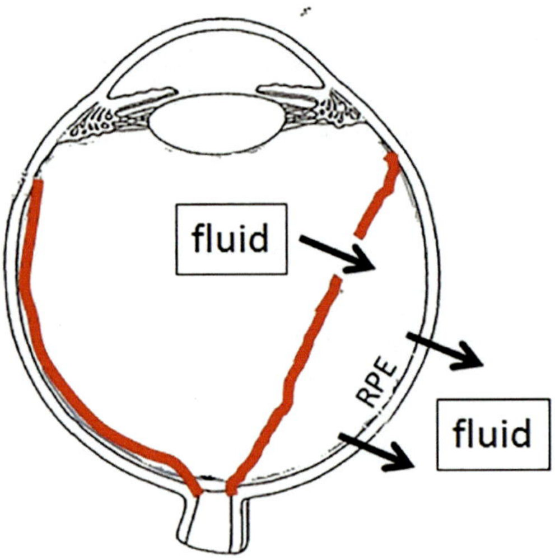

Fig. 15.2 Fluid flows through the rupture into the subretinal space and at the same time subretinal fluid is pumped outside the eye with the RPE

In short: (1) Cryopexy of the tear. (2) Application of a segmental buckle. Drainage only in highly bullous cases. No encircling band is necessary.

The complete surgery is performed with a microscope. We use the microscope with BIOM instead of a helmet with binocular ophthalmoscopy. For endoillumination a chandelier light is inserted.

Why? Today vitreoretinal surgeons are more used to the microscope. It is easier for a vitreoretinal surgeon to inspect the retina with a microscope than with binocular ophthalmoscopy. In addition, suturing of the silicone sponge is easier under a microscope than with a helmet. This is especially the case for long myopic eyes.

Choice of buckle (Table 15.1)

The choice of buckle is dependent on the size of the retinal break. If the break is 1 mm in size, then the sponge must be at least 3 mm in size. We have only 5 mm and 7 mm sponges and choose therefore in this case a 5 mm sponge. If the break is 4–5 mm in size, we choose a 7 mm sponge. If the break is larger than 5 mm we place the 5 mm or 7 mm buckle circumferential. See Table 15.1.

Table 15.1 Choice of silicone sponge depending on the size of the break

Break	Sponge	Suture
1 mm	5 mm radial	7 mm
2 mm	5 mm radial	7 mm
3 mm	5 mm radial	7 mm
4 mm	7 mm radial	9 mm
5 mm	7 mm radial	9 mm
6 mm	circumferential	7 mm (in case of 5 mm sponge)

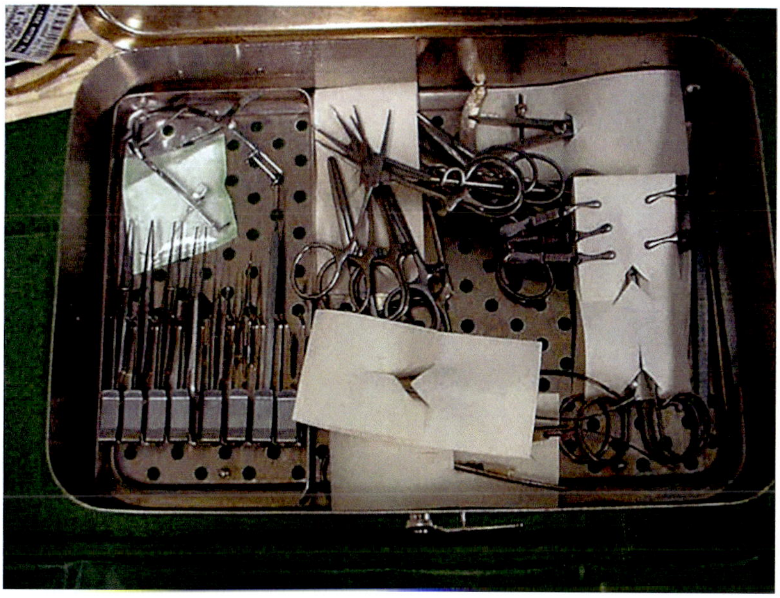

Fig. 15.3 Episcleral buckling instrument set

15.2 Instruments

Here you will find all the details of our episcleral buckling instrument set, which we use at the University Hospital of Uppsala (Fig. 15.3). The instruments vary, of course, from hospital to hospital. The instruments in **bold** are absolutely necessary.

Blepharostat

1 × Williams open adult

Cannulas

1 × rough curved

Forceps

2 × anatomical forceps

2 × forceps claw 1 × 2

1 × forceps Bonn

Scissors

1 scissors eyes straight sharp

1 scissors eyes bent sharp

1 scissors Westcott Geuder 19,750, (Fig. 15.4)

1 scissors straight Vannas **Geuder 19,760**

Clamping scissors

2 clamping scissors bent Halstedt

2 clamping scissors Hartman straight

1 clamping scissors Crile straight 14 cm

Needle holders

1 needle holder Barraquer without lock

1 needle holder Snowdon pencer with lock

Orbital spatula

1 orbital spatula Helvestone

1 orbital spatula Sautter Geuder 15,740, (Fig. 15.5), **alternative: Arruga spatula**

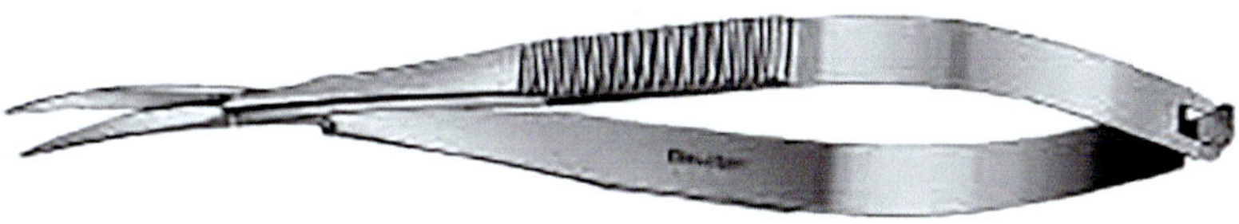

Fig. 15.4 Westcott scissors

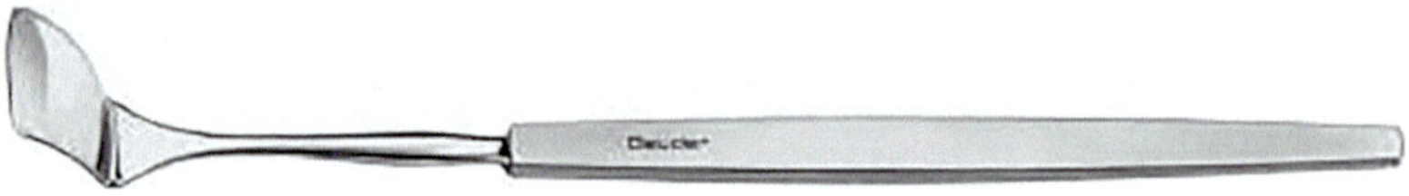

Fig. 15.5 Orbital spatula

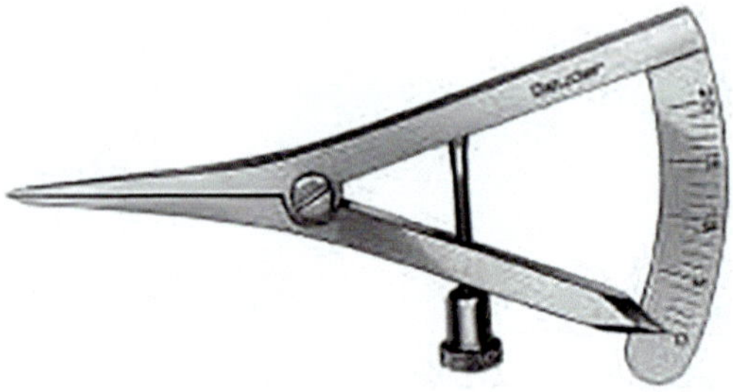

Fig. 15.6 Caliper

Knot holder
2 Knot Holder Rapp

Other
1 Caliper Castroviejo Straight 1–20 mm Geuder 19,135, (Fig. 15.6)
1 ruler
4 clamp Diefenbach 2
1 depressor scleral with or without marker
1 strabismus hook Bonn 1 mm hole, Geuder 15,821, (Fig. 15.7).

15.3 Material

1. Silicone sponge: (Fig. 15.8)
   (1) 5 × 3.77 mm partial thickness sponge (Labtician, Canada). Our most commonly used is silicone sponge. Indication: Ora dialysis, all normal size breaks. This sponge requires a 7 mm marking.
   (2) 7.0 × 5.28 mm partial thickness sponge (Labtician, Canada). Less commonly used is silicone sponge. Indication: Big breaks. This sponge requires a 9.0 mm marking.
2. Surgical skin marker with ultra-fine tip (Many companies, for example: 1456XL SR-100, Viscot Medical LLC, USA).
3. Supramid suture 4–0 (REF SP151399, Serag Wiessner, Germany), alternative: Polyester 5–0 (Alcon).
4. Silk suture 3–0 (Ethicon).

Main surgical steps:
(1) 180° limbal peritomy
(2) 2 or 3 traction sutures
(3) Insertion of a chandelier light
(4) Search for the retinal break with scleral depressor
(5) Cryopexy of the break
(6) Scleral marking of the break
(7) Marking of sutures
(8) Apply the sutures
(9) Paracentesis, release aqueous from anterior chamber
(10) Fasten the sponge
(11) Inspect the retina
(12) If sponge covers the break fasten the sponge permanently. If sponge does not cover the break, then replace the sponge.
(13) Remove the chandelier light and suture the sclerotomy with a Vicryl 8–0 suture.
(14) Remove the traction sutures and close the conjunctiva with Vicryl 6–0.

The surgery step-by-step: (Figs. 15.9, 15.10, 15.11, 15.12, 15.13, 15.14, 15.15, 15.16, 15.17, 15.18, 15.19, 15.20, 15.21, 15.22, 15.23, 15.24, 15.25 and 15.26)

1. **180° limbal peritomy**
2. **2 or 3 traction sutures**

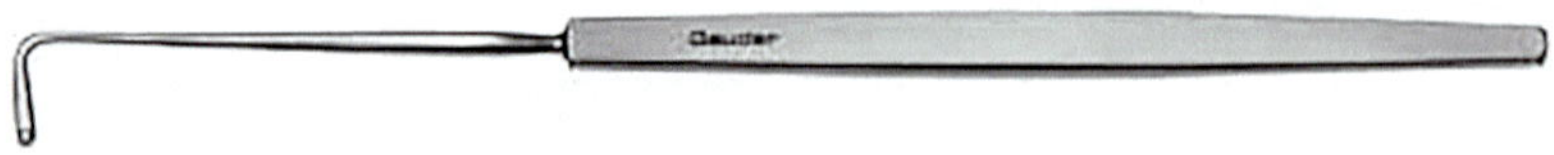

Fig. 15.7 Strabismus hook

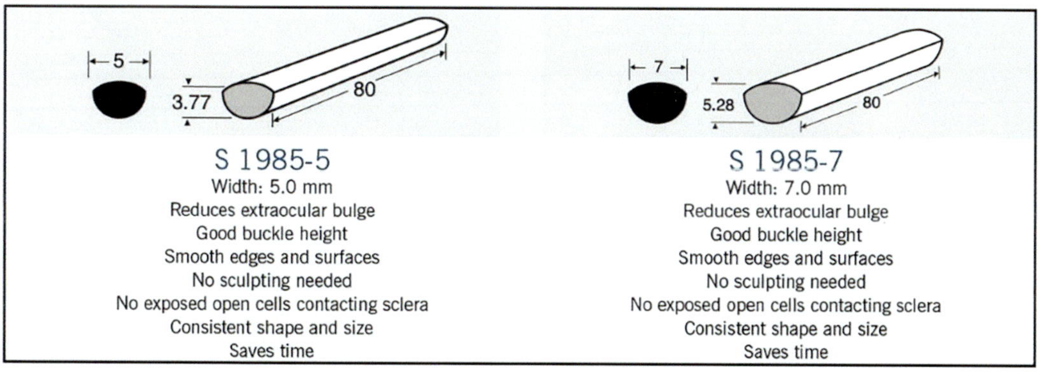

Fig. 15.8 Silicone sponge

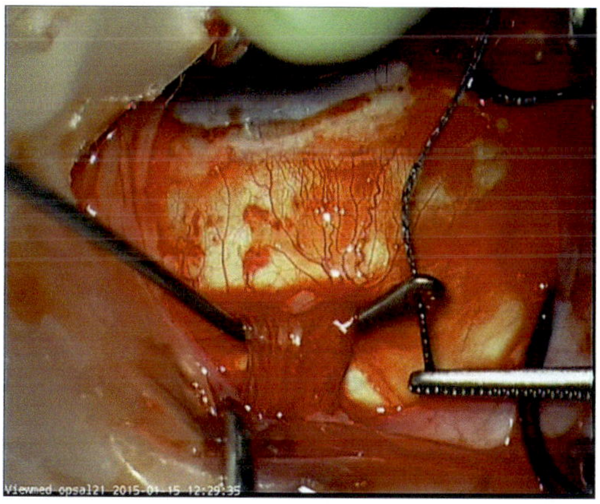

Fig. 15.9 Place a strabismus hook with hole under the complete muscle and insert a silk suture

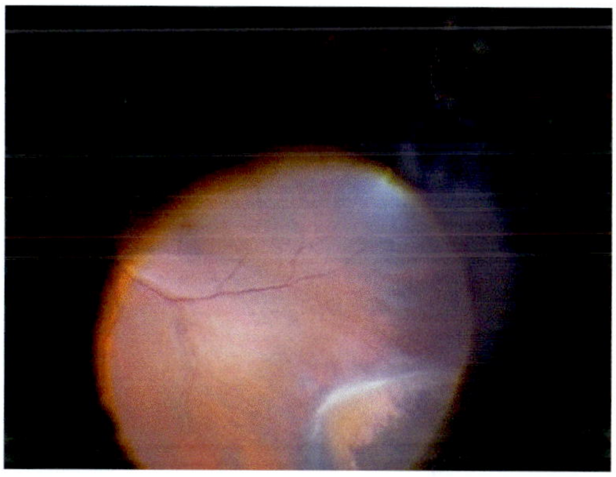

Fig. 15.11 It is easy to examine the retina with the microscope and a viewing system

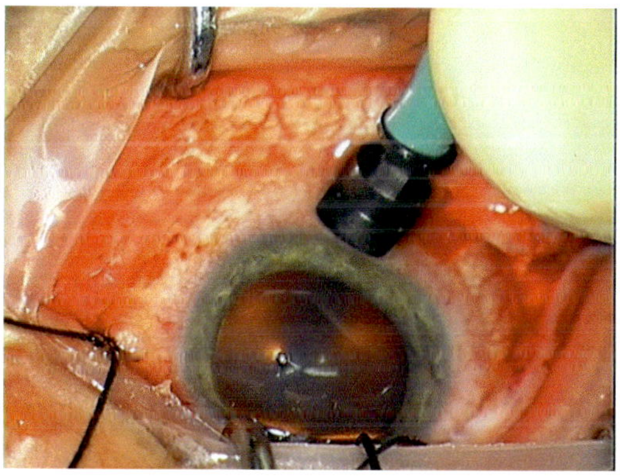

Fig. 15.10 Insert a chandelier light at 6 o'clock opposite to a break at 12 o'clock

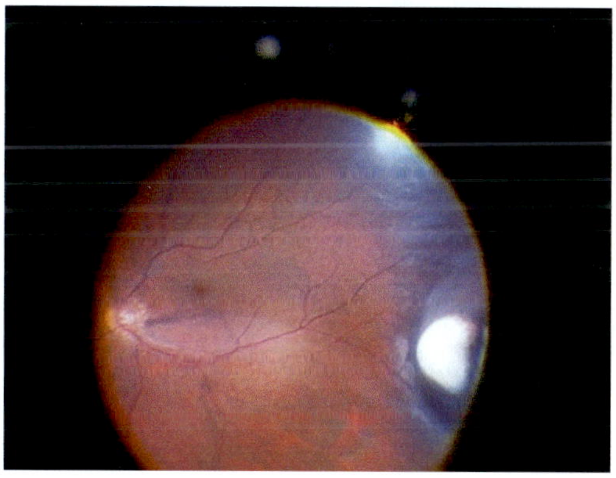

Fig. 15.12 Freeze the retinal break with the cryopexy handpiece

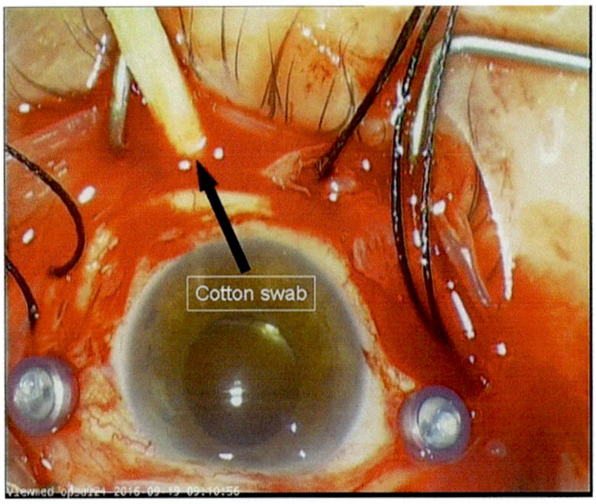

Fig. 15.13 Locate the retinal break with a cotton swab or scleral depressor

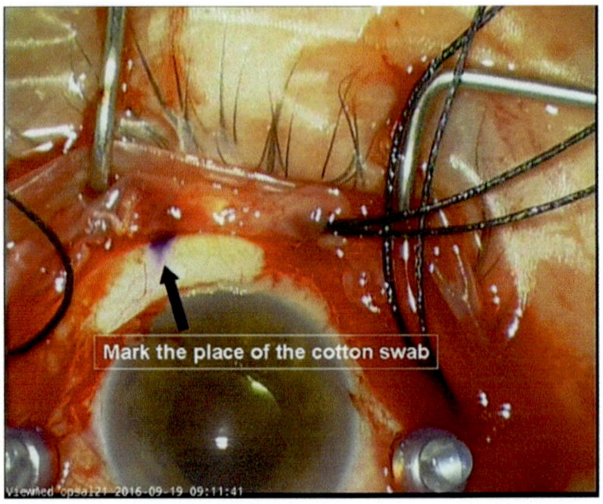

Fig. 15.14 Then mark the sclera or limbus at the position of the cotton swab

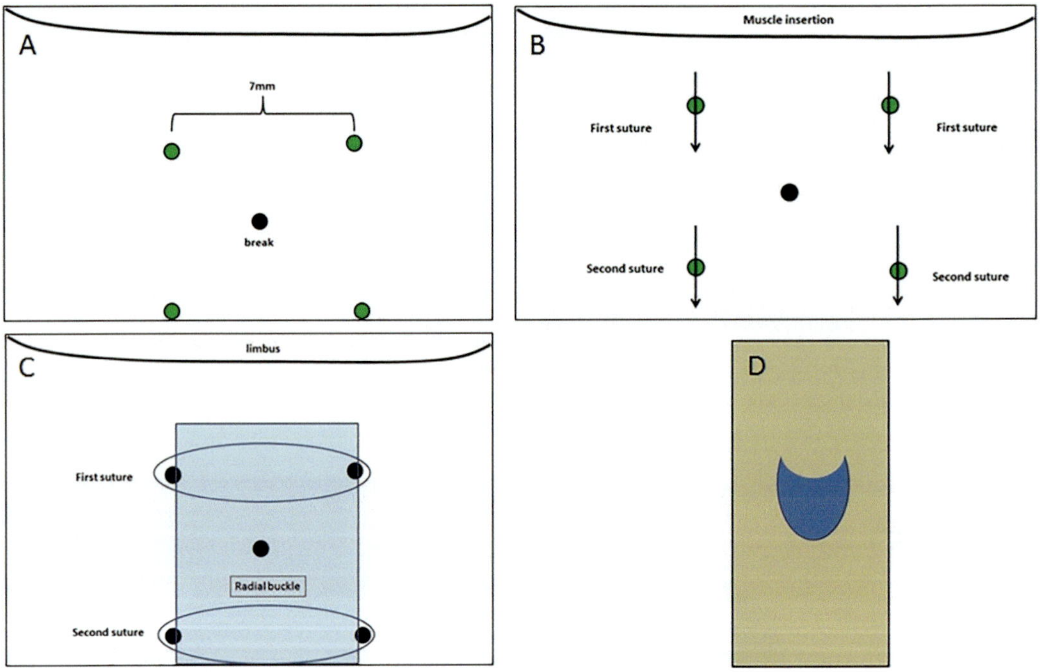

Fig. 15.15 **A, B, C, D:** A radial sponge. **A** Mark 7 mm anterior and posterior of the break. **B** Move the needle as depicted for the first and second suture. **C** After complete surgery. **D** The break is located in the middle of the radial sponge. No fish mouthing is possible

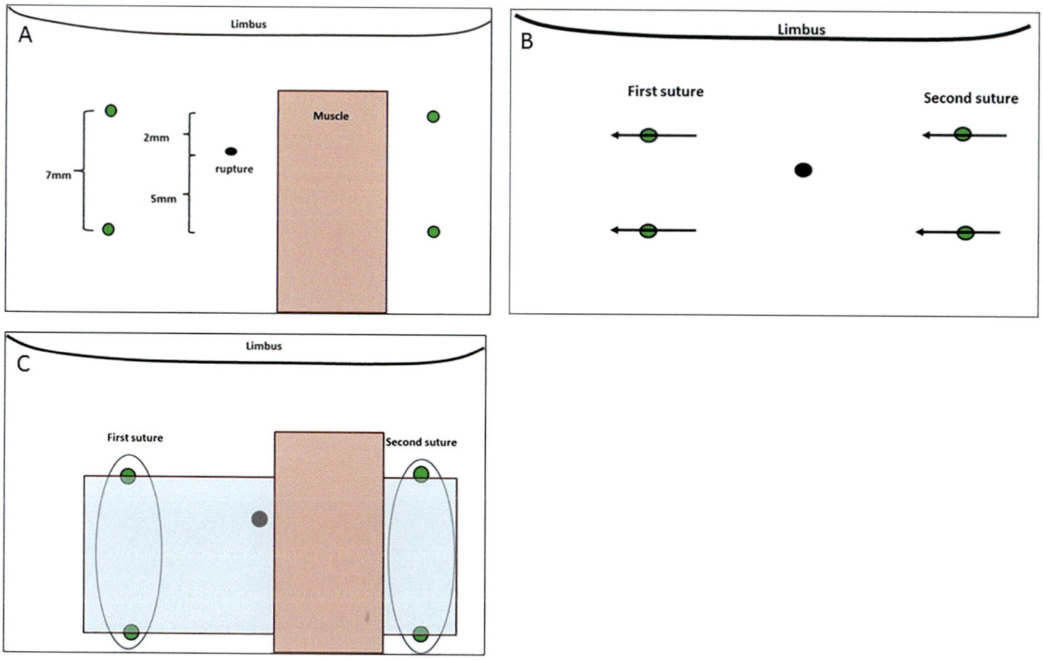

Fig. 15.16 **A, B, C:** A circumferential sponge. **A** Mark again 7 mm so that the retinal break is located in the upper half of the buckle. If the break is close to the muscle, then place the sponge under the muscle. **B** Place the first suture as depicted and then the second suture **C** Then place the sponge under the suture and tighten the knot with 2–1-1 throws (Supramid or Mersilene suture)

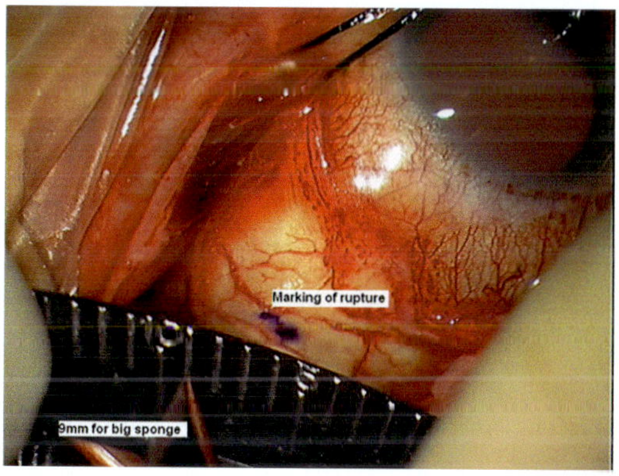

Fig. 15.17 Set the caliper to 9 mm for a big sponge and to 7 mm for a normal sponge

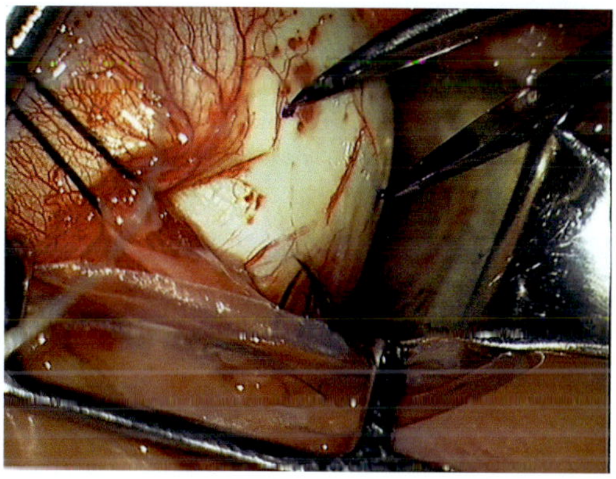

Fig. 15.18 Then mark the sclera with the caliper

The limbal peritomy and the 3 traction sutures are placed according to the location of the break. If the break is located at 12 o'clock then the lateral rectus, medial rectus and the superior rectus require traction sutures and the limbal peritomy is located from 9 o'clock over 12 o'clock to 3 o'clock.

If the break is located at 1:30 then a limbal peritomy from 12:00 to 3:00 is performed and two holding sutures are placed under the superior and lateral rectus muscle.

Perform a limbal peritomy and place a strabismus hook with hole behind a straight muscle. Confirm that you grabbed the whole muscle

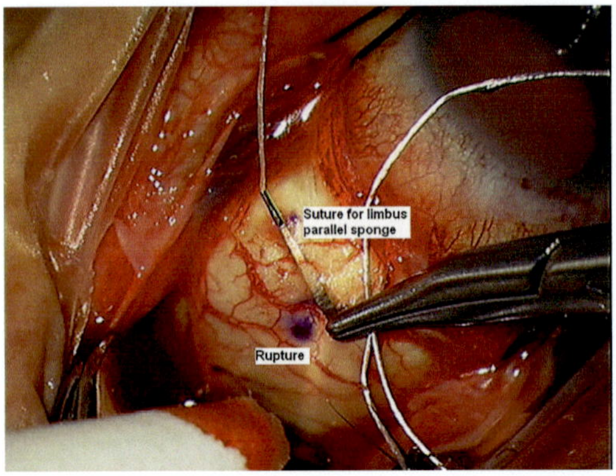

Fig. 15.19 Place the first scleral bite for limbus parallel (=circumferential) buckle

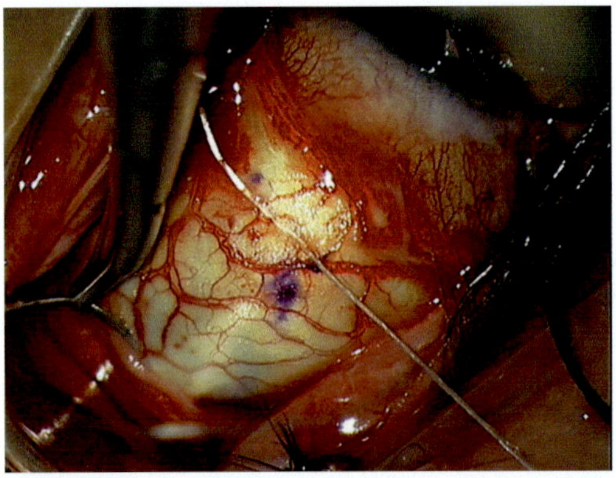

Fig. 15.20 Place the second scleral bite at the second marking

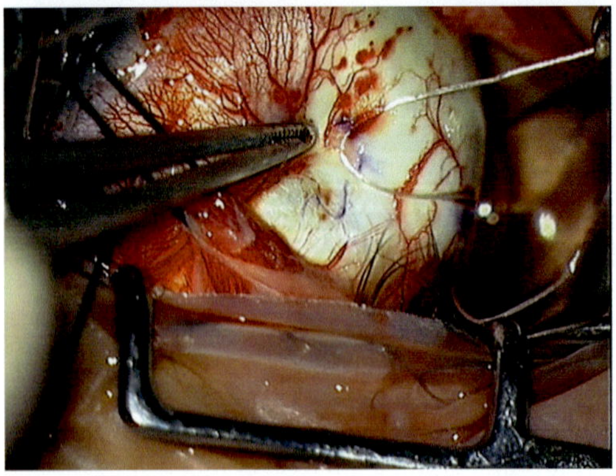

Fig. 15.21 The first suture is done

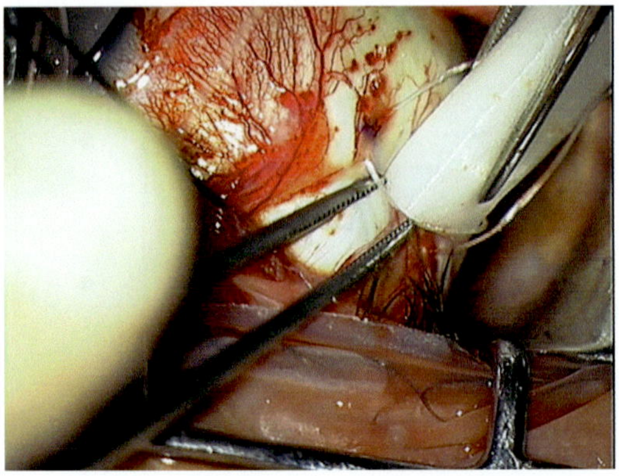

Fig. 15.22 Place the sponge under the suture

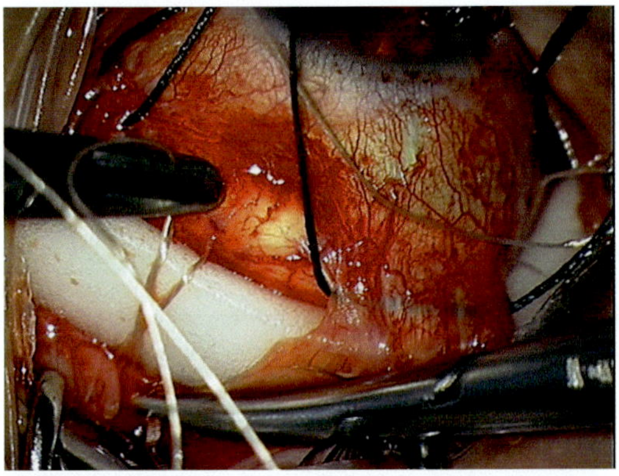

Fig. 15.23 Close the suture with 2–2-1 throws

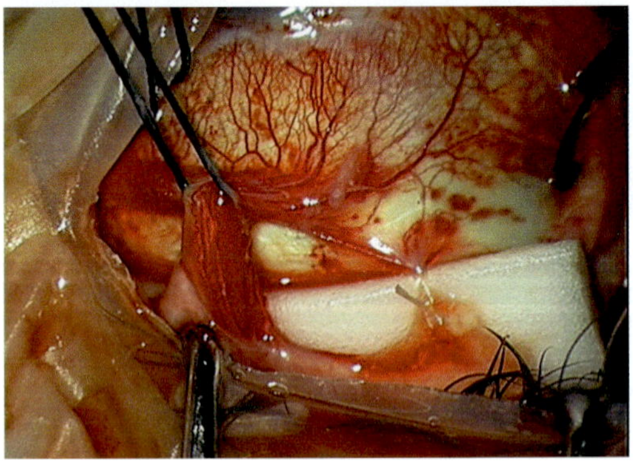

Fig. 15.24 Fasten the suture on both sides

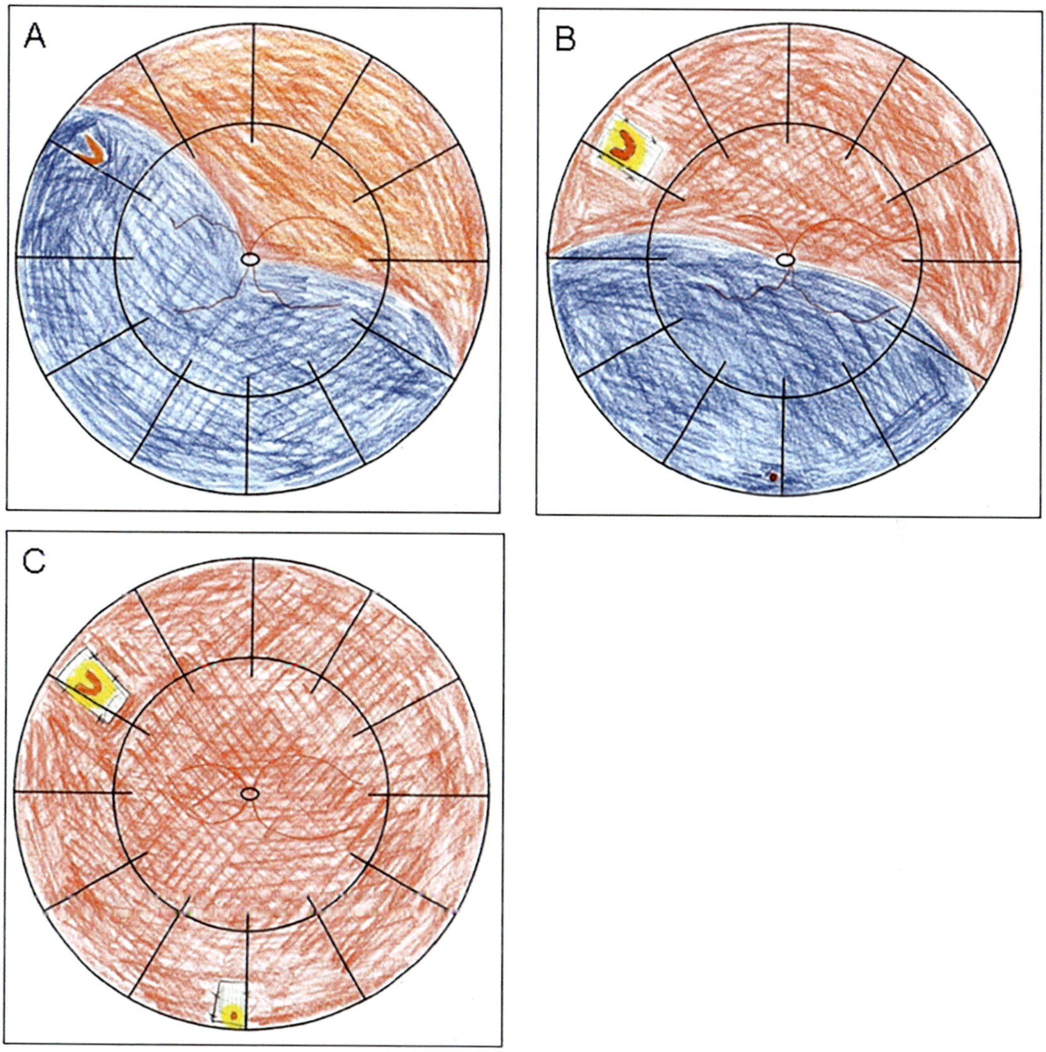

Fig. 15.25 **A** A superotemporal detachment with a rupture at 2 o'clock and at a second rupture at 6:15. **B** A residual detachment. The silicone sponge is placed on the break and the break is dry. But the silicone sponge at 6 o'clock is wrongly placed and the break at 6:15 is still detached. The buckle is 5 mm wide so you must replace the buckle 2,5 mm to the right side. **C** The sponge is replaced 2,5 mm and one day later the retina is reattached and the rupture is located now on the buckle

because you may place a sponge beneath the muscle. Insert the silk suture into the hole and retract the hook with the suture (Fig. 15.9). Tie a knot into the suture. Repeat this procedure with the two other straight muscles.

3. **Insertion of a chandelier light** (Fig. 15.10)

Continue with insertion of the chandelier light. The best location is opposite to the break. If the break is located superiorly then insert the chandelier light inferiorly.

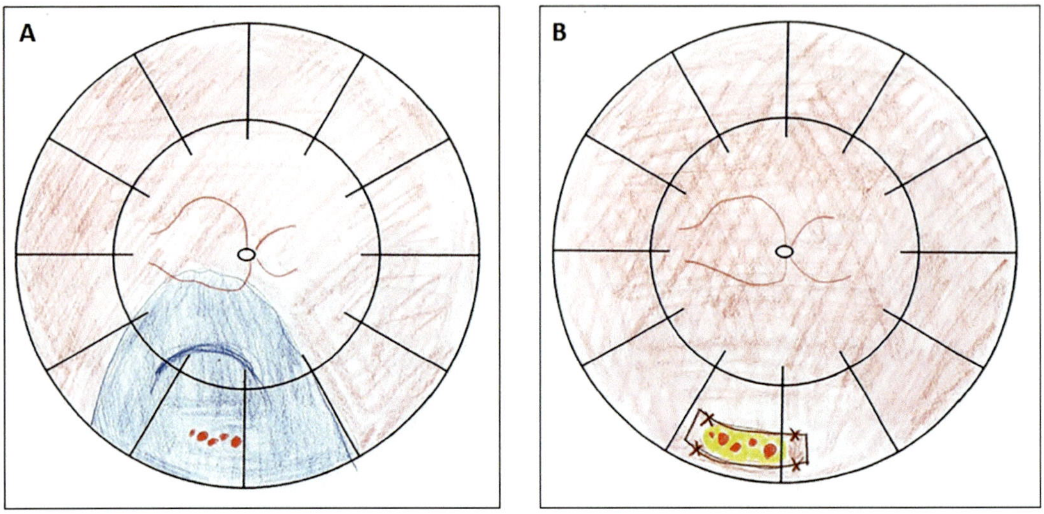

Fig. 15.26 **A** A young myopic patient with several retinal breaks at 6–7 o'clock. **B** A circumferential buckle is placed from 5:30 to 7:00 and the retina is reattached one day later

4. **Search for the break with scleral depressor** (Fig. 15.11)

Flick in the BIOM and search for the break. This maneuver is a bit more difficult compared to vitrectomy because the globe is more difficult to rotate. The search for a retinal hole goes like this: For example, a retinal detachment from 6:00 to 10:00: Place the scleral depressor at 10:00 and move it slowly in a straight line from the ora serrata towards the posterior pole. Look for a hole or a hole flap. Then continue placing the depressor at 9:30 and move it in a straight line towards the posterior pole; and so on. It is like mowing a lawn.

5. **Cryopexy of the break** (Fig. 15.12)
6. **Scleral marking of the break** (Figs. 15.13 and 15.14)

Freeze now the break (Fig. 15.12), keep the cryopexy hand piece in place, flick out the BIOM, rotate the globe, the assistant inserts an orbital spatula between tenon/conjunctiva, and sclera to identify the freezing spot. Dry the freezing spot with a cotton swab and mark it with the surgical marker pen (Figs. 15.13 and 15.14). The sclera must be absolutely dry that you can mark it.

7. **Marking of sutures** (Figs. 15.15 and 15.16)

Decide now whether you want to apply a radial sponge or a limbus parallel (circumferential) sponge (Figs. 15.15 and 15.16). If the break is located under a muscle an ora parallel (=circumferential) approach is advisable because it is difficult to suture under the muscle. Paint the tips of the caliper with the surgical skin marker pen. Mark the sclera with the caliper (Geuder). How wide? Two millimeters more than the width of the sponge. If the sponge is 5 mm wide, then mark 7 mm.

Where to mark? In case of a radial sponge hold the caliper so that the hole is in the middle (Fig. 15.15) Make two marking approximately two millimeters anterior to the break and two millimeters posterior to the break.

In case of an ora parallel (circumferential) sponge and a retinal break at 6:30 place two markings at 5:30 and two markings at 7:00 (Fig. 15.16). Place the silicone sponge under the inferior rectus muscle. The muscle force will help to indent the sponge.

8. **Apply the sutures** (Figs. 15.17, 15.18, 15.19, 15.20 and 15.21)

You need one suture with one needle for 2 markings. Cut the suture in two halves so that you have two sutures with one needle each. How to suture? The suture is the most dangerous maneuver in the complete surgery because you can perforate the sclera. Move the needle less deep but a long way through the sclera. The needle must be visible through the sclera. Repeat this maneuver at the second marking (Figs. 15.20 and 15.21).

Surgical pearls no. 70
Retinal tear under a muscle. Alternatively, to an ora parallel (=circumferential) sponge you can apply a radial sponge. If you want to apply a radial sponge under the muscle, then remove the muscle, suture the sponge and suture the muscle back to place. Or suture the sponge onto the muscle. If the patient experiences diplopia after surgery you can remove the sponge after approximately 3–4 weeks.

9. **Paracentesis, release aqueous from anterior chamber**

You need a soft globe to achieve a proper indentation of the sponge. Perform a paracentesis and release aqueous from the anterior chamber.

10. **Fasten the sponge** (Figs. 15.22, 15.23 and 15.24)

Place the silicone sponge under the sutures (Fig. 15.22), make two throws, tighten the suture a little bit, then release tension on the traction sutures and then tighten the suture again (Figs. 15.23 and 15.24). The knot has 2–1-1 throws. Perform the same maneuver with the second suture. Important: Do not pull the traction sutures while tying the sponge in order to achieve a good indentation.

11. **Inspect the retina**

Flick in the BIOM and inspect the retina. If the sponge does not cover the break, then reposition the sponge. The repositioning surgery goes usually faster than the first surgery.

12. **Remove the chandelier light**
13. **Remove the traction sutures and close the conjunctiva with Vicryl 6–0.**

Remove the chandelier light and suture the sclerotomy with a Vicryl 8–0 suture. Continue with cutting the traction sutures and remove them. Replace the conjunctiva and close it with Vicryl 6–0 or 8–0.

15.4 Complications

Scleral perforation (see video: Complication during episcleral buckling)
A scleral perforation can be seen by leakage of intraocular fluid. Redraw the needle, freeze the leakage site with cryopexy and repeat the suture at a different location.

Repositioning of a buckle
It is no problem and in fact technically quite easy to reposition a wrongly placed buckle. In some cases, the perioperative visualization of the hole on the buckle is not easy. One day later at the slit lamp the visualization is, however, in the most cases better. If the hole is located aside the buckle and not on the buckle, then try to estimate how many millimeters the hole is aside. Keep in mind that the buckle is 5 mm wide. If, for example, the hole is located at 5:30 and the buckle at 6:00, then remove the old sponge, place new sutures 2,5 mm next to the old sutures, and refasten the same sponge.

15.5 FAQ

Can I place a silicone sponge during vitrectomy?
Yes. If you want to buckle, for example, a break at 6 o'clock then place a limbus parallel (=circumferential) silicone sponge under the inferior rectus.

What about episcleral buckling in a vitrectomized eye?
This is no problem. It is easier because the impression of the sponge is more pronounced due to the absent vitreous body. In case of a focal recurrent detachment we often place a segmental buckle. Often the retinal break is difficult to find and often it is a laser necrosis which causes a tiny break. Place a sponge on this laser treated break and the retina will be attached the next day.

Is it difficult to reposition a silicone sponge?
It is no problem and in fact technically easy to reposition a wrongly placed buckle, as well during the first surgery as during a second surgery. For more see chapter "Buckle with chandelier".

What to do if the rupture is located under a muscle?
If a rupture is located under a muscle then place the silicone sponge directly on the muscle. An alternative is an ora parallel buckle. But remember: The best buckle is a radial buckle!!

15.6 Case Reports

First case report: Persistent retinal detachment
A superotemporal detachment was treated with a radial buckle at 10:00 (Fig. 15.25A). One day postoperative, the detachment around the break at 10:00 was attached but a persistent detachment is present. Why? Remember: The retina reacts logical. What kind of detachment is now present? It is a non-bullous inferior detachment Lincoff type 3. There must be a break between 6:30 and 9:00. After a new examination a break at 6:30 was found (Fig. 15.25B). A second buckle was placed on the break and the retina attached completely (Fig. 15.25C).

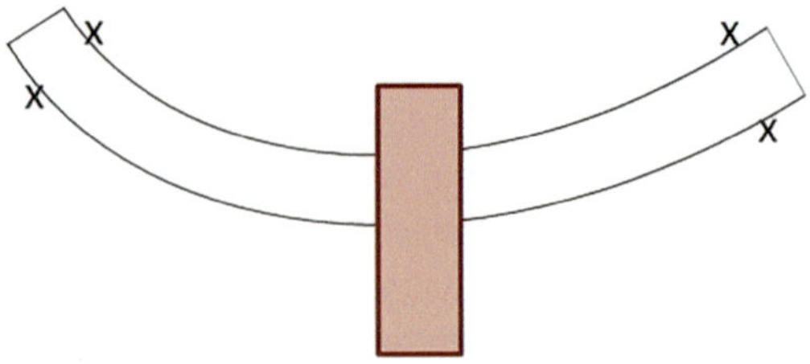

Fig. 15.27 A 90° buckle is placed under one rectus muscle

Seconds case report: 90° circumferential buckle
Young *myopic eyes* with an *inferior RD* are a good indication for episcleral buckling surgery (Fig. 15.26A, B). A 90 deg circumferential buckle under one rectus muscle is required (Fig. 15.27). We employ always segmental buckles in these cases.

Example: 27 y/o male patient with −3.5sph = 0.4 and an inferior detachment with 6 holes at 6–7 o'clock. Cryopexy and segmental buckle from 5 to 8 o'clock (under inferior rectus muscle).

Part III
Special Cases

All videos of this part are found in a playlist on my youTube channel:
https://youtube.com/playlist?list=PL0dKYclPD7yMn861X0g-aHCS6KZ5NcH1N
Chapter 16: No video
Chapter 17: **Recurrent Retinal Detachment**
Recurrent retinal detachment operated with 27G
Aphakia and inferior redetachment: Inferior buckle and Artisan IOL
Traumatic PVR redetachment
Chapter 18: No video
Chapter 19: **Rhegmatogenous Retinal Detachment in Children**
Retinal detachment secondary to Stickler syndrome (1)
Retinal detachment secondary to Stickler syndrome (2).

16 Special Cases—Giant Tear, Ora Dialysis, Young Myope, Chronic Detachments

Zoran Tomic and Ulrich Spandau

16.1 Giant Tear

A giant tear is defined as a tear of ≥ 3 clock hours. For *giant tears* vitrectomy is the method of choice (Fig. 16.1). We recommend combined phaco vitrectomy with a silicone oil tamponade because the risk for slippage is high. We do not recommend the Stockholm technique because the encircling band is not necessary and gas has a high risk for slippage. The same argument applies for the Moorfield technique.

Surgery of a giant tear

After vitrectomy you instill PFCL up to the ora serrata. Then proceed with a laser photocoagulation of the giant tear. This takes time. The next step is the difficult fluid against air exchange. Switch to air and aspirate until the fluid reaches the inferior edge of the giant tear. Then perform a thorough fluid aspiration at the giant tear until both edges are attached. Repeat this maneuver (aspiration of PFCL and aspiration at giant tear) several times. After complete removal of PFCL some slippage may occur. This does not matter because the silicone oil tamponade will take care of this problem and replace the retina—without creating macular folds. If you want to push back the retina, then use a silicone tip Charles flute needle. Place the silicone tip to the inferior edge of the sipped break and pull it towards ora serrata.

An alternative is a PFCL against silicone oil tamponade. This procedure reduces the slippage but is technically more difficult. As tamponade we recommend 1000 or 5000 csts silicone oil. Do not use gas because the risk for a slippage and retinal folds is increased.

16.2 Young Myopic RD and Ora Dialysis

In the United States, there are two remaining indications for episcleral buckling: Young myopic and ora dialysis.

Retinal detachments in patients <40 years we operate with episcleral buckling. The posterior vitreous is attached and the optical media are clear. A typical example are young myopes. *Myopic eyes* with an *inferior RD* are a good indication for episcleral buckling surgery. Encircling bands and segmental buckles may be used for this pathology. An encircling band causes a myopic shift of approximately 3D and a segmental buckle cause astigmatism. In both cases, the buckle can be removed after 4 weeks so that the globe can regain its original shape. We employ always segmental buckles in these

Z. Tomic
Milos Klinika, Belgrade, Serbia

U. Spandau (✉)
St. Eriks Hospital, University of Stockholm, Stockholm, Sweden
e-mail: ulrich_spandau@yahoo.de

U. Spandau et al. (eds.), *Retinal Detachment Surgery and Proliferative Vitreoretinopathy*,
https://doi.org/10.1007/978-3-031-11946-0_16

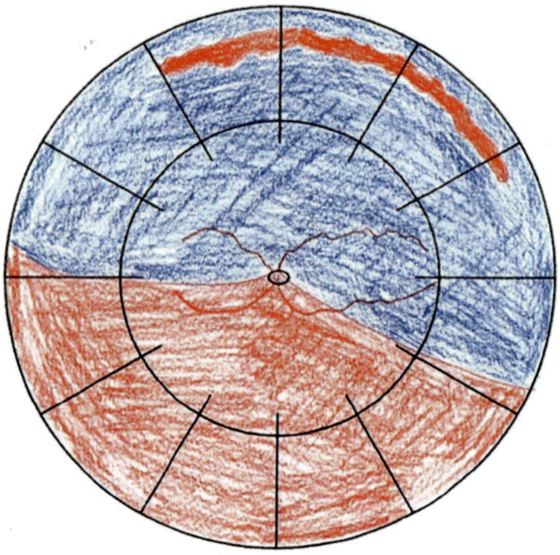

Fig. 16.1 A giant retinal tear has a length of 90° and more. A good candidate for vitrectomy

cases. This technique is explained in detail in Chapt. 15.

Example: A 27 y/o male patient with −3.5sph = 0.4 and an inferior detachment with 6 holes at 6–7 o'clock. Cryopexy and segmental buckle from 5:30 to 7:30 (under inferior rectus muscle) was performed (Fig. 16.2A, B).

16.3 Ora Dialysis

The *ora dialysis* is another pathology where a episcleral buckling is recommended because the success rate of reattachment for ora dialysis is 99% with episcleral buckling. If you choose to operate an ora dialysis with vitrectomy you need to achieve the same reattachment rate.
Example: 42 y/o male patient with ora dialysis at 6–7 o´clock and chronic inferior detachment due to trauma. A cryopexy and segmental buckle from 5 to 8 o'clock (under inferior rectus muscle) was performed (Fig. 16.3).

16.4 Chronic Detachments

Old detachments are difficult detachments. Young patients may present with an old and peripheral detachment. These eyes are often myopic and no symptoms are present. If no PVR is present and a break is visible we would operate these eyes with episcleral buckling. But in case of an old detachment with intravitreal PVR and retinal traction, we would choose a vitrectomy with encircling band. See treatment algorithm (Fig. 16.4). The episcleral buckling technique is explained in Chapt. 15.

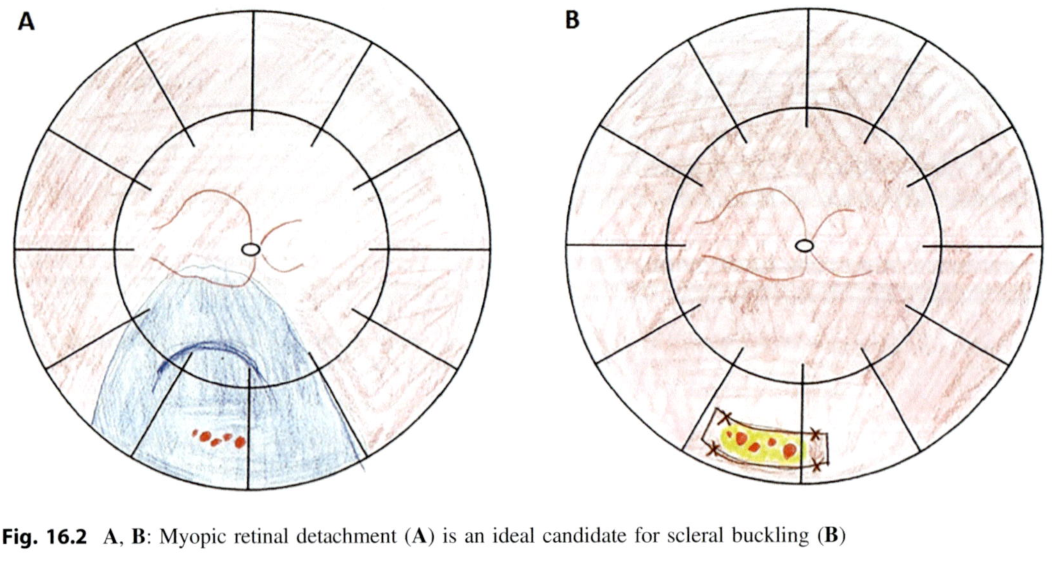

Fig. 16.2 **A**, **B**: Myopic retinal detachment (**A**) is an ideal candidate for scleral buckling (**B**)

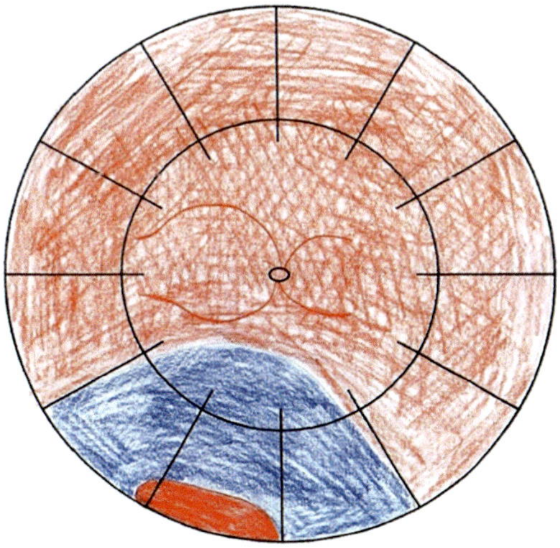

Fig. 16.3 An ora dialysis from 6:00 to 7:15

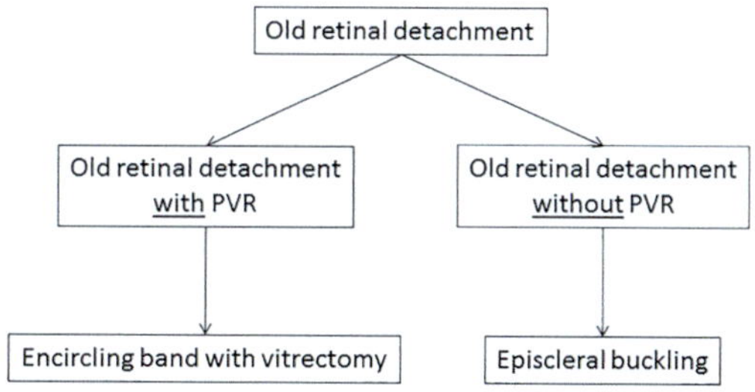

Fig. 16.4 Treatment algorithm from our University hospital for old detachments

16.4.1 Old Retinal Detachment Without PVR

The *chronic detachment* is definitely a complicated detachment. But in case of a clear break situation without PVR and the employment of episcleral buckling this complicated detachment becomes easy. Subretinal strands may be present but in the most cases they need not to be removed. Vitrectomy would be much more difficult. Why? The pigment epithelium in the detached area is weak and the subretinal proliferations enhance the detachment. In case of vitrectomy you need to remove the subretinal proliferations and then instill a gas tamponade to press the retina against the pigment epithelium. A buckle, however, creates an excellent impression between the weak pigment epithelium and the retina and seals the hole.

Case report 1

A 34 y/o female patient with superotemporal quadrant detachment, subretinal proliferations, and a retinal tear at 10:30 (Fig. 16.5A). Cryopexy and scleral buckling of a radial sponge was performed (Fig. 16.5B). The retina attached after 1 day.

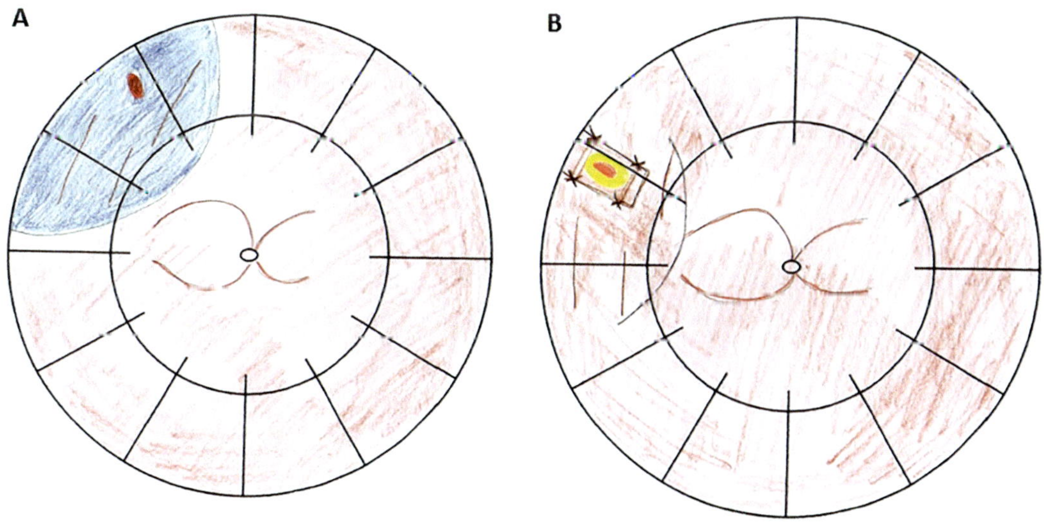

Fig. 16.5 **A, B**: A chronic and asymptomatic retinal detachment in a young patient. The vitreous is attached. A vitrectomy is difficult and attachment is difficult to achieve because the RPE in this area is weak. A scleral buckling is easier and the permanent indentation of the radial buckle seals the tear and reattaches the retina

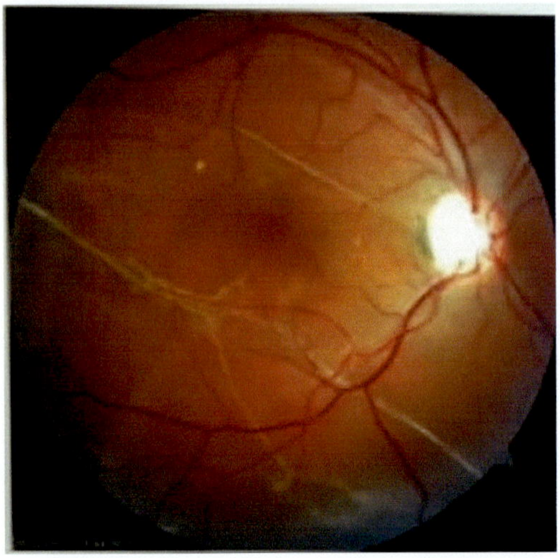

Fig. 16.6 Attached retina after episcleral buckling for chronic retinal detachment with subretinal bands

Case report 2

A 25 y/o female patient presents with a superotemporal retinal detachment. The macula is off. Several subretinal bands are present. No intravitreal or retinal PVR can be observed. A horse shoe rupture at 10 o´clock is present. A cryopexy with a radial buckle is performed. The 1-week follow-up shows an attached retina (Fig. 16.6).

16.4.2 Chronic Retinal Detachment with PVR

The surgery of a *chronic macula-off detachment* with PVR is unthankful because the surgery is very difficult and often several surgeries are necessary to achieve a final attachment. The visual outcome remains poor. Therefore, even if you succeed in reattaching the retina, the most patients will not praise you for your surgical excellency. We, therefore, do not operate chronic retinal detachments older than 1 year. For surgical management see Chapter: Vitrectomy for PVR stage C and Vitrectomy for PVR stage D.

17 Recurrent Retinal Detachment

Zoran Tomic and Ulrich Spandau

Is a recurrent detachment 18 months after primary surgery a recurrent detachment or a new detachment? There are different definitions of time interval until a redetachment occurs. The different time intervals until redetachment may be 3 months, 6 months, or 12 months. The most recurrent detachments occur in the first three months. We use therefore the 3-month interval for our definition of recurrent detachment. A later redetachment is considered as a new primary detachment.

The main question when examining the retina of a recurrent detachment is: What is the cause for the redetachment? Is there a new retinal break? If a new tear is present, we would operate the eye as a primary detachment. See treatment algorithm, Fig. 17.1. But in many cases a retinal break cannot be found. In this case, a mini rupture must be searched for. This mini rupture is often a laser necrosis and located at the edge of a laser scar. In order to localize the rupture, you must remember the Lincoff rules and use the following trick: Inject PFCL posterior to the suspected rupture and look for Schlieren. Schlieren is subretinal fluid which enters the vitreous cavity through the rupture. Search for the rupture using a light fiber and scleral depressor.

In the most cases of recurrent detachment, however, a break cannot be found and PVR is present. We recommend for these cases an encircling band, removal of membranes, and a silicone oil tamponade. See treatment algorithm. Another alternative for a redetachment is anterior PVR. This pathology is discussed in detail in a later chapter. Remark: In rare cases, the cause for a redetachment is an attached and contracted posterior hyaloid. The removal of posterior hyaloid results in mobilization of the retina and an reattachment.

We have three main scenarios (Fig. 17.1):

(1) In case of detachment without PVR and clearly visible new tears we prefer vitrectomy with gas.
(2) In case of a PVR redetachment we recommend encircling band, removal of membranes, ILM peeling, and silicone oil tamponade.
(3) If no PVR is present and no break can be found, we recommend an encircling band with silicone oil tamponade.

Surgical technique for recurrent detachment:
Scenario 1: New retinal rupture: Vitrectomy, laser or cryopexy and gas

Z. Tomic
Milos Klinika, Belgrade, Serbia

U. Spandau (✉)
St. Eriks Hospital, University of Stockholm, Stockholm, Sweden
e-mail: ulrich_spandau@yahoo.de

U. Spandau et al. (eds.), *Retinal Detachment Surgery and Proliferative Vitreoretinopathy*,
https://doi.org/10.1007/978-3-031-11946-0_17

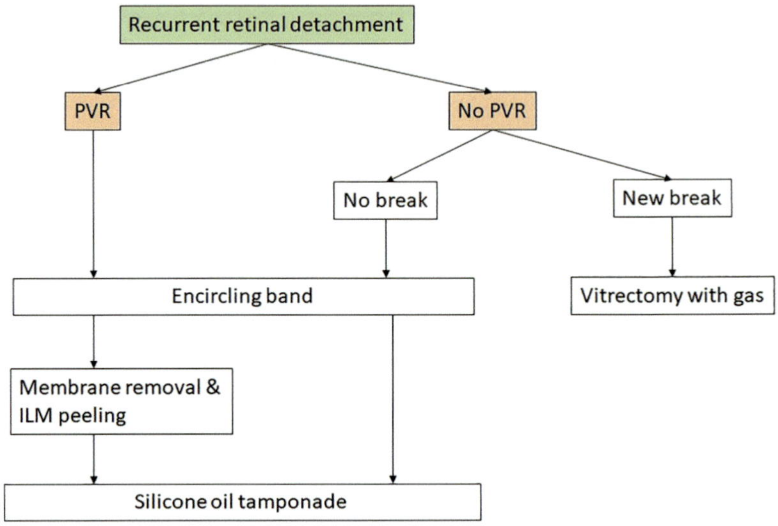

Fig. 17.1 Our treatment algorithm for a recurrent retinal detachment

Scenario 2: PVR: Encircling band, ILM peeling, vitreous base shaving, laser, and C3F8

Main surgical steps for scenario 2:

(1) Encircling band
(2) Injection of PFCL to find unknown rupture
(3) Staining with trypane blue to visualize PVR membranes
(4) Removal of central membranes and ILM peeling
(5) Partial PFCL injection
(6) Stain the vitreous base with triamcinolone acetonide
(7) Vitreous base shaving
(8) Laser photocoagulation
(9) Gas or silicone oil tamponade

The surgery in detail:

(1) Encircling band
(2) Injection of PFCL to find unknown rupture

Place four holding sutures and suture an encircling band on height of the equator. Insert trocar cannulas and a chandelier light. Search with the light fiber and scleral depressor for a retinal rupture. Examine thoroughly the edges of the old laser spots if a tear is present. Then inject slowly PFCL and look for Schlieren.

(3) Staining with trypane blue to visualize PVR membranes
(4) Removal of central membranes and ILM peeling
(5) Partial PFCL injection

Inject trypane blue to visualize PVR membranes. If this is the case then start with an ILM peeling at the posterior pole. Then remove all centrally located PVR membranes with an end-gripping forceps. In a next step inject PFCL so that the posterior pole is covered. This PFCL bubble stabilizes the posterior pole and creates a counterpressure if you remove the membranes in the periphery. Remove then all PVR membranes up to the equator. Add more PFCL and remove then all membranes up to ora serrata.

(6) Stain the vitreous base with triamcinolone acetonide
(7) Vitreous base shaving

Then inject triamcinolone acetonide to stain the vitreous base. Indent the sclera with the scleral depressor and remove the residual vitreous base. Search again for a small rupture.

(8) Laser photocoagulation
(9) Gas or silicone oil tamponade

Inject PFCL up to anterior edge of the rupture. Continue with laser photocoagulation. Proceed with a fluid against air exchange. In case of a superior RD, we recommend long-lasting gas or light silicone oil and in case of an inferior RD we recommend Densiron Xtra tamponade.

Tips and tricks:

Laser photocoagulation in a detached retina without tears: If you do not find a tear then laser treat the retina along the cerclage impression. If no cerclage is present, lasertreat according to the Lincoff rules.

18 Schisis Detachment Associated with Rhegmatogenous Retinal Detachment

Zoran Tomic and Ulrich Spandau

Retinoschisis is most frequently found in the infero-temporal periphery and does not develop a pigment demarcation line over time. In the majority of cases, it is asymptomatic and non-progressive and does not require treatment unless complicated by an outer layer detachment. Confusion of the retinoschisis elevation with rhegmatogenous retinal detachment does occur and results in unnecessary laser or surgical intervention (Lincoff and Kreissig 2012).

Progressive rhegmatogenous retinal detachment (RRD) associated with retinoschisis in which breaks of both the inner and outer layers allow intraocular fluid to access the subretinal space. Surgical treatment of posterior schisis detachment and progressive RRD requires closing the outer wall breaks using vitreoretinal surgical techniques.

Pars plana vitrectomy and/or scleral buckle may be used to repair the RRD. Factors favoring pars plana vitrectomy include posterior location of outer wall breaks and presence of PVD. Anterior location of outer wall breaks and absence of PVD favor scleral buckle. When performing pars plana vitrectomy, a drainage retinotomy in the inner wall overlying the outer wall may be created to drain subretinal fluid. Alternatively, the inner wall of the schisis cavity may be resected entirely and the detached retina was treated with a scatter laser.

View this surgical video: https://www.youtube.com/watch?v=fIrvNjo6qJ0.

Case report

A 68 y/o female patient was operated with vitrectomy and gas for a temporal retinoschisis detachment (Fig. 18.1). Two weeks postoperative a retinal redetachment was observed (Fig. 18.2). In a second surgery, a retinectomy of the complete inner retinal layer and a silicone oil tamponade was performed. Two months postoperative the silicone oil was removed and the retina remained attached.

Main surgical steps

(1) Endodiatermy of schisis edge
(2) Retinectomy
(3) Scatter laser photocoagulation
(4) Tamponade

Z. Tomic
Milos Klinika, Belgrade, Serbia

U. Spandau (✉)
St. Eriks Hospital, University of Stockholm, Stockholm, Sweden
e-mail: ulrich_spandau@yahoo.de

U. Spandau et al. (eds.), *Retinal Detachment Surgery and Proliferative Vitreoretinopathy*,
https://doi.org/10.1007/978-3-031-11946-0_18

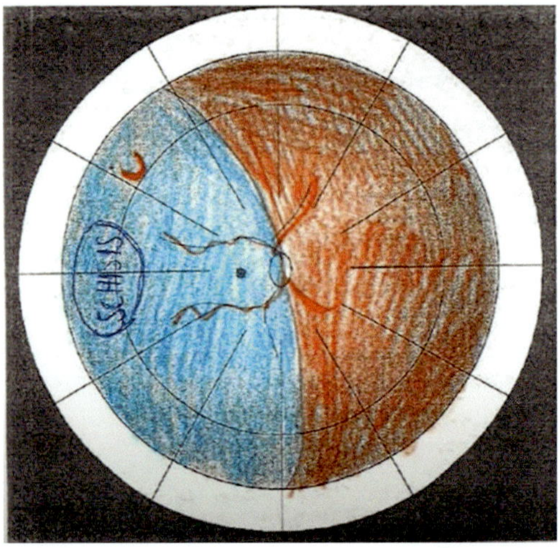

Fig. 18.1 Retinal detachment during primary investigation

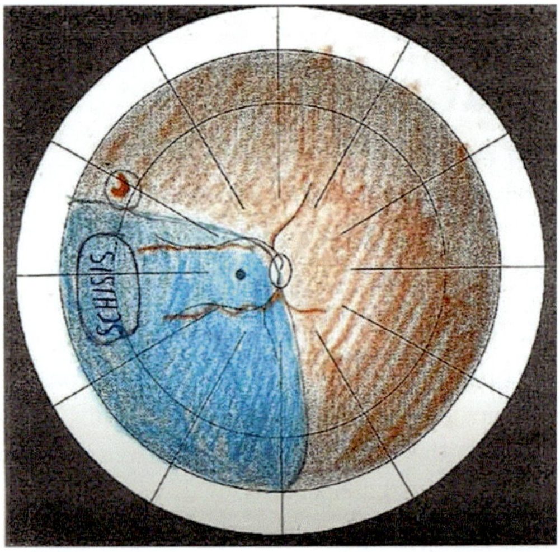

Fig. 18.2 Redetachment after vitrectomy. Note that the break at 10 o'clock is attached

The surgery in detail

(1) Endodiatermy of schisis edge
(2) Retinectomy

Cauterize the edge of the retinal schisis (Figs. 18.3 and 18.4). Then remove the inner retinal layer with the vitreous cutter (Fig. 18.4).

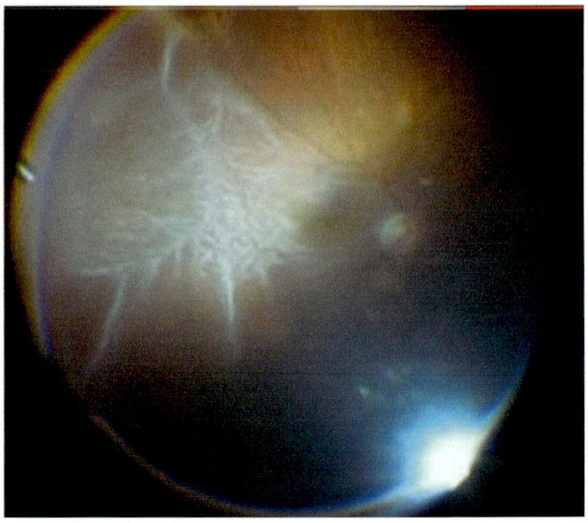

Fig. 18.3 Preoperative fundus. Note the retinal schisis

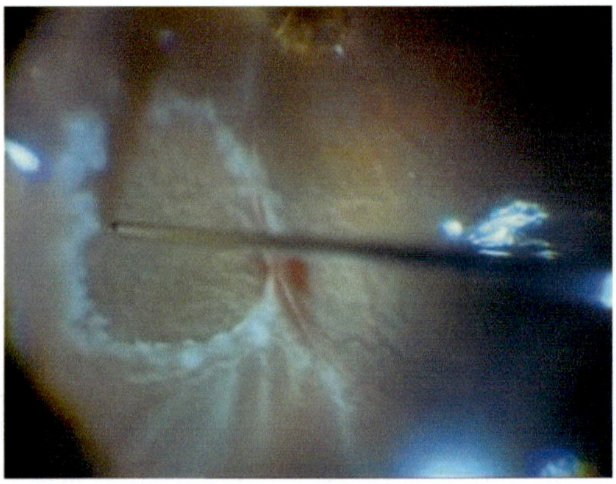

Fig. 18.4 After endodiathermy the inner layer is removed

The settings are 200–400 cuts/min and 300 mmHg aspiration. Then inject PFCL up to the ora serrata in order to attach the schisis.

(3) Scatter laser photocoagulation
(4) Tamponade

The next step is a scatter laser photocoagulation of the outer layer (Fig. 18.5). Continue with a fluid x air exchange. We recommend a C_3F_8 gas tamponade or alternatively a silicone oil tamponade (Fig. 18.6).

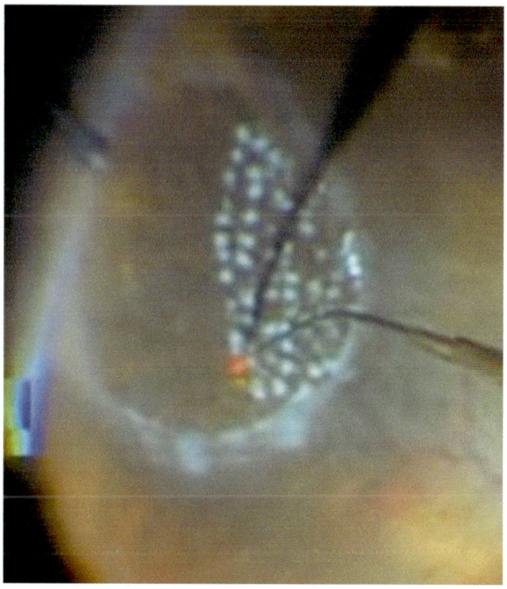

Fig. 18.5 Laser photocoagulation of the outer layer

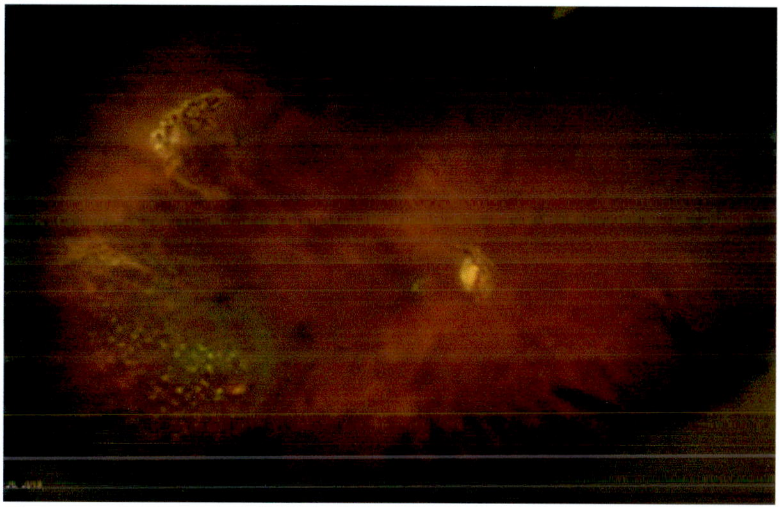

Fig. 18.6 Fundus 2 weeks after surgery. Note that some laser effects are still white. The retina is attached and remained attached

Reference

1. Lincoff H, Kreissig I. The misdiagnosis of retinoschisis. Acta Ophthalmol. 2012;90(5):492–4. https://doi.org/10.1111/j.1755-3768.2011.02301.x. (Epub 2011 Dec 13 PMID: 22151582).

Rhegmatogenous Retinal Detachment in Children

19

Ulrich Spandau and Zoran Tomic

Vitrectomy for primary repair of retinal detachment has become the preferred choice for vitreoretinal surgeons. Several studies, however, reveal the importance of avoiding a primary vitrectomy in the majority of pediatric RRD cases [1–3]. A recent study demonstrates the unfavorable outcome and increased PVR rate of vitrectomy for pediatric RRD surgery [4].

The most retinal detachments in children are caused by trauma or myopia. The vast majority of these detachments can be operated with an episcleral buckling. The vitreous in children is intact and attached. The silicone sponge reattaches the retinal tear and the pediatric vitreous serves as a good tamponade. Removing the vitreous in a vitrectomy means the loss of this tamponade plus an increased risk for PVR because the vitreous has to be removed completely including the posterior hyaloid. The complication spectrum and PVR risk for episcleral buckling is low.

Conclusion: The preferred technique for pediatric retinal detachment is episcleral buckling. If this is not possible then vitrectomy is required. Vitrectomy requires always an encircling band and induction of a complete PVD.

19.1 Episcleral Buckling

The surgery of traumatic RD in children using vitrectomy technique is very difficult, the risk of PVR redetachment is high, the likelihood of several surgeries is also high and the outcome is poor. In contrast, the surgery of traumatic RD using episcleral buckling is easier and the outcome in almost all cases excellent. Why? A common retinal finding after trauma is an ora dialysis. Ora dialysis has a 100% attachment rate with scleral buckling. Other common pediatric detachments are giant tears with more or less focal detachments. The vitreous may be detached at the area of a giant tear and removing this attached vitreous with vitrectomy creates only problems and complications. The vitreous in children is dense and attached. It serves as a scaffold for growth of scaring tissue and its occurrence is common. In buckling surgery, the vitreous is not removed. Place a buckle on the sclera and seal the retinal break, that's all.

The surgical technique

For children, we use the conventional surgical technique with panophthalmoscope because the view of retina in children is excellent. The cornea, the lens, and the vitreous are clear. For the suturing of the silicone sponge, we use the microscope.

U. Spandau (✉) · Z. Tomic
Department of Ophthalmology, Uppsala University Hospital, Uppsala, Sweden
e-mail: ulrich_spandau@yahoo.de

Z. Tomic
e-mail: zorannos@yahoo.se

U. Spandau et al. (eds.), *Retinal Detachment Surgery and Proliferative Vitreoretinopathy*,
https://doi.org/10.1007/978-3-031-11946-0_19

The surgery step by step:

1. **Limbal peritomy**
2. **3 holding sutures**
3. **Cryopexy of the retinal break**
4. **Marking of the break**
5. **Choice of silicone sponge regarding on a retinal break size**
6. **Suturing of the silicone sponge**
7. **Inspection of retina**
8. **In case of detached retinal edges inject 0,5 ml air.**

Material: Silicone sponge:

(1) 5 × 3.77 mm partial thickness sponge (Labtician, Canada). Our most commonly used is silicone sponge. Indication: Ora dialysis, all normal size breaks. This sponge requires a 7 mm marking.

(2) 7.0 × 5.28 mm partial thickness sponge (Labtician, Canada). Less commonly used is silicone sponge. Indication: Large breaks. This sponge requires a 9.0 mm marking.

The surgery step by step:

1. **Limbal peritomy**
2. **3 holding sutures**

This part is done under the microscope: Start with limbal peritomy and dissect the thick Tenon's capsule from the sclera. Then place three holding sutures on the recti muscles closest to the break.

3. **Cryopexy of the retinal break**
4. **Marking of the break**
5. **Choice of silicone sponge regarding a retinal break size**

This part is done with the panophthalmoscope: Place a cryopexy on the retinal break until you see a white bleaching of the retina. Leave the cryopexy tip on the sclera, insert an orbita spatula behind the cryopexy tip, and rotate the globe towards you. Dry the sclera around the cryo tip, remove it, and mark the sclera. In children, the sclera is often bluish after cryopexy. Continue with cryopexy and marking of the complete retinal break. At the end, the retinal break is marked on the sclera and you can choose a silicone sponge. If you are insecure then measure how wide the break is with help of a caliper. If the break is 3 mm wide then a 5 mm wide sponge is sufficient. If the break is 5 mm wide, then a 7 mm wide sponge is required.

Tipps & tricks

A cryopexy is also diagnostic for finding a retinal break: When the retina becomes white from cryopexy, then you see the dark break inside the white retina.

6. **Suturing of a silicone sponge**

This part is done under the microscope: Suture the sponge onto the sclera so that the sponge covers the complete break. Mark first the location of the sutures with the caliper. Tipp: Mark the tips of the caliper with the pen so that the sclera is marked by the caliper.

Then place two sutures. Before placing the sponge, we need a hypotensive globe. Take a syringe with 30G cannula and remove aqueous from the anterior chamber. If you use a paracentesis knife then you must suture the paracentesis because this is a child's eye.

Then place the sponge and tie the knot with 2-1-1 throws in case of Supramid suture and 3-1-1 in case of Mersilene.

7. **Inspection of retina**
8. **In case of detached retinal edges inject 0,5 ml air.**

This part is done with the panophthalmoscope: Observe if the sponge covers the break and observe if the retinal edges are very elevated. If the latter is the case, then inject 0.5 ml air into the eye. Remark: Air is inside the eye for 3–5 days and this is sufficient to tamponade the break. SF_6 is not necessary because it stays too long time in the eye, causes ocular irritation and PVR and may result in a tractive detachment.

Example: Case 1: (Figs. 19.1 and 19.2)

An 18 y/o male patient was hit in his left eye by a hockey stick. Due to the visual acuity decrease he visited an optician the following week. The optician stated a visual acuity decrease to 0.2 uncorrected and submitted him to the local eye clinic. Three weeks later he was examined at the local eye clinic and a PVR detachment with a large ora dialysis was detected. The macula was shallowly detached and the retinal edges of the ora dialysis were rolled in. The visual acuity was + 3.0sph = 0.1 and the IOP was 0 mmHg. He was consequently submitted to us for surgery (Fig. 19.1A).

The operation was performed with binocular indirect ophthalmoscope, cryopexy and the 9 × 5,77 sponge from Labtician, Canada (Fig. 19.2) was used. The intraoperative retinal inspection showed small tear at 11:45, large ora dialysis from 12 to 3 o'clock, and subretinal PVR from 3 to 6 o'clock. The segmental buckle was placed under the superior and lateral recti muscles sutured at 11:30, 1:30, and 3:30. The suture at 1:30 was necessary to achieve sufficient impression. A 0.3 cc vitreous tap (puncture) was done. 0.5 ml air was injected to attach the enrolled retinal edges. In addition, triamcinolone was injected subconjunctivally to reduce the risk of PVR and to increase the IOP.

The 3-day follow-up showed a completely attached retina, VA was 0.2 without correction, 20% of the vitreous cavity was filled with air and IOP was 18 mmHg. The enrolled edges persisted, and the choroid was visible (Fig. 19.1B).

The 1-month follow-up showed a completely attached retina, VA was 0.2 with −3.0D an IOP was 16 mmHg. The retina was completely attached. The enrolled edges persisted.

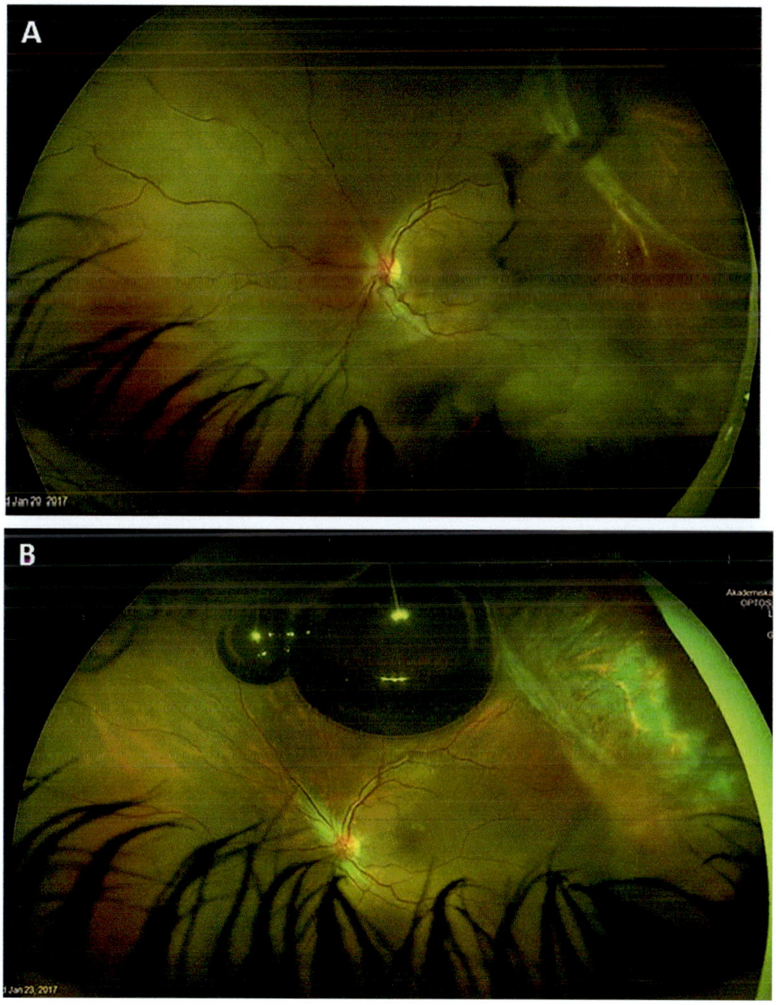

Fig. 19.1 **A**: A 18 y/o male patient with a 4-weeks old traumatic retinal detachment secondary to an ora dialysis with rolled edges. **B**: 4 days postoperative view to fundus. Operated with scleral buckle and air injection

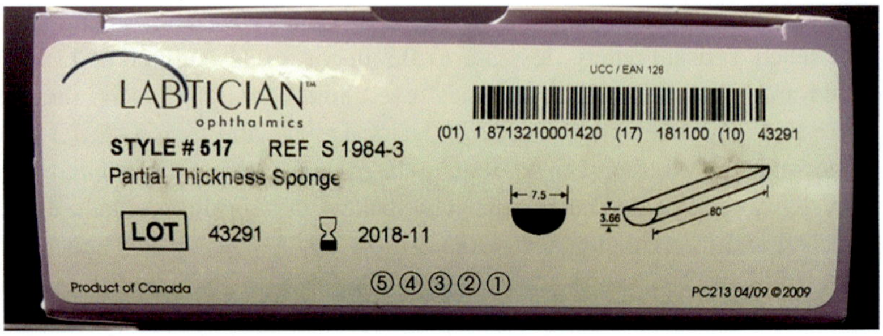

Fig. 19.2 A 7,5 mm wide silicone sponge was used for this case

Case 2: (Figs. 19.3, 19.4 and 19.5)
A 5 y/o boy was injured with a stick. At examination, an inferior detachment with a large tear from 5 to 7 o´clock was detected. A cryopexy of the retinal edges was performed and a silicone sponge was placed from 7:30 to 9:15. The upper edge of the silicone sponge was 1–2 mm below the muscle insertion. The retina was reattached within 2 days. If one chooses a vitrectomy the surgery becomes difficult. Why? (1) The risk of natural lens opacification. If you remove it then the eye will become severe amblyopic. (2) The removal of the dense pediatric vitreous which serves as a scaffold may result in inferior PVR detachment.

Case 3: (Figs. 19.6, 19.7, 19.8 and 19.9)
A 11 y/o boy was hit in left eye by a football. Ophthalmological examination revealed an ora dialysis. A silicone sponge was placed under the inferior rectus muscle. The upper edge of the sponge was in height with the muscle insertion. No drainage was necessary.

19.2 Vitrectomy of a Pediatric Retinal Detachment

In our experience, vitrectomy for retinal detachment in children has two essential steps: (1) Encircling band and (2) PVD. For PVD, we stain the posterior hyaloid with triamcinolone to be

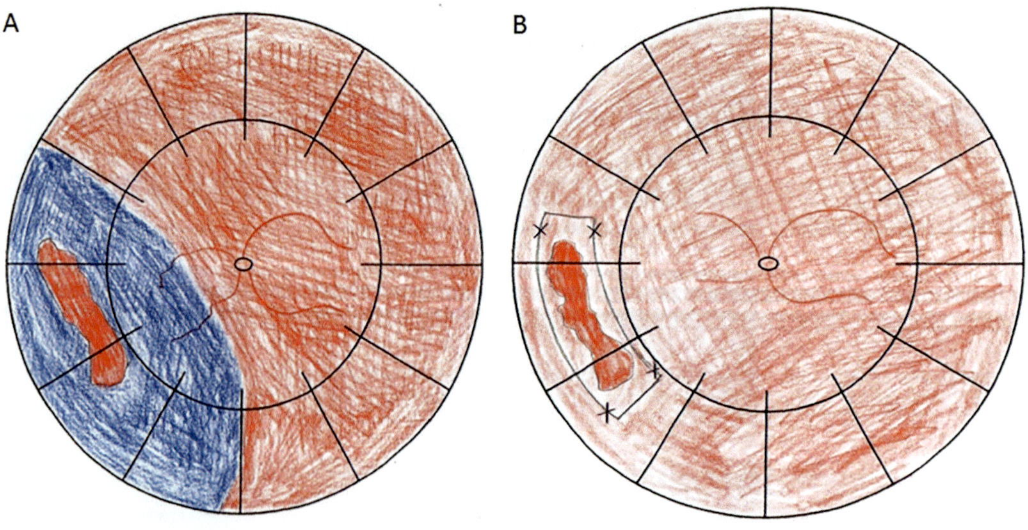

Fig. 19.3 **A**, **B**: A 4 y/o boy with traumatic retinal detachment (**A**). A giant tear from 7:30 to 9:15. A vitrectomy in this case is very diffcult and has a large complication spectrum. Try first a scleral buckle and in the most cases you will succeed with one surgery. The retina was attached after 2 days (**B**)

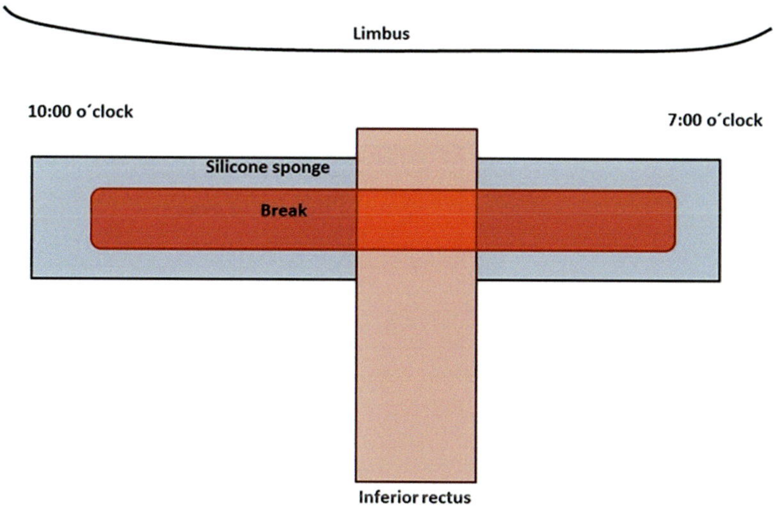

Fig. 19.4 The silicone sponge was placed under the rectus muscle

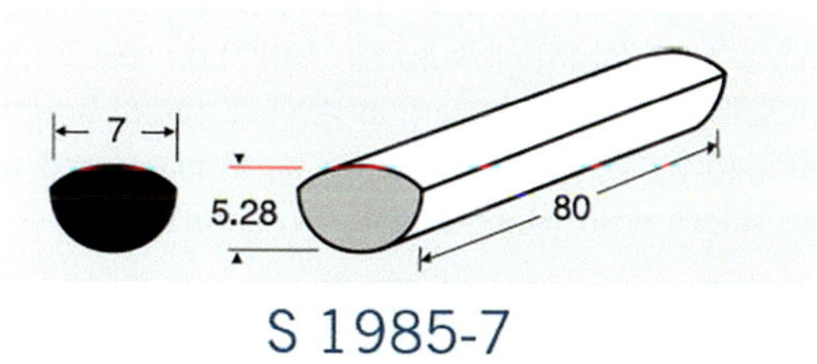

Fig. 19.5 This silicone sponge was used (Labtician, Canada)

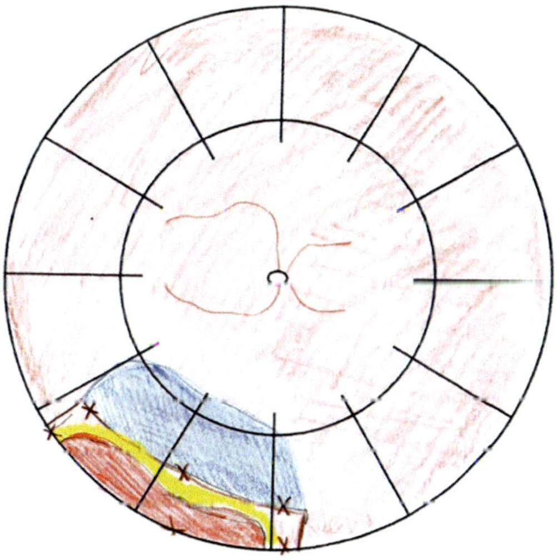

Fig. 19.6 A 8 y/o boy with ora dialysis secondary to a football

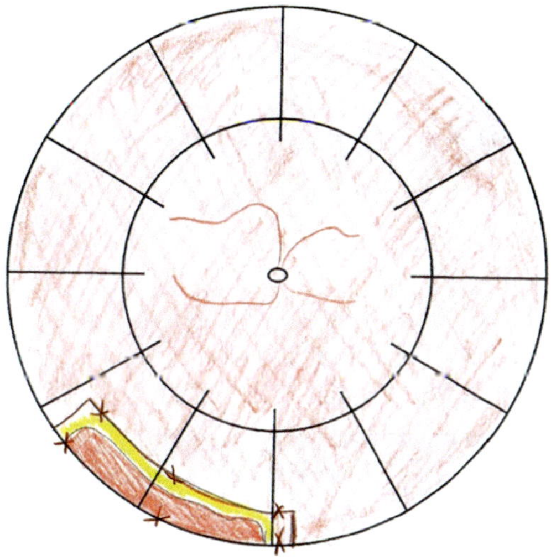

Fig. 19.7 The retina is attached after 2 days

completely sure that a complete PVD was induced. Otherwise the risk for PVR is 70%. A PVD is performed with vitreous cutter and 27G endgripping forceps. In case of a fresh retinal detachment, we prefer to preserve the natural lens and choose a tamponade with gas and not silicone oil. In case of an old detachment, we prefer phaco/IOL and a silicone oil tamponade.

In children with an age under 2 years, the encircling band must be removed or cut after 6 months. Otherwise, a grave myopia will develop.

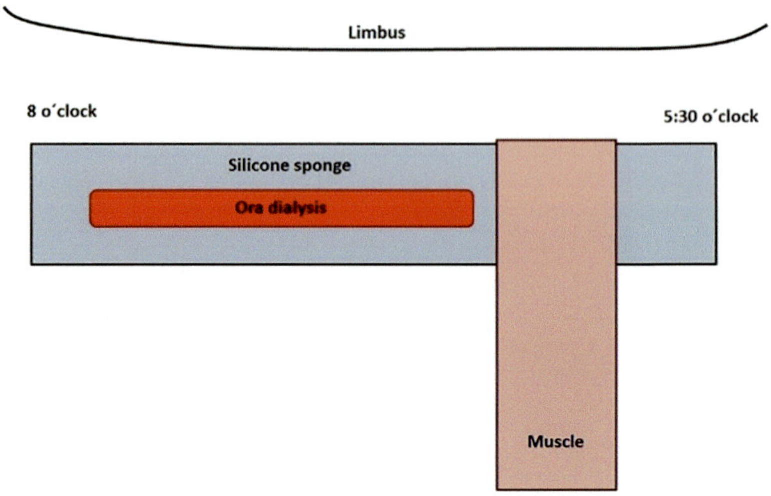

Fig. 19.8 The silicone sponge was placed under the inferior rectus muscle. The muscle indents the sponge

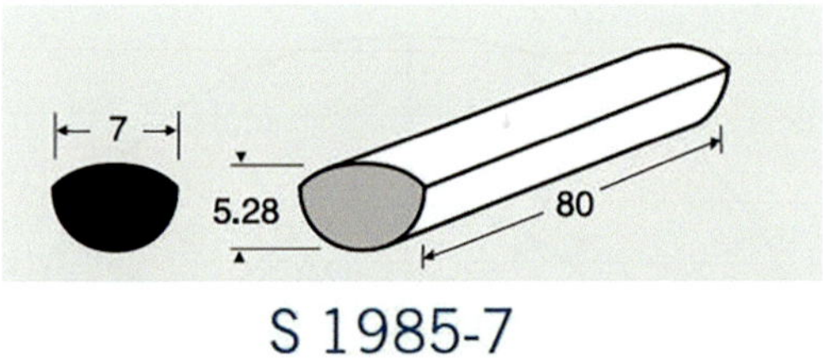

Fig. 19.9 This silicone sponge was used (Labtician, Canada)

The surgery step by step:

(1) Limbal peritomy
(2) Encircling band
(3) 25G or 27G trocar cannulas with chandelier light
(4) Lens sparing vitrectomy
(5) Staining with triamcinolone
(6) Induction of complete PVD with vitreous cutter and end-gripping forceps
(7) Endodiathermy of retinal tear edges
(8) Injection of PFCL
(9) Laser photocoagulation
(10) Fluid/air exchange with removal of PFCL and aspiration of subretinal fluid.
(11) Gas tamponade.

The surgery in detail:

(1) Limbal peritomy
(2) Encircling band

We start with a 360° limbal peritomy. Then place four holding sutures (silk) on the recti muscles. Mark the sclera at AXL/2 (axial length divided by 2). The encircling band is sutured to the sclera with Mersilene 4–0 (Alcon).

(1) 25G or 27G trocar cannulas with chandelier light
(2) Lens sparing vitrectomy

We recommend 25G or 27G trocar cannulas. Insert also a chandelier light because bimanual surgery is required. The next step is a lens sparing core vitrectomy. The posterior hyaloid is usually firmly attached in children. Try to induce central PVD with the vitreous cutter. Try to continue with PVD to the vitreous base.

(3) Staining with triamcinolone
(4) Complete PVD with vitreous cutter and end-gripping forceps
(5) Endodiathermy of retinal tear edges

Then stain the vitreous with triamcinolone. Complete PVD with 27G end-gripping forceps. You may need to stabilize the central retina with PFCL. Remember: A complete PVD is crucial for a successful surgery. Then mark the retinal tear edges with endodiathermy.

(6) Injection of PFCL up to ora serrata
(7) Laser photocoagulation

PFCL is injected bimanually. The dominant hand holds the syringe and the other hand the back-flush cannula. The syringe cannula is placed close to the retina, and PFCL is slowly injected. As the PFCL bubble grows the syringe cannula is pulled backwards towards the lens, and the cannula remains always at the top part of the bubble. Continue with laser photocoagulation.

(1) Removal of PFCL and aspiration of subretinal fluid
(2) Gas tamponade

Continue with a fluid/air exchange. Aspirate the subretinal fluid through the retinal tear. We prefer a 15% C_2F_6 tamponade rather than SF6 20%.

References

1. Drenser K. Pearls for managing pediatric retinal detachments. Ophthalmology. 2019;126(9):1271–2. https://doi.org/10.1016/j.ophtha.2019.03.022 PMID: 31443787.
2. Carranza-Casas M, Quiroz-González E, Hernández-Reyes A, Matsui-Serrano R, Ariza-Camacho E, Graue-Wiechers F. Pediatric rhegmatogenous retinal detachment: predictors of anatomic and functional success. Int Ophthalmol. 2021;41(8):2777–88. https://doi.org/10.1007/s10792-021-01834-w Epub 2021 Apr 11 PMID: 33840049.
3. Smith JM, Ward LT, Townsend JH, Yan J, Hendrick AM, Cribbs BE, Yeh S, Jain N, Hubbard GB 3rd. Rhegmatogenous retinal detachment in children: clinical factors predictive of successful surgical repair. Ophthalmology. 2019;126(9):1263–70. https://doi.org/10.1016/j.ophtha.2018.11.001. Epub 2018 Nov 10. PMID: 30419297; PMCID: PMC6510644.
4. Rejdak R, Nowakowska D, Wrona K, Maciejewski R, Junemann AG, Nowomiejska K. Outcomes of vitrectomy in pediatric retinal detachment with proliferative vitreoretinopathy. J Ophthalmol. 2017;2017:8109390.

Part IV
PVR Detachment

All videos of this part are found in a playlist on my youTube channel:
https://youtube.com/playlist?list=PL0dKYclPD7yMn861X0g-aHCS6KZ5NcH1N
Chapter 20: No video
Chapter 21: **Vitrectomy for PVR Detachment Stage C**
PVR detachment
Membrane peeling in ARN
Cerclage
Cerclage removal
Extraction of a sponge and cerclage
Phacoemulsification
Iris retractors
Core vitrectomy
Vitreous base shaving
Staining with trypan blue
PVR peeling short
PVR peeling detailed
Peeling techniques for PVR detachment
Removal of peripheral membranes
Subretinal peeling
Removal of Subretinal membranes
PFCL injection
Ando iridectomy
Silicone oil injection
Dislocated IOL and one-year-old retinal detachment
Chronic PVR detachment
Chapter 22: **Vitrectomy for PVR Stage D**
PVR stage D
Retinotomy
Laser for retinotomy
Vitrectomy for total retinal detachment secondary to morning glory
Chapter 23: **Special Surgical Techniques for PVR Detachment**
180° retinotomy

How to Approach Surgical Treatment of PVR

20

Marco Mura and Antonella D'Aponte

In this chapter Marco Mura and Antonella D'Aponte provide a comprehensive theoretical practical overview about PVR detachment.

Key concept:

1. **Proliferative vitreoretinopathy** (**PVR**) is a disease that develops as a complication of rhegmatogenous retinal detachment
2. The accumulation of fluid in the subretinal space and the tractional force of the vitreous on the retina result in rhegmatogenous retinal detachment
3. The RPE cells lay down fibrotic membranes while they migrate and these membranes contract and pull at the retina
4. For a successful management of posterior PVR is important: localization of all retinal breaks, release of the traction through membrane peeling and dissection.
5. Retinectomy implies the complete excision of the entire complex formed by the vitreous base, anterior membranes, and shortened retina.

20.1 Introduction

Proliferative vitreoretinopathy (**PVR**) is a disease that develops as a complication of rhegmatogenous retinal detachment. PVR complicates approximately 5% to 10% of all retinal detachment repairs. Typically, PVR occurs after primary retinal detachment repair; however, it can occur in longstanding primary detachments and in traumatic retinal detachment. PVR can be treated with surgery to reattach the detached retina but the visual outcome of the surgery is unpredictable [1, 2]. PVR was originally referred to as **massive vitreous retraction** and then as **massive periretinal proliferation**. The term "proliferative retinopathy" was coined in 1983 by the Retina Society Terminology Committee. In 1989, the classification was amended by the Silicone Study Group before being most recently modified in 1991 to its current classification. The name is derived from *proliferation* (by the retinal pigment epithelial and glial cells) and *vitreo retinopathy* to include the tissues which are affected, namely the vitreous and the retina [3]. There is inconsistent and limited use of the current PVR classifications. The two most used classifications are reported in Tables 20.1 and 20.2; in Table 20.3, we report a 1993 morfological classification by Robert Machemer that has important surgical implications.

During rhegmatogenous retinal detachment, fluid from the vitreous enters a retinal hole. The

M. Mura (✉)
The King Khaled Eye Specialist Hospital, Riyadh, Kingdom of Saudi Arabia
e-mail: mmura1@jhmi.ed

A. D'Aponte
Wilmer Eye Institute, Johns Hopkins University, Baltimore, MD, USA
e-mail: adaponte@kkesh.med.sa

U. Spandau et al. (eds.), *Retinal Detachment Surgery and Proliferative Vitreoretinopathy*,
https://doi.org/10.1007/978-3-031-11946-0_20

Table 20.1 The Retina Society Terminology Committee (1983)

Grade and type	Clinical signs
A (minimal)	Vitreous haze and pigment clumps
B (moderate)	Surface retinal wrinkling, rolled edge of retinal, retinal stiffness, and vessel tortuosity
C (marked) (i) C1 (ii) C2 (iii) C3	Full-thickness fixed retinal folds in (i) one quadrant (ii) two quadrants (iii) three quadrants
D (massive) (i) D1 (ii) D2 (iii) D3	Fixed retinal folds in four quadrants that result in (i) a wide funnel shape (ii) a narrow funnel shape (iii) closed funnel without view of optic disc

accumulation of fluid in the subretinal space and the tractional force of the vitreous on the retina result in rhegmatogenous retinal detachment. During this process, the retinal cell layers come in contact with vitreous cytokines. These cytokines trigger the ability of the retinal pigmented epithelium (RPE) to proliferate and migrate. The process involved resembles fibrotic wound healing by the RPE cells. The RPE cells undergo epithelial-mesenchymal transition (EMT) and develop the ability to migrate out into the vitreous. During this process, the RPE cell layer-neural retinal adhesion and RPE-ECM (extracellular matrix) adhesions are lost. The RPE cells lay down fibrotic membranes while they migrate and these membranes contract and pull at the retina. All these finally lead to secondary retinal detachment after primary retinal detachment surgery. A number of studies have also shown that arachidonic acid metabolic cascade (one of the major inflammatory cascades) is important in the development of PVR. COX-2 expression was found in human idiopathic epiretinal membranes [4]. Phospholipase A2 and cyclooxygenase blocking reduced structural abnormalities of the rat retina in concanavalin model of PVR [5].

The RPE cells migrate out into the vitreous, proliferate excessively, and lay down ECM on both sides of the detached retina. The ECM laid on the vitreous side of the retina are referred to as epiretinal or preretinal membranes (ERM) and those laid down between the RPE layer and the photoreceptors are referred to as subretinal or retroretinal membranes (SRM). The two membranes differ in composition; the ERM is composed of RPE cells, glial cells, macrophages, and fibrocytes, while the SRM is rich in RPE cells. The subretinal membranes are of two types. One forms as diffuse sheets, which are not contractile and either lack or contain very little ECM. The presence of this type of membrane does not usually affect retinal reattachment surgery. The retina can be reattached even with the membrane in place. The other type forms as very thick contractile membranes which pull at the retina. These are opaque and block the light falling on the retina so the retinal reattachment surgery needs to be performed after manually peeling the membrane off [7, 8]. A number of cytokines such as tumor necrosis factor alpha (TNFα), transforming growth factor beta 2 (TGFβ_2), platelet derived growth factor (PDGF), and interleukins have been shown to play a role in PVR progression.

TGFβ_2 levels have been shown to be elevated up to three times the normal during the progression of PVR. TGFβ_2 is the most predominant isoform in the eye and is secreted as a latent inactive peptide into the vitreous by epithelial cells of the ciliary body and the lens epithelium and is also produced by the RPE cells and the Muller cells of the retina. TGFβ_2 is known to induce EMT in RPE cells and fibrosis in the eye [9]. Expression of PDGF in particular PDGF-AA is triggered during ocular injury and contributes to PVR pathology [10]. RPE cells express the receptor for hepatocyte growth factor (HGF).

Table 20.2 The Updated Retina Society Classification (1991)

Grade and type	Clinical signs
A	Vitreous haze, pigment clumps, and pigment clusters on inferior retina
B	Wrinkling of inner retinal surface, retinal stiffness, vessel tortuosity, rolled and irregular edge of retinal break, and decreased mobility of vitreous
CP(posterior) (i) Type: – a Focal – b Diffuse – c Subretinal	Full-thickness retinal folds or subretinal strands posterior to equator (1–12 clock hours involvement) (i) Starfolds posterior to vitreous base (ii) Confluent starfolds posterior to vitreous base; optic disc hat may not be visible (iii) Proliferation under the retina Annular strand near disc; linear strands; moth-eaten-appearing sheets
CA (anterior) (i) Type: – a Circumferential – b Anterior	Full-thickness retinal folds or subretinal strands anterior to equator (1–12 clock hours involvement), anterior displacement, and condensed vitreous strands Retina contraction inwards at the posterior edge of the vitreous base; with central displacement of the retina; peripheral retina stretched; posterior retina in radial folds (i) Anterior contraction on the retina at vitreous base; ciliary body detachment and epiciliary membrane; iris retraction

Table 20.3 Proliferative Vitreoretinopathy classification of Machemer

Proliferative Vitreoretinopathy(PVR) Classification of Mechemer
Full thikness fold, Type:
1. Focal starfold posterior to equator
2. Diffuse multiple folds posterior to equator
3. Subretinal proliferation "napkin" ring around disc "motheaten" sheets
4. Circumferential contraction contraction along posterior edge of vitreous base with central displacement of retina peripheral retina streched posterior retina in radial folds
5. Anterior displacement vitreous base pulled anteriorly peripheral retinal trough ciliary processes streched or covered iris retracted

HGF stimulates RPE cell migration and its presence is also strongly detected in retinal membranes. Interleukin 6 levels are elevated in the vitreous humor during PVR [11]. About 15% of all retinal detachment are traumatic, they are much more common in the young individuals and more prone to develop rapidly severe PVR [14]. Blunt trauma, with and without rupture of the globe, and penetrating trauma can cause retinal detachment. RRD is more important in the setting of a closed-globe blunt trauma or contusion blunt trauma represents about 70–85% of all traumatic retinal detachment [15–17]. In the case of blunt trauma with rupture and penetrating trauma, TRD secondary to fibrous ingrowth and intraocular proliferation is more prominent [18–26].

Complete PVR removal is essential in the treatment of chronic and recurrent rhegmatogenous retinal detachment and in traumatic retinal detachment. Epiretinal and subretinal membrane removal allow apposition of the contracted retina to the retinal pigment epithelium and reestablishment of the RPE pump function with consequent retinal attachment.

For a successful management of posterior and anterior PVR, the following steps need to be taken into consideration:

1. Surgical setup and identification of all retinal breaks and membranes
2. Release of vitreoretinal traction, membrane peeling, and dissection
3. Drainage of subretinal fluid (SRF), sealing of retinal breaks, and tamponade

20.2 Surgical Setup and Identification of Retinal Breaks and Membranes

Intraoperative identification of the retinal breaks is made easy using wide field visualization systems such as BIOM (Oculus, Wetzlar Germany), RESIGHT (Carl Zeiss, Germany), EIBOS (Haag-Streit,Wedel Germany), and scleral depression.

These devices allow the surgeon to acquire a panoramic view on the surgical field up to 120/130 degrees without the help of a surgeon assistant; auxiliary chandelier light illumination is mandatory in PVR cases to allow bimanual dissection and membrane removal in anterior and posterior PVR.

The gauge choice is dependent on the severity of the pathology, the extension, and location of the PVR. In PVR cases up to grade C, 27 and 25 gauge are our choice; in cases of PVR D or in post-traumatic cases, where the membranes are more fibrotic, large gauge with broader surface of action such us 23 and sometimes 20, are more often used. We routinely use a 4 port approach with a chandelier light located in the infero-nasal quadrant. This location is particularly advantageous because the chandelier light fiber can easily be taped in place on the patient's nose bridge minimizing the risk of displacement.

All our PVR cases are done bimanually. We prefer to use a combination of end-gripping forceps (Eckardt type), curved horizontal scissors, serrated forceps, diamond dusted Tano scraper, and illuminated pick. To help identifying residual vitreous, we standardly use triamcinolone acetonide (Kenalog 40 mg/ml) undiluted. Epiretinal membrane are in our practice better stained with membrane blue dual (Dorc, Zuidland,The Netherlands). This combination of 0.15% Trypan blue, 0.025% of BBG (brillant blue G), and 4% PEG (polietileneglicosate) has the advantage of staining both internal limiting membrane and epiretinal membrane without the need to exchange fluid for air.

In PVR cases, the use of Perfluorocarbon liquid (PFCL) has multiple functions: it helps the surgeon to flatten the posterior retina while working more anteriorly (third hand effect), facilitates the peeling of posterior membranes in mobile detached retina and/or internal limiting membrane in detached retina, and gives indirect signs of traction release. Among the PFCLs we prefer to use PFO (perfloro-octane) because being lighter than PFD (perfluoro-decalin) gives the surgeon a better feeling of the residual traction present; also, being PFO volatile, the chance of retained heavy liquids in the vitreous cavity after surgery is very small because the small droplets left after PFO-air exchange can freely evaporate.

20.2.1 Release Of Vitreoretinal Traction, Membrane Peeling, and Dissection

The first step in dealing with PVR cases is to stain the possible residual vitreous with Triamcinolone acetonide. We inject triamcinolone through the valved trocar cannula, and we facilitate the dispersion of the crystals inside the vitreous cavity. This is achieved by increasing infusion pressure up to 60 mmHg, aspirating and shaking the eye or blasting water into the Kenalog with the back-flush cannula. The triamcinolone crystals will stick to the residual vitreous and to the vitreous cortex, if present, allowing the surgeon to detach and remove the vitreous cortex with a Tano scraper or end-gripping forceps completely. After doing this maneuver or in case no vitreous remnants are identified we proceed with a second staining, injecting membrane-blue-dual (MBD). We usually take care that the MBD is injected in the posterior pole and in the peripheral retina and we usually leave the dye in contact with the retina for 1 min and 30 s before aspirating. Because of the heavy nature of the staining molecules, the dye will sink to the posterior pole; to facilitate the staining of the peripheral membranes, we first remove the posterior membranes and then, when the retina is mobile, we inject PFO up to the edge of the anterior membranes. At this stage MBD can be re-injected; the dye now will stay at the top of the PFO bubble allowing the staining of the peripheral anterior membranes (PFO assisted staining). We usually start peeling the membranes using end-gripping (Eckardt type) forceps because we can use their tips as pick instrument.

With forceps open we use one of the branches to engage the edge of the starfolds from inside out. The lifting of the edge of the membranes sometimes can be challenging and can be facilitated with the use of a Tano scraper or a pick.

When the adherence of the membranes to the retina surface is very strong, the membranes are very fibrotic or the retina is very thin (especially in the proximity of the ora serrata), to avoid iatrogenic retinal breaks due to the peeling maneuver, bimanual delamination with a blunt spatula and forceps or dissection with forceps and scissors can be performed. A useful technique in these cases is also the bimanual stretching maneuver with two forceps. Using serrated jaws and an end-gripping forceps, we grasp the edges of the membrane keeping the forceps next to each other and then we move them a part in the opposite direction. With this maneuver, we can shred the epiretinal tissue avoiding traction on underlying retina.

We generally tend to remove the epiretinal tissue completely from the retinal surface. When this is not possible due to intra-retinal extension of the epiretinal tissue or when the traction is still present, we can opt for two solution:

- circumferential encircling buckle
- retinectomy

20.2.2 Circumferential Encircling Buckle

We routinely use the circumferential buckle, 240 band with 70 sleeve, taking care of placing the band posterior to the residual traction. When this is not possible because of the posterior location of the pathology or the excessive circumferential traction with fixed folds or because of excessive scleral thinning, we opt to perform a retinectomy.

20.2.3 Retinectomy

Retinectomy implies the complete excision of the entire complex formed by the vitreous base, anterior membranes, and shortened retina, sometimes involving the pars plana. Much attention is paid to the anatomy surrounding old sclerotomy sites: often anterior traction is present at these sites, and if so, these areas are included in the retinectomy. The circumferential extent of anterior PVR dictated the minimal circumferential extent of the retinectomy, but often a larger circumferential extent of the retinectomy is carried out. We believe that a retinectomy of at least 6 clock hours, preferably covering the area between the 3 and the 6 o'clock meridian, has the greatest chance of relieving circumferential traction. The anteroposterior extent of the retinectomy is dictated by the individual pathologic features. The lower edge of the retinectomy is aimed to lie between the equator and the lower vascular arcade, preferably closer to the equator than to the vascular arcade. After completion of the retinectomy and coagulation of cut vessels, we use PFO to flatten the entire retina. Laser retinopexy is applied in 4 rows along the entire edge of the retinectomy. The spots are placed in a confluent pattern leading to a total width of the barrage of 1500 to 2000 mm. We consider the starting and the ending points of retinectomy incision as crucial and most vulnerable, and therefore often secured these locations with 5 rows of laser coagulates. We did not apply 360-° laser as standard procedure[31]. At the end, silicon oil is infused after fluid-air exchange or during direct perfluorocarbon liquid-silicone oil exchange. In aphakic cases, a peripheral iridectomy is made with the vitrectomy probe in the inferior quadrants.

Large retinectomies are often the best approach to remove large posterior subretinal membrane complexes. Chronic and traumatic RRDs are complicated by subretinal membrane formation. These can present as linear or circumferential bands creating a tenting effect on the retina. In more advance case, these membranes can further contract giving the retinal detachment a posterior closed funnel configuration due to napkin ring formation. In these cases, retinotomy, subretinal bands, and ring removal are mandatory to achieve full retinal reattachment. Linear subretinal bands and/or limited membrane networks can be better removed with minimal approach through punch-through retinotomies. Using a serrated type forceps the subretinal band is pinched and grabbed together with a small portion of overlying retinal tissue.

The band is then pulled anteriorly creating a small retinotomy. The subretinal band can then be rotated around the shaft of the forceps for a better grip or grasped with another forceps from the contralateral side to avoid losing the more elastic membranes.

20.2.4 Drainage of SRF, Sealing of Retinal Breaks, and Tamponade

Subretinal fluid prevents the retina from reattaching and must be removed from the subretinal space.

We tend to drain the SRF from the preexisting break using the back-flush cannula during fluid-air exchange (FAX). If more breaks are present, we choose the more posterior one to avoid shifting of SRF posteriorly. We typically set the air infusion to 40 mmHg. We mark the break with endo-diathermy to be able to identify the break under air. We reduce or switch off the chandelier light to reduce the glare and we bring the back-flush cannula on the top of the retinal break, holding it still in position until all the SRF has been aspirated and the retina is flattened. In some cases when the breaks are very anterior, subretinal fluid removal through the preexisting break can be challenging and may result in an uncomplete SRF removal. In these cases when SRF is very significant a postoperative retinal fold can occur.

To avoid this problem we usually inject PFO under air up to the edge to the primary break to let the fluid egress from the subretinal space. To perform this technique we use the chandelier light; from one side we inject PFO and from the other side we passively aspirate the SRF with the back-flush cannula from the break (AIR/PFO exchange).

In the retinectomy cases to avoid accumulation of fluid behind the retina with consequent slippage, we use the following strategies:

1. slow fluid-air exchange
2. direct PFO-oil exchange

20.2.5 Slow Fluid-Air Exchange

With this maneuver, we generally set the air infusion at 40 mmHg and we take care of aspirating the fluid present between the PFO bubble and the air bubble until we are sure no more BSS and/or subretinal fluid is present. Contact between PFO and air is in our experience evident when no more fluid comes out from the back-flush cannula placed at the edge of the PFO interface, and by change in reflection at the PFO-air interface (droplet effect).

20.2.6 Direct PFO-Oil Exchange

When the retinectomy is very anterior, complete fluid aspiration can be challenging and BSS can seep behind the retina creating slippage of the anterior edge of the retinectomy. This can be avoided with direct PFO-oil exchange. We connect the silicone oil syringe directly to the infusion line, and we set the VFC injection of the constellation (Alcon, Fort Worth, USA) to 26/30 PSI and the extrusion vacuum to 650 mmHg. We let the oil flow into the vitreous cavity through the infusion cannula, until the oil bubble gets in contact with the BSS. At this stage, we have three different layers: PFO inferiorly, silicone oil superiorly, and BSS in the middle. At this point, while we inject the silicone oil we can passively aspirate the BSS from the interface avoiding retina slippage. Once the retina is flattened, we need to seal all retinal breaks or the retinectomy edge with laser photocoagulation; we prefer to do that either under PFO or air. When we do it under PFO, the whole vitreous cavity needs to be filled with the heavy liquid; the presence of subretinal fluid around the breaks or at the retinectomy edges will, in fact, not allow laser uptake and efficient sealing. When the beaks are posterior, we prefer to laser under air to avoid fluid entrapment in the periphery (donut effect) or PFO migration in the subretinal space. Sometimes, in cases with persistent retinal folds after PVR membrane peeling and retinectomy, we prefer to inject silicone oil in the vitreous cavity and defer the laser treatment to a second surgery 2–4 weeks after the folds have been resolved or new PVR has occurred. This delay allows the retina to regain the original position and gives us the chance to re-operate the patient avoiding a more posterior retinectomy if new PVR develops.

In PVR cases, most of the times, we tamponade with silicone oil or long-acting gas (C3F8 12%). Recurrent cases and when retinectomies are performed our tamponade of choice is silicone oil 1000–5000 cs. Our injection method calls for a maximal vitreous cavity filling; we take particular attention to the complete removal of any subretinal fluid and to achieve full contact of the oil bubble to the retinal surface. We always vent one of the trocar cannulas, and we care to inject oil until we appreciate the silicone oil egressing from the vent itself. In this way, we minimize the risk of any underfilling.

In cases of anterior PVR with membrane at the level of pars plana and ciliary processes, circumferential contraction of the fibrotic membranes can generate ciliary body detachment. In these cases, anterior dissection might become challenging due to the presence of the crystalline lens. We prefer to remove the lens and the capsule via pars plana in these cases to avoid reproliferation along the posterior lens capsule with consequent hypotony. Lensectomy can be performed with the vitreous cutter in young patients with relatively soft lenses or with a 20 g fragmatome after opening one of the superior ports. We usually set the u/s at 30 and the vacuum at 200 mmHG using the constellation. The lens capsule is first opened at the equator with a sharp MVR blade, then hydrodissection can be performed to facilitate the detachment of the lens from its capsule and afterwards the nucleus can be removed. We generally tend to remove completely the anterior and posterior lens capsule with the vitreous cutter or with serrated forceps, paying particular attention to the remnants that could stay attached at the zonules. These need also to be removed because they can contract and give recurrent detachment of retina or ciliary body detachment. Inferior iridectomy is then performed a 6 o'clock to avoid pupillary block in case silicone oil is used as tamponade.

References

1. Leaver PK. Proliferative vitreoretinopathy. Br J Ophthalmol. (1995);79(10):871–2. https://doi.org/10.1136/bjo.79.10.871. PMC 505283. PMID 7488570.
2. "Proliferative Vitreoretinopathy". Retina and Vitreous of Texas. Retrieved 2009–05–28.
3. Ceron OM, Arroyo JG. Better outcomes may be ahead for PVR. Rev Ophthalmol. (2009);16:1. Retrieved 2009–05–29.
4. Kase S, Saito W, Ohno S, Ishida S. Cyclo-oxygenase-2 expression in human idiopathic epiretinal membrane. Retina. (2010);30:719–23. https://doi.org/10.1097/IAE.0b013e3181c59698. PMID 19996819
5. Erdiakov A, Gavrilova S. Influence of lornoxicam and triamcinolone on the dynamics of eye remodeling in concanavalin model of inflammation. Acta Ophthalmologica. (2014);92.https://doi.org/10.1111/j.1755-3768.2014.F077.x
6. Spirn MJ, Regillo C. Proliferative vitreoretinopathy. Retinal Physician. (2008). Retrieved 2009–05–29.
7. Hiscott P, Grierson I. Subretinal membranes of proliferative vitreoretinopathy. Br J Ophthalmol. 1991;75(1):53. https://doi.org/10.1136/bjo.75.1.53. PMC 504108. PMID 1991089
8. Casaroli-Marano RP, Pagan R, Vilaró S. Epithelial–mesenchymal transition in proliferative vitreoretinopathy: intermediate filament protein expression in retinal pigment epithelial cells. Investigat Ophthalmol Visual Sci. (1999);40(9):2062–72. PMID 10440262.
9. Connor TB, Roberts AB, Spom MB, Danielpour D, Dart LL, Michels RG, Bustros SD, Enger C, Kato H, Lansing M, Hayashi H, Glaser BM. Correlation of fibrosis and transforming growth factor-β Type 2 levels in the eye. J Clin Investig. 1989;83(5):1661–6. https://doi.org/10.1172/JCI114065. PMC 303874. PMID 2708527
10. Andrews A, Balciunaite E, Leong FL, Tallquist M, Soriano P, Refojo M, Kazlauskas A. Platelet-derived growth factor plays a key role in proliferative vitreoretinopathy. Investigat Ophthalmol Visual Sci. (1999);40(11):2683–89. PMID 10509666.
11. Kauffmann DJ, van Meurs JC, Mertens DA, Peperkamp E, Master XC, Gerritsen ME. Cytokines in vitreous humor: interleukin-6 is elevated in proliferative vitreoretinopathy. Investigat Ophthalmol Visual Sci. (1994);35(3):900–6. PMID 8125753.
12. Kon CH, Asaria RH, Occleston NL, Khaw PT, Aylward GW. Risk factors for proliferative vitreoretinopathy after primary vitrectomy: a prospective

study. Br J Ophthalmol. 2000;84(5):506–11. https://doi.org/10.1136/bjo.84.5.506. PMC 1723478. PMID 10781515.
13. Kon CH, Tranos P, Aylward GW. Risk factors in proliferative vitreoretinopathy. In: Kirchoff B, Wong D, editors. Vitreo-retinal surgery. Springer Berlin Heidelberg. (2005). p. 121–34. ISBN 978-3-540-20044-4.
14. Balles MW. Traumatic retinopathy. In: Albert DM, Jakobiec FA, editors. Principles and practice of ophlhnlmoltigy. WB Saunders: Philadelphia. (1994), Vol 2, p. 1029–31.
15. Giovinazzo VJ, Yannuzzi LA. Soreiison JA et nl. The ocular complications of boxing Ophthalmology. 1987;94:587–96.
16. Goffestein R, Burton TC. Differentiating traumatic from nontraumatic retinal detachment. Ophthalmology. 1982;89:361–8.
17. Malbran E, Dodds R, Hulsbus R. Traumatic retinal detachment Mod Probl Ophthal. 1972;10:479–89.
18. Cleary PE, Ryan SJ. Histology of wound, vitreous, and retina in experimental posterior penetrating eye injury in the rhesus monkey. Am j Ophthalmol. 1979;88:221–31.
19. Cleary PE, Ryan SJ. Method of production and natural history of experimental posterior penetrating eye injury in the rhesus monkey. Am } Ophthalmol 1979;88 212–20
20. Gregor Z, Ryan SJ. Combined posterior contusion and penetrating injury in the pig eye. I. A natural history study. Br J Ophthalmol 1982;66:793–8.
21. Cleary PE, Ryan SJ. Experimental posterior penetrating eye injury in the rabbit. I. Method of production and natural history. Br J Ophthamol 1979,63.306–11.
22. Cleary PE, Ryan SJ. Experimental posterior penetrating eye injury in the rabbit. II. Histology of wound, vitreous, and retina. Br f Ophthalmol 1979;63:312–21.
23. Cleary PE, Ryan SJ. Vitrectomy in penetrating eye injury. Results of a controlled trial of vitrectomy in an experimental posterior penetrating eye injury in the rhesus monkey. Arch Ophthalmoi 1981;99:287–91.
24. Gregor Z, Ryan SJ. Complete and core vitrectomies in the treatment of experimental posterior penetrating eye injury in the rhesus monkey. I Clinical features Arch Ophthalmol. 1983;101:441–5.
25. Gregor Z, Ryan SJ. Complete and core vitrectomies in the treatment of experimental posterior penetrating eye injury in the rhesus monkey, II. Histologic features. Arch Ophthalmol. 1983;101:446–50.
26. Hsu HT, Ryan SJ. Natural history of penetrating ocular injury with retinal laceration in the monkey. Graefe's Arch Clin Exp Ophthalmol. 1986;224:1–6.
27. Cox MS. Retinal breaks caused by blunt nonperforating trauma at the point of impact. Trans Am Ophthalmol Soc. 1980;78:414–66.
28. Cox MS, Schepens CL, Freeman HM. Retinal detachment due to ocular contusion. Arch Ophthalmol. 1966;76:678–85.
29. Scott JD. Retinal dialysis. Trans Ophthalmol Soc UK. 1977;97(1):33–5.
30. Zion VM, Burton TC. Retinal dialysis. Arch Ophthalmol. 1980;98(11):1971–4.
31. Tan HS, Mur M, Oberstein SY, de Smet MD. Primary retinectomy in proliferative vitreoretinopathy. Am J Ophthalmolo. 2010;149(3):447–52.

21 Vitrectomy for PVR Detachment Stage C

Ulrich Spandau and Zoran Tomic

21.1 Introduction

The name *proliferative vitreoretinopathy* was provided in 1989 by the Silicone Oil Study group (1). The name is derived from *proliferation* of the retinal pigment epithelial and glial cells and *vitreoretinopathy* to include the tissues which are affected, namely, the vitreous and the retina.

The **current management is t**he surgical relief of vitreal, preretinal and subretinal tractions. The final aim is the re-establishment of retinal attachment and visual function.

The **principles of management** are (1) closure of all retinal breaks, (2) relief of traction and (3) long-term retinal stabilisation. The following Table 21.1 shows the principles and surgical procedures for PVR detachment.

Regarding the **timing of surgery,** an early surgical treatment is favourable because it preserves the loss of photoreceptors and improves a favourable visual outcome. A delayed surgical treatment (after 6 weeks) is unfavourable for the visual function but surgery is easier; the proliferative membranes become "mature" and are therefore surgically easier to remove.

Indication: Feasible pathologies for this surgery are the first surgery of PVR detachments grade C2, C3 and D.

The surgical spectrum in general varies from 360° retinotomy with radial cuts and silicone oil tamponade to encircling band and C_3F_8 gas tamponade. Our approach is as follows: We inform the patient that in the most cases 2–3 surgeries are necessary to achieve retinal reattachment.

Surgically we would choose an encircling band with vitrectomy and silicone oil tamponade. In some cases, an inferior redetachment occurs. In this case, the silicone oil will be removed and exchanged against Densiron Xtra. See treatment algorithm in Fig. 21.1.

21.2 Instruments for PVR detachment

Membrane removal:

- # Trypane blue
- # 27G End-gripping forceps
- # 27G DORC wide grip forceps (1286. WRD04)
- # knob spatula or
- # membrane pic
- # Atkinson cannula
- # straight scissors

U. Spandau · Z. Tomic (✉)
Department of Ophthalmology, Uppsala University Hospital, Uppsala, Sweden
e-mail: zorannos@yahoo.se

U. Spandau et al. (eds.), *Retinal Detachment Surgery and Proliferative Vitreoretinopathy*,
https://doi.org/10.1007/978-3-031-11946-0_21

Table 21.1 Principles and surgical procedures for PVR detachment

Principle	Surgical procedure
Closure of all retinal breaks	• Identification • Closure
Relief of traction	• Membrane dissection • Retinotomy/retinectomy
Long-term retinal stabilisation	• Laser photocoagulation • Scleral buckle • Intraocular tamponade

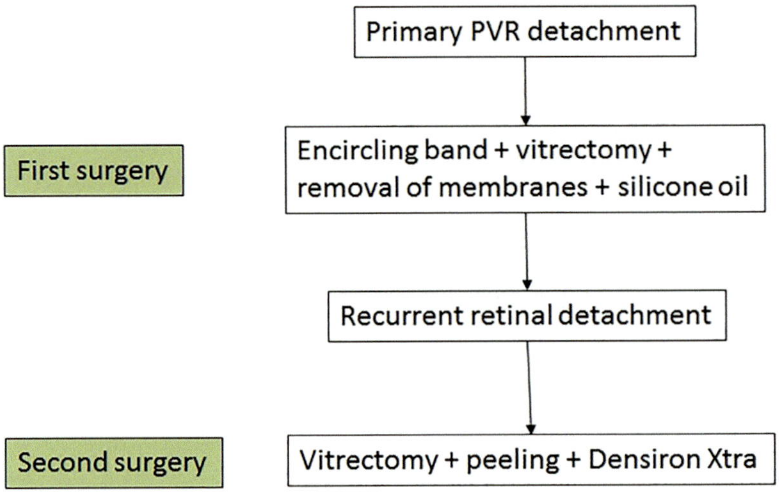

Fig. 21.1 Treatment algorithm for PVR stage C

21.3 The Main Surgical Steps

(1) **Encircling band (cerclage)**
(2) **Phacoemulsification and IOL implantation**
(3) **Pars plana vitrectomy**
(4) **Vitreous staining with triamcinolone**
(5) **Vitreous base shaving**
(6) **Staining of membranes with trypane blue**
(7) **Removal of epiretinal membranes**
(8) **Removal of subretinal membranes**
(9) **180 deg retinotomy**
(10) **Instillation of PFCL**
(11) **Laser photocoagulation**
(12) **Prepare the anterior chamber**
(13) **Tamponade**

21.4 Every Surgical Step in Detail

(1) **Encircling band (cerclage) (see video)**

Introduction: An encircling band relieves traction at the vitreous base. It facilitates also the closure of peripheral retinal breaks. And finally, an encircling band supports the vitreous base during anterior dissection. An encircling band is used less nowadays. We place an encircling band in PVR stage C3 and in PVR redetachments.

The surgery of an encircling band is described in detail in Chap. 17.1.

(2) **Phacoemulsification and IOL implantation**

For vitrectomy of PVR detachment, we recommend regardless of the age phacoemulsification with IOL implantation in the bag. The lens removal allows the visualisation of the vitreous base and assessment of anterior PVR and it allows more importantly the surgical access to the vitreous base. We avoid a (pars plana) lensectomy because the lens capsule is absent which serves otherwise as a scaffold between the posterior and anterior chamber. For example, in case of a silicone oil tamponade, the oil may prolapse into the anterior chamber and cause anterior chamber complications.

Surgical pearls no. 88

Management of miotic pupil: A miotic pupil may be a major obstacle for PVR surgery because the pathology is often located in the periphery. In many cases an intracameral injection of Adrenaline (1:10) is sufficient. Adrenaline may also be given during surgery. If posterior synechiae are present, then a synechiolysis is recommended. This can be achieved through iris stretching. Insert two Sinskey hooks through the paracenteses and stretch the pupil (Fig. 21.2). Alternatively, iris retractors with four-point fixation or a Malyugin ring can be implanted (Figs. 21.3 and 21.4).

(3) **Pars plana vitrectomy**

A main step in pars plana vitrectomy is the removal of the core vitreous resulting in relief of transvitreal traction.

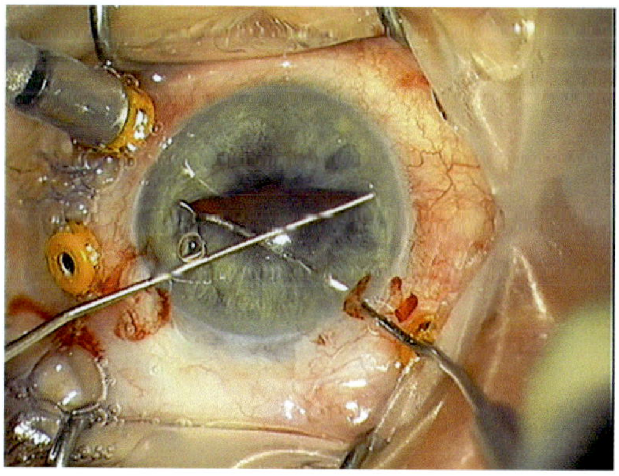

Fig. 21.2 Iris stretching with Sinskey hooks

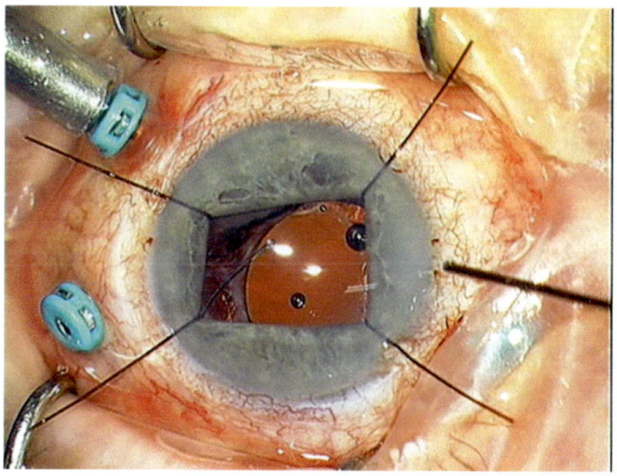

Fig. 21.3 Iris retractors

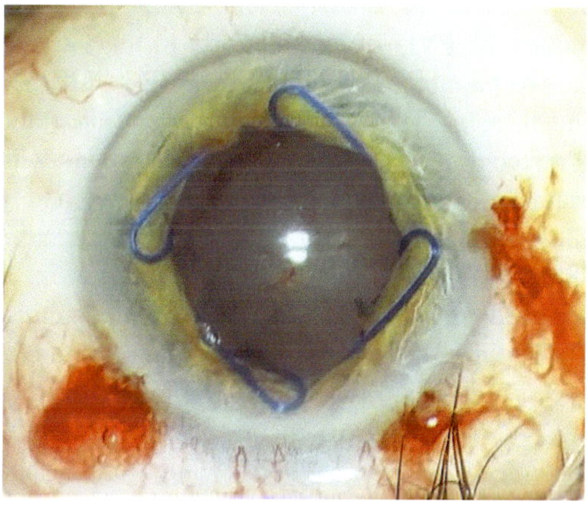

Fig. 21.4 Malyugin ring

We use a standard three-port PPV with 25G trocars. We use 25G and not 23G because smaller trocars require smaller instruments and this results in less traumatic surgery and less leakage from the trocars. In case of pseudophakia, the sclerotomies are placed 3.5 mm behind the limbus and in case of a natural lens 4.0 mm. Insert the infusion line in a quadrant without anterior traction. Otherwise the infusion will be located subretinally. In complicated vitrectomies, we insert always a chandelier light (four-port PPV) which allows for bimanual dissection of membranes, bimanual injection of PFCL and injection of silicone oil under view to retina.

A vital point for successful and complication-free vitrectomy is a good visualisation. Wide-angle viewing systems have a viewing field of 60 to 130°. They allow for anterior dissection and limit the need of scleral depression. The visualisation in an air-filled eye is improved. The stereopsis is however reduced. The conventional contact lens system has a viewing field of only 20 to 30° and requires scleral depression. We use the Resight Biom system from Zeiss together with a Zeiss Lumera microscope.

(4) **Vitreous staining with triamcinolone**
(5) **Vitreous base shaving**

A posterior vitreous detachment (PVD) is usually present in idiopathic PVR. In contrast, a PVD is not present in diabetic and traumatic PVR. Induce the PVD as far anteriorly to the vitreous base as possible. The vitreous in PVR is inflamed and therefore a thorough removal is important. We recommend the staining of the vitreous with triamcinolone to assess if a PVD is present and to allow a meticulous shaving of the vitreous base. "Shaving" means that the vitreous cortex is removed to the surface of the peripheral retina. The settings of the vitreous cutter are a high clip rate (5000–7500 cuts/min) and a low aspiration rate (200 mmHg). Crucial for a successful shaving is a wide-angle viewing system and scleral depression. Ideally, the scleral depression is performed bimanually under illumination of a chandelier light.

(6) **Membrane dissection (see video)**

In general: The removal of preretinal membranes results in relief of preretinal traction. All**epi**retinal membranes must be removed. Even in case of retinotomy remove all membranes up to the retinotomy edges. If you leave epiretinal membranes, then they will continue to proliferate and cause a tractive detachment. In contrast, remove **sub**retinal proliferation *only* if the posterior retina is not flattened under PFCL. Begin with the removal of the membranes located at the posterior pole and continue with membrane dissection in the peripheral retina (Fig. 21.5).

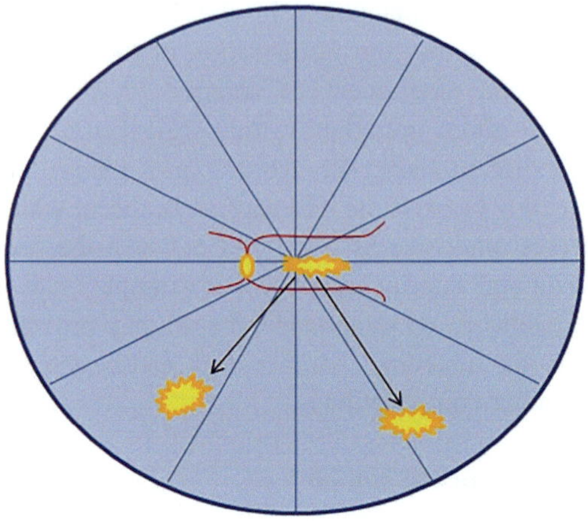

Fig. 21.5 In PVR detachment membrane dissection starts in the central posterior pole and continues in the periphery

Technique of membrane staining: In PVR detachments, the membranes are located centrally and peripherally. It is easy to stain central membranes in a BSS-filled eye because the dye falls down on the posterior pole. This manoeuvre is, however, difficult for peripherally located membranes.

We stain, therefore, in an air-filled eye. In an air-filled eye, the contact between membrane and dye is longer and more concentrated before the dye falls down on the posterior pole. Perform a fluid x air exchange and drop a few drops of the dye directly on the membranes (Figs. 21.6 and 21.7). Wait 30 s, aspirate first the dye from the posterior pole and then continue with an air x fluid exchange. With this method, a higher

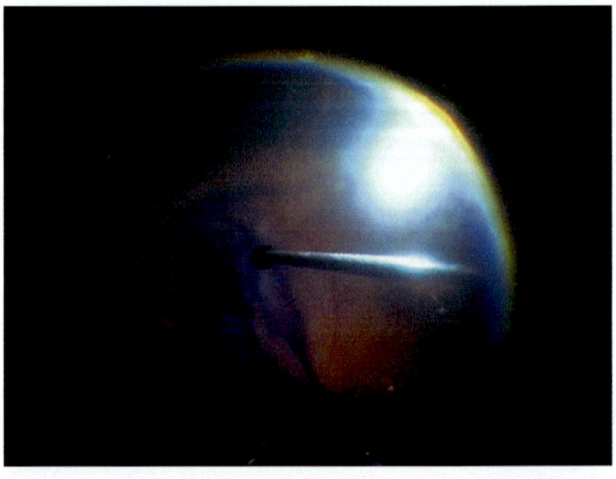

Fig. 21.6 The dye is dropped on the membrane

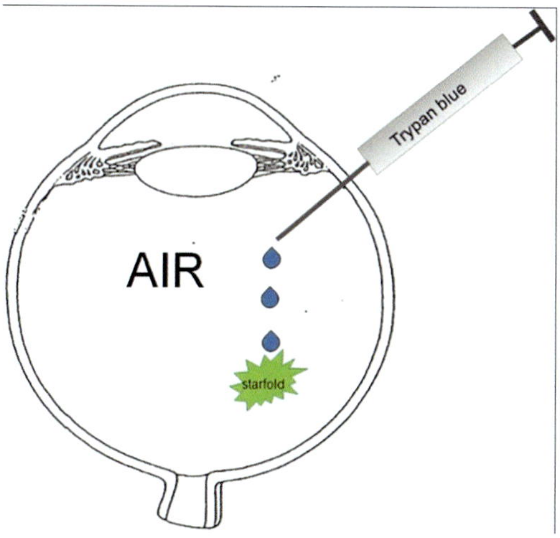

Fig. 21.7 The vitreous cavity is filled with air. This method increases the concentration of the dye and enables the staining of peripheral membranes

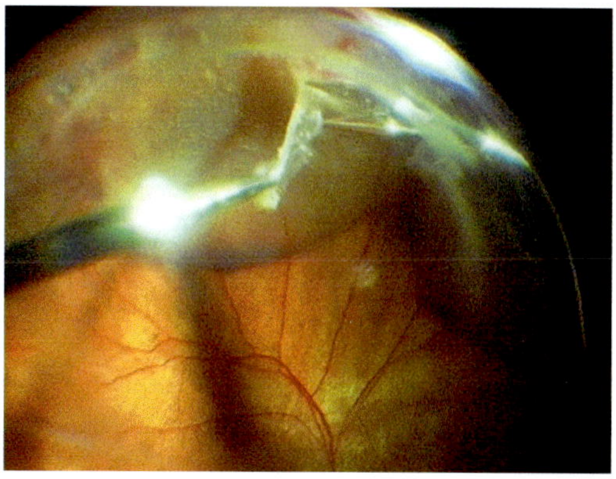

Fig. 21.8 Removal of peripheral membranes with end-gripping forceps and straight scissors

concentration of the dye is achieved and therefore a better staining of the membranes.

Technique of membrane removal: The peeling of PVR membranes is technically very difficult. It requires patience, good visualisation and good instruments. Centrally located membranes can be removed with one hand but peripherally located membranes require bimanual peeling. Our setup is a 4 port PPV with 3 trocars and one chandelier light.

21.5 Removal of Epiretinal Membranes (Fig. 21.8) (See Video)

A successful membrane removal depends on a large amount of the instrument; even if you are an experienced vitreoretinal surgeon. You need good delamination instruments and good forceps. Test therefore many different peeling forceps to find the one which suits you best.

For delamination of the membrane, we use a 25G or 27G blunt retrobulbar cannula (Atkinson, Beaver Visitec); alternatively, you can use a membrane pic (DORC). For dissection of membranes, three different forceps from DORC are available. In our experience, the 27G end-gripping forceps (DORC) are suitable for every tissue from ILM to thick membranes. Membranes with strong adhesions require stronger forceps such as the serrated jaws forceps or strong end-gripping forceps. Vitreoretinal tractions can be cut with straight 25G microscissors (Fig. 21.8) (DORC, NL and Eye Tech, UK) and curved 27G microscissors (DORC).

The most difficult surgical manoeuvre for removal of PVR membranes is the delamination of the membranes from the retina. This manoeuvre is even more difficult in eyes after a silicone oil tamponade. After a silicone oil tamponade, the membranes are even more adherent to the retina. Delaminate the membrane with an Atkinson cannula and create an opening between membrane and the retina. Then lift the membrane here with forceps and move at the same time the delamination cannula or alternatively a 25G knob spatula (Eye Tech, UK) backward and forward through the opening.

The peripheral membranes are very difficult to remove because the retina is detached and because the membranes are difficult to reach with the instruments. Instil PFCL to stabilise the posterior retina and facilitate membrane removal (*PFCL assisted membrane removal*). In addition, perfluorocarbon liquids (PFCLs) draw the vitreous base more posteriorly. This effect facilitates anterior dissection and reduces the chances of retina or vitreous incarceration in a sclerotomy site. Furthermore, it facilitates drainage of subretinal fluid through anterior retinal breaks. Important: All breaks must be *freed of traction* before they come in contact with the PFCL. Otherwise, there is a risk that the PFCL tracks subretinally.

Subretinal proliferations are present in nearly half of the cases of PVR but rarely prevent retinal reattachment. Must all proliferations be removed? No, only the significant ones. A significant subretinal membrane is one that will preclude flattening of the retina unless it is removed. Their significance becomes obvious when PFCL is instilled. Remove a subretinal proliferation *only* if the posterior retina is not flattened under PFCL. A special case of a subretinal proliferation is a "napkin ring". A napkin ring is a tight annular band near the optic disc. Its removal requires a 360 deg retinotomy. See chapter "Traumatic PVR".

21.6 Removal of Subretinal Proliferations (See Video)

Before removing subretinal membranes perform a complete posterior and anterior epiretinal dissection.

The complete surgery is shown step by step in Chap. 23.

21.7 Retinotomy

Video 13.13: Retinotomy

The relaxing retinotomy consists of three main surgical steps:

1. Ora parallel diathermy
2. Retinotomy
3. Removal of anterior retina (retinectomy)

The complete surgery is shown step by step in Chap. 23.

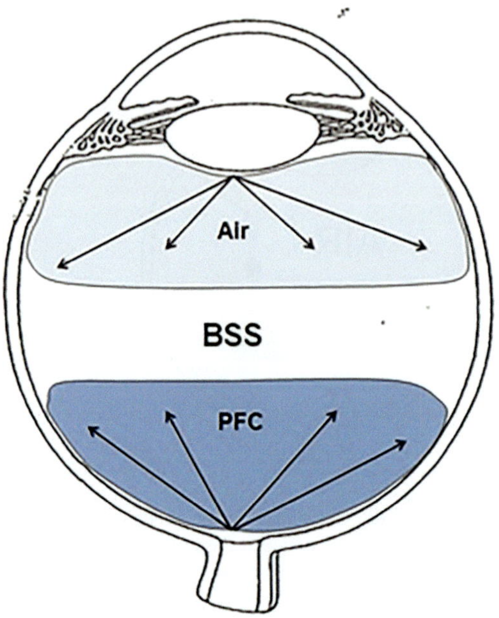

Fig. 21.9 Opposite mechanisms of action of PFCL and air in a BSS-filled eye. Air fills the globe from anterior to posterior. PFC fills the globe from posterior to anterior

21.8 Instillation of PFCL

As the next step, we perform an **attachment test:** Fig. 21.9. For an attachment test, you can use PFCL or air. PFCL attaches the retina with its gravity. Air attaches the retina with its surface tension pressure. If the retina is attached under PFCL, then perform a PFCL against air exchange and check if the retina is also attached under air. If this is the case, then the retina will also be attached under a gas tamponade. BUT: The retina is not necessarily attached under a silicone oil tamponade because the surface tension pressure of silicone oil is lower than the surface tension pressure of air.

Injection of PFCL: We inject PFCL bimanually; one hand holds the PFCL syringe and the other hand holds the Charles flute needle. Hold the tip of the PFCL cannula in the middle of the

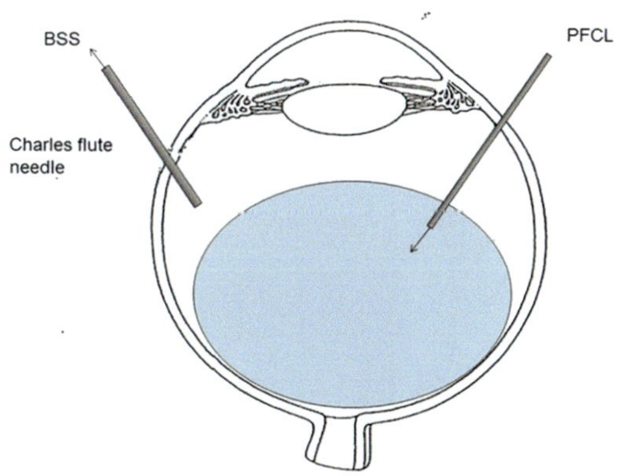

Fig. 21.10 Work bimanual. The left hand releases BSS with a backflush instrument and the right hand injects PFCL

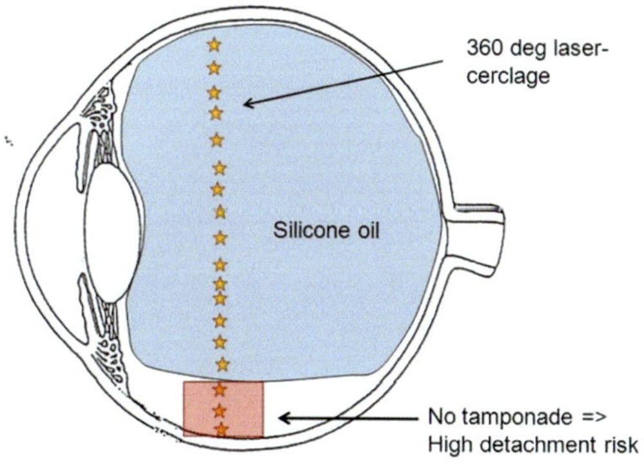

Fig. 21.11 In case of a 360 deg lasercerclage there is a risk of a laser necrosis at the inferior pole due to a lack of tamponade

vitreous cavity and inject a little bit. Then start to inject the PFCL at the posterior pole and keep the tip of the cannula always in the PFCL bubble in order to prevent small bubbles (Fig. 21.10). Aim never towards the macula or a retinal break. The PFCL bubble becomes bigger and bigger; pull the PFCL cannula slowly backwards but the tip remains constantly inside the bubble.

21.9 Laser Photocoagulation

The aim of laser photocoagulation is a long-term stabilisation of the reattached retina. Laser photocoagulation causes less RPE cell dispersion than cryotherapy and consequently less PVR. In addition, laser photocoagulation induces no disruption of the blood aqueous barrier.

Technique of laser photocoagulation
Laser photocoagulation can be performed in the PFCL-filled eye or in the air-filled eye. Apply the laser effects confluently surrounding all retinal breaks. Our laser power for retinal breaks with an argon laser (Iridex, CA) is Power: 100–300 mW, Duration: **200** ms, Interval: 300 ms.

Surgical pearls no. 89

Laser cerclage ≠ encircling band (Fig. 21.11). Both, an encircling band and a laser cerclage, create a barrier for tears located anterior to the barrier. In addition, an encircling band creates an indentation of the retina which results in a relaxation of the shortened retina. A laser cerclage, however, does not create an indentation and can therefore not help in relaxing a shortened retina. This is important for PVR detachments with intraretinal PVR and a shortened retina.

Surgical pearls no. 90

Cryopexy versus laser photocoagulation: Cryopexy creates PVR; this is especially the case if the posterior hyaloid is detached. In vitrectomy for retinal detachment surgery, laser photocoagulation is recommended because it induces less PVR.

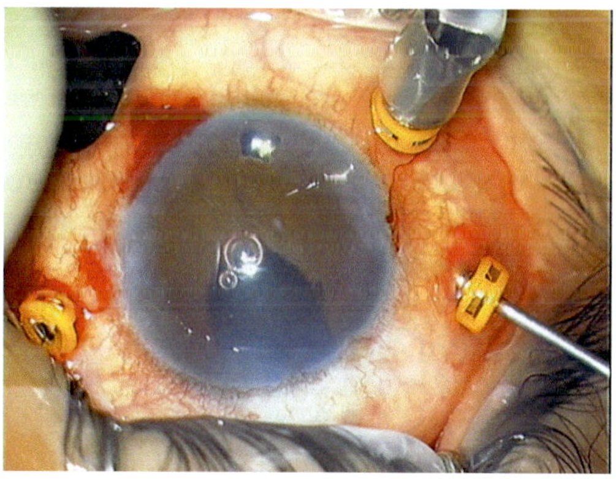

Fig. 21.12 Ando iridectomy with vitreous cutter

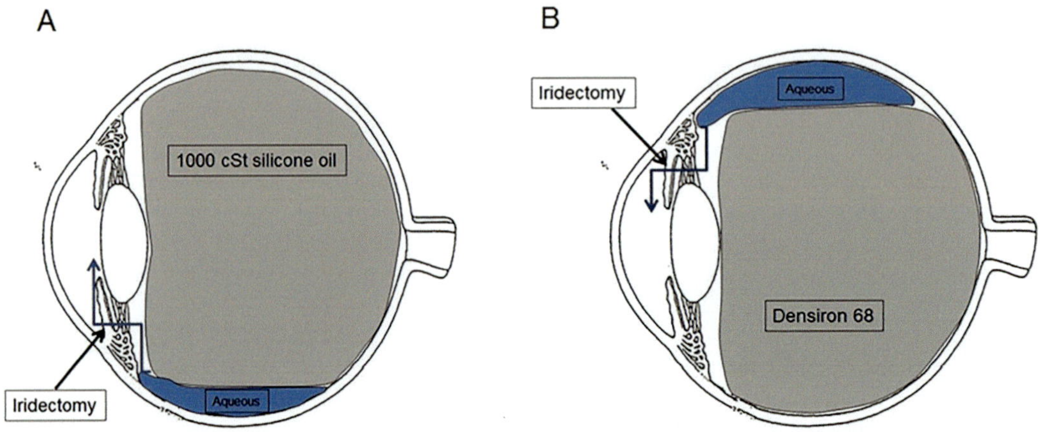

Fig. 21.13 An inferior (**A**) or superior (**B**) iridectomy depending on the silicone oil

21.10 Prepare the Anterior Chamber (See Video)

Before finalising surgery with the intraocular tamponade, **the anterior segment must be prepared** (Figs. 21.12 and 21.13). In case of 1000 or 5000 csts silicone oil, an inferior Ando iridectomy is performed to enable a flow of aqueous from the inferiorly located aqueous phase in the posterior chamber to the anterior chamber. In case of a Densiron 68 tamponade, a superior iridectomy is performed to enable the flow of aqueous from the superior located aqueous phase in the posterior chamber to the anterior chamber. Not in all cases an iridectomy must be performed. In a normal pseudophakia situation an iridectomy is not necessary. An iridectomy is however necessary in aphakia, in 360 deg posterior synechiae and in partial zonular lysis. In the aphakic eye, the inferior peripheral iridectomy prevents a pupil block by the anterior surface of silicone oil. Face-down positioning for the first 24 h is necessary to ensure the reformation of the anterior chamber.

In addition, you can inject methylcellulose into the anterior chamber to prevent an immediate postoperative flow from silicone oil into the anterior chamber. The methylcellulose causes no IOP increase in case of a silicone oil tamponade.

21.11 Tamponade

PFCL removal and tamponade
For gas tamponades, a PFCL x air exchange is routine. For silicone oil tamponades two surgical techniques exist: (1) A PFCL against silicone oil exchange and (2) a PFCL against air and then an air against silicone oil exchange. We use a PFCL against silicone oil exchange in traumatic retinal detachments. Otherwise, we use always a PFCL against air exchange.

Slippage is a complication which occurs in giant tears or retinotomies. If subretinal fluid is present at the posterior pole and the eye is filled with gas and the patient is located face down, then a slippage at the posterior pole with macular folds may occur. To avoid the slippage, use PFCL and perform a thorough aspiration of fluid at the giant tear edges and avoid face down positioning directly after surgery. In silicone oil, slippage with macular folds does not occur. The reason for this is that the surface tension pressure of silicone oil is too low to press away the fluid at the posterior pole; the fluid is resorbed by the pigment epithelium and the retina slowly reattaches.

PFCL against silicone oil exchange: (Fig. 21.14). For this step, a chandelier light is not required. If you exchange PFCL against silicone oil one hand aspirates the PFCL and the

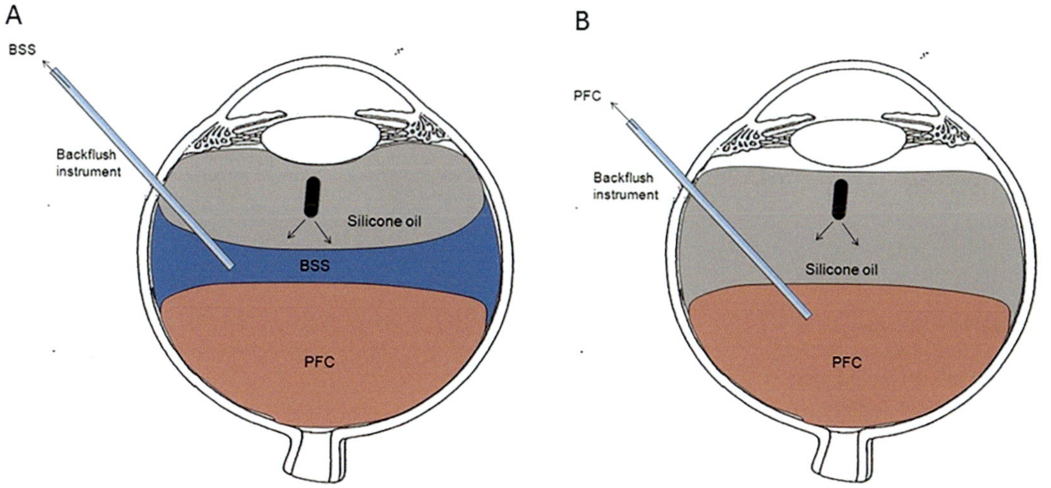

Fig. 21.14 PFCL against silicone oil exchange: In a first step (**a**) silicone oil is injected and fills the eye from anterior to posterior. Aspirate first the BSS phase. After removal of BSS (**b**) hold the flute needle into the PFCL phase and remove it

other hand holds the light fibre while the silicone oil is injected with the infusion line.

Intraocular tamponade

Gas or silicone oil: According to the silicone oil study C_3F_8 is superior (higher reattachment rate and better visual outcome) to SF_6 in complicated detachments. The silicone oil study does not compare C_3F_8 with silicone oil. The advantages and disadvantages of C_3F_8 are listed in Table 21.2 and of silicone oil in Table 21.3. For complicated retinal detachments, we prefer silicone oil. The main reason is that the recurrent detachment risk in complicated RD´s is higher than in easy detachments. And a recurrent detachment under silicone oil is better than a recurrent detachment under gas. Why? A recurrent detachment under gas develops fast into a PVR detachment. A recurrent detachment under silicone oil develops slowly. Under gas an immediate surgery is required. Under silicone oil you can postpone and plan surgery.

Gas tamponade: Gas has two great advantages over silicone oil. The surface tension pressure of gas is much higher than for silicone oil which enables a more effective sealing of retinal holes. Secondly, the gas is a temporary tamponade. Long-term damages of gas are therefore not existent compared to silicone oil.

Injection of gas: SF_6, C_2F_6 and C_3F_8 are due to the fluorine atoms heavier than air. The gases sink therefore to the ground, whereas the lighter air stays above. Hold the Charles flute needle behind the lens to aspirate the air and the gases

Table 21.2 The pros and cons of C_3F_8

Advantages of C_3F_8	Disadvantages of C_3F_8
Disappears spontaneously	Only temporary tamponade
High surface tension pressure	Specific head positioning (not for children, disabled)
	Air travel must be postponed (risk of expansion)
	Vision is restricted (not for monocular patients)
	Cataractogenic

Table 21.3 The pros and cons of silicone oil

Advantages of silicone oil	Disadvantages
"Non-temporary" longer tamponade	Need for a second operation
Does not require positioning	Scaffold for reproliferation (?)
Earlier visualisation (option for monocular patients)	Cataractogenic
Air-travel is possible	Low surface tension pressure
Lower risk of hypotony	

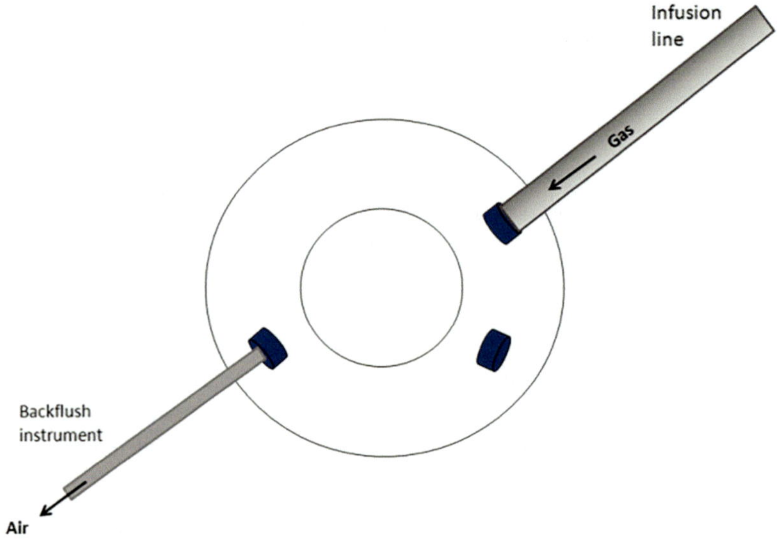

Fig. 21.15 The setup for a gas injection. The gas is injected through the infusion line and the flute needle evacuates the air

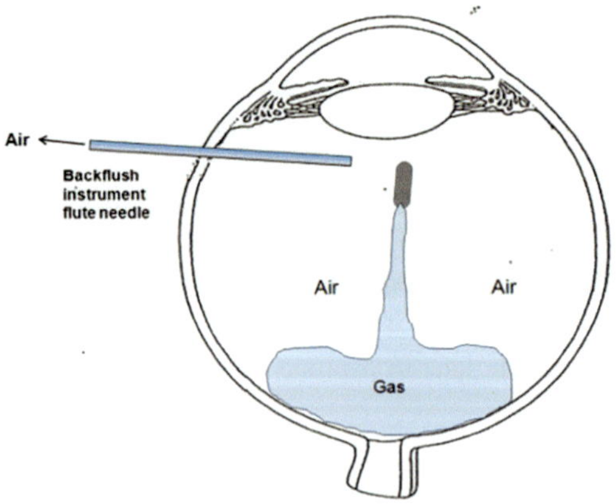

Fig. 21.16 The heavy gas fills the vitreous cavity from posterior to anterior and the flute needle aspirates the light air

can fill the vitreous cavity from posterior to anterior (Figs. 21.15 and 21.16).

Surgical pearls no. 91.

Shake the 50 cc gas syringe before injection because the gas sinks to the bottom of the syringe resulting in a wrong concentration of the gas in the eye.

Silicone oil tamponade (see video).

Silicone oil is an excellent temporary tamponade but a very bad permanent tamponade. It causes high IOP, emulsifies and the final result is an optic atrophy. Silicone oil should be avoided in fresh and primary detachments. Silicone oil is

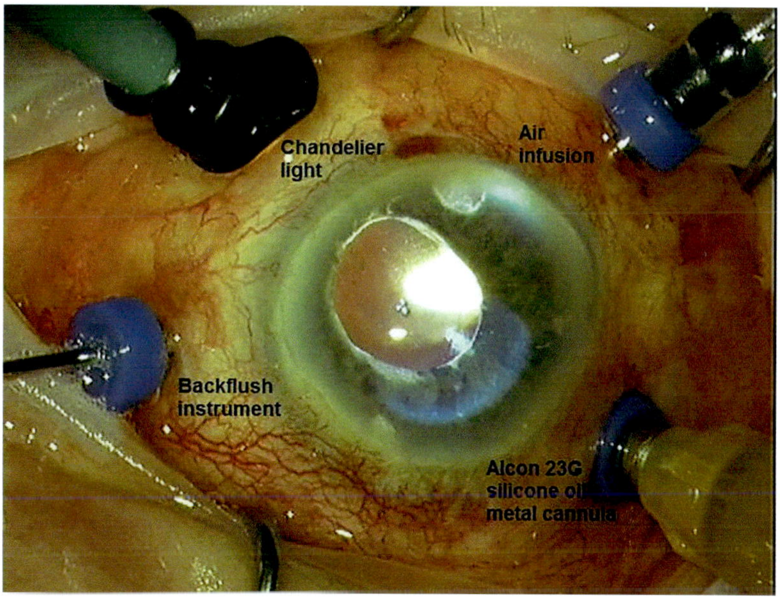

Fig. 21.17 Silicone oil injection **under** view to retina. Note that a chandelier light is required

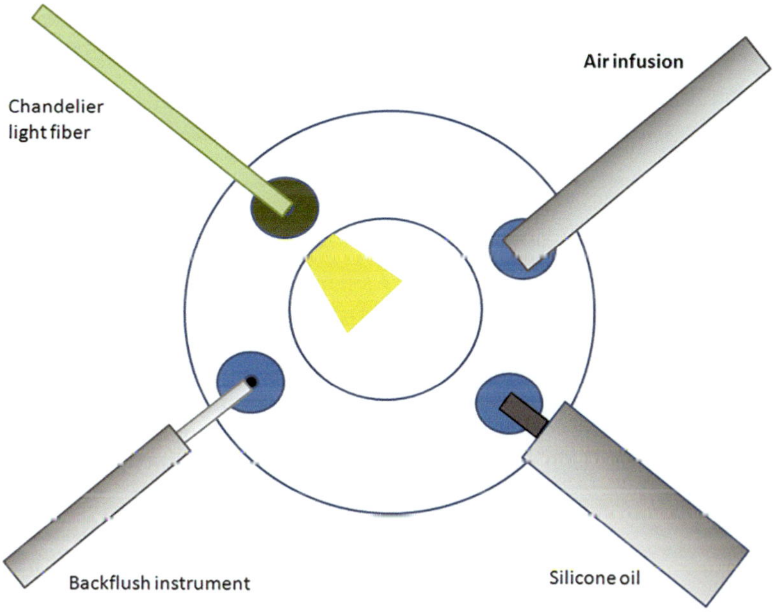

Fig. 21.18 Setup for oil injection with view to retina

Fig. 21.19 You work bimanual in order to inject the silicone oil under view to retina

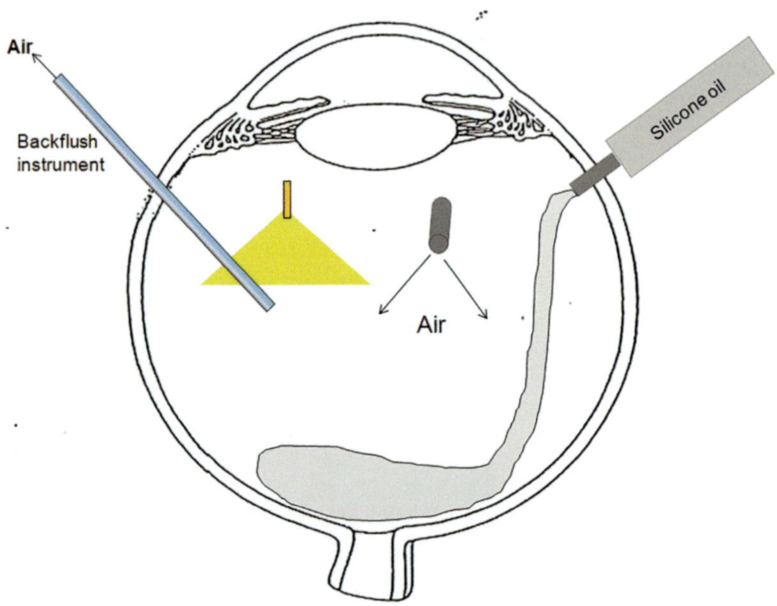

Table 21.4 The duration of a silicone oil tamponade at the University of Uppsala

Duration of silicone oils	Normal case	Young patient	Trauma case (with low IOP)
1000/1300 csts silicone oil	1,5 to 3 months	6-8 weeks	6 months to ∞
5000 csts silicone oil	3 months to ∞	6-8 weeks	6 months to ∞
Densiron 68	1,5 to 3 months	6-8 weeks	Exchange to 5000 csts silicone oil

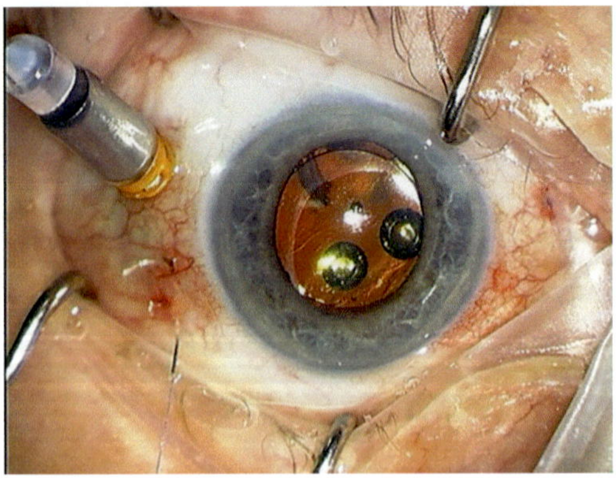

Fig. 21.20 Cut the infusion line after silicone oil injection so that excessive oil can flow out

indicated in recurrent detachments, in complicated PVR detachments and in diabetic tractive detachments. But even in these cases try to remove the silicone oil after three months.

Silicone oil injection (Figs. 21.17, 21.18 and 21.19):

1000 csts or 5000 csts silicone oil: 5000 csts induces less IOP increase and less emulsification. If you plan a long silicone oil tamponade (longer than 6 months) then use 5000 csts silicone oil. If you plan a short duration (shorter than 6 months) then use 1000 csts silicone oil. The duration of the silicone oil is listed in Table 21.4.

Surgical pearls no. 92.

Silicone oil overfill (Fig. 21.20): Cut the infusion line with scissors so that the excessive silicone oil can escape. An IOP of approximately 10 mmHg is fine or wait so long until no more oil escapes from the infusion line.

Referencess

1. Vitrectomy with silicone oil or sulfur hexafluoride gas in eyes with severe proliferative vitreoretinopathy: results of a randomized clinical trial. Silicone Study Report 1. Arch Ophthalmol. 1992;110(6):770–9.
2. Kreissig I. A practical guide to minimal surgery for retinal detachment. Thieme, Germany ISBN 9783131606914.

Vitrectomy for PVR Stage D

22

Zoran Tomic and Ulrich Spandau

22.1 Introduction

In this chapter the surgical management of a PVR stage D is described step-by-step. PVR stage D with a closed funnel without a view to the optic disc (Fig. 22.1) is surgically the most demanding and most difficult pathology within PVR detachments. The retina is stiffened with full-thickness retinal folds. A circumferential traction leads to a purse string funnel detachment. The surgical aim is to remove these tractional forces and mobilize the retina.

PVR stage D detachment cannot be treated with scleral buckling due to the extensive circumferential traction. A PVR stage D detachment is a clear indication of vitrectomy. A PVR stage D vitrectomy includes in many cases a 180–360° retinotomy. In most cases, a 270° retinotomy is required. The advantage of a 270° retinotomy over a 360° retinotomy is that a macular rotation is impossible.

Alternatively, you can use an encircling band. In our experience, an encircling band does not create a sufficient impression to attach the stiffened retina. We usually do not place an encircling band in PVR stage D detachment.

Prognosis: The visual prognosis is low and we, therefore, operate only PVR stage D detachments with less than 1 year of duration.

22.2 Surgery

Instruments:
1. Peeling instruments
2. Retinotomy instruments
3. PFCL
4. 5000 cSt silicone oil.

The main surgical steps:

1. **4-port vitrectomy with chandelier light**
2. **Vitrectomy with complete removal of vitreous base**
3. **Removal of epiretinal membranes from posterior pole to ora serrata**
4. **Ora parallel (circumferential) endodiathermy**
5. **270–360° retinotomy**
6. **Meticulous cautery of retinal edge bleeding**
7. **Retinectomy of anterior retina**
8. **Removal of subretinal membranes**
9. **Instillation of PFCL**
10. **Flattening of retinal edges**
11. **Attachment test and rotation test**
12. **Laser treatment**
13. **PFCL against silicone oil exchange**.

Z. Tomic
Milos Klinika, Belgrade, Serbia

U. Spandau (✉)
St. Eriks Hospital, University of Stockholm, Stockholm, Sweden
e-mail: ulrich_spandau@yahoo.de

U. Spandau et al. (eds.), *Retinal Detachment Surgery and Proliferative Vitreoretinopathy*,
https://doi.org/10.1007/978-3-031-11946-0_22

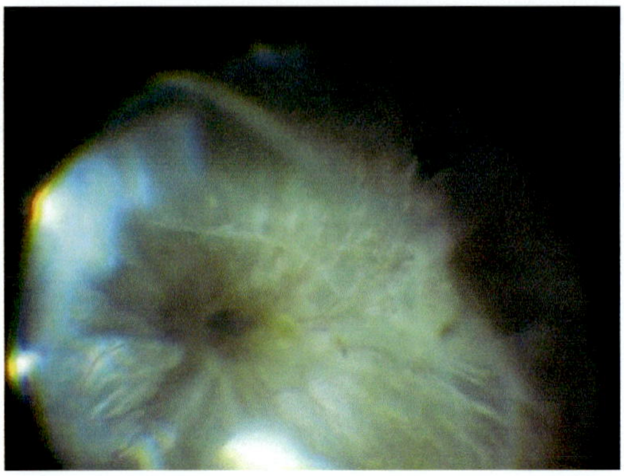

Fig. 22.1 A funnel detachment without view to optic disc. Start with a core vitrectomy

The surgery in detail:

1. **4-port vitrectomy with chandelier light**
2. **Vitrectomy with complete removal of vitreous base**

A 3-port vitrectomy with chandelier light is recommended. Start with a core vitrectomy and continue with a peripheral vitrectomy (Figs. 22.1 and 22.2).

3. **Removal of epiretinal membranes from posterior pole to ora serrata (Figs.** 22.3 **and** 22.4)

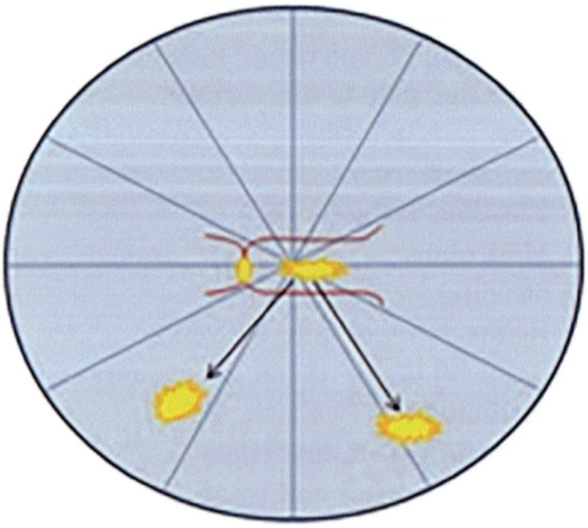

Fig. 22.2 In PVR detachment start with a central peeling and continue with a peripheral peeling

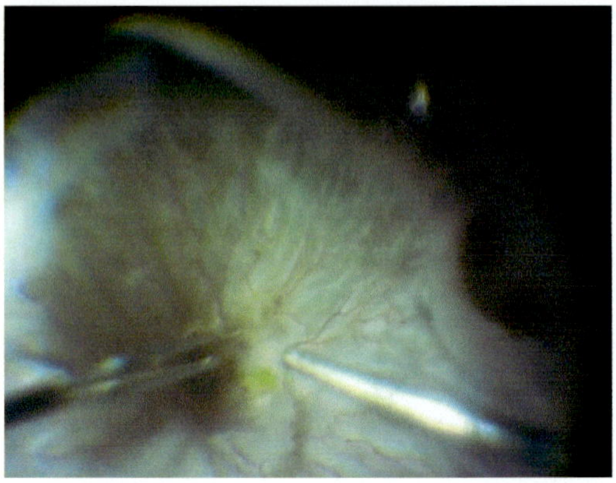

Fig. 22.3 Start with removal of central membranes

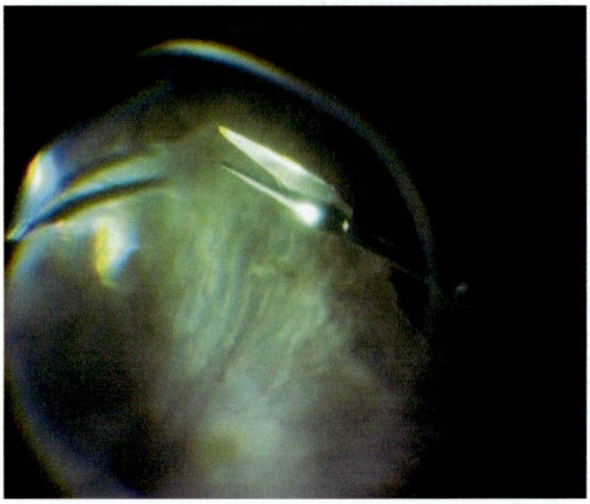

Fig. 22.4 Continue with removal of peripheral membranes

This step is VERY time-consuming. A complete posterior and anterior dissection of epiretinal membranes is required in order to mobilize the foreshortened retina. Stain the membranes with trypan blue or triamcinolone. Start with membrane dissection at the posterior pole (Fig. 22.3) and continue towards the ora serrata. Work bimanual with an endgripping forceps, a delamination instrument (knob spatula, Atkinson cannula, pic) and curved or straight scissors (Fig. 22.4).

4. **Ora parallel (circumferential) endodiathermy**
5. **270–360° retinotomy (Fig.** 22.5)
6. **Meticulous cautery of retinal edge bleeding**

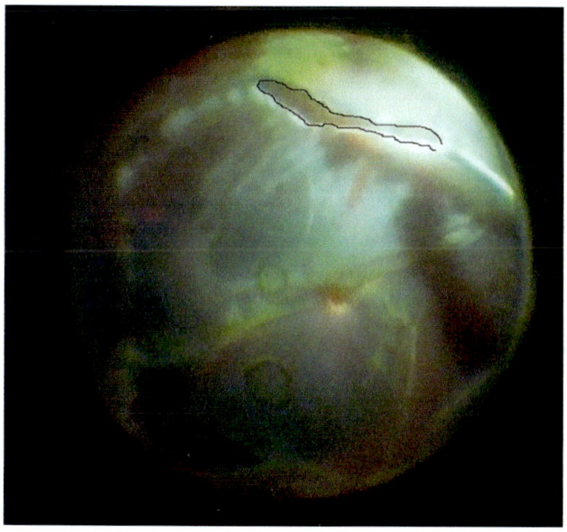

Fig. 22.5 Retinotomy with 25G cutter

After removal of all epiretinal membranes, continue with diathermy. Cauterize the peripheral retina with an ora parallel, circumferential row of diathermy spots. If the retina cannot be cauterized, then vitreous is present. Remove the vitreous and then cauterize the retina again. The same applies to residual membranes. The next step is a retinotomy. Use vertical forceps or even better a 25G and even better a 27G vitreous cutter to perform the retinotomy along the cauterized retina (Figs. 22.5 and 22.6). Starting first with a meticulous cautery of haemorrhages at the retinal edge is necessary in order to prevent recurrent

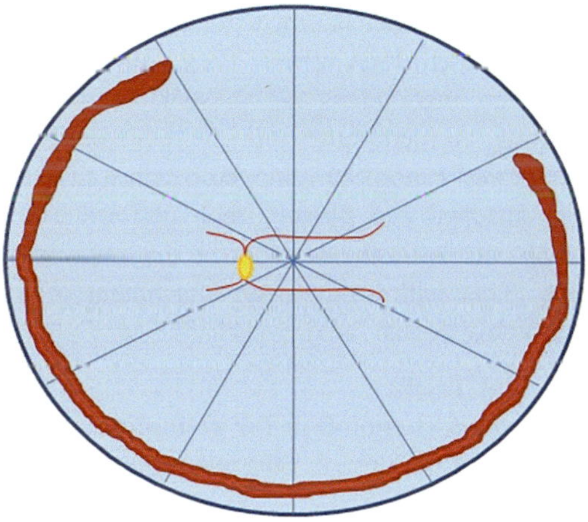

Fig. 22.6 In PVR stage D, a 270 retinotomy is often required

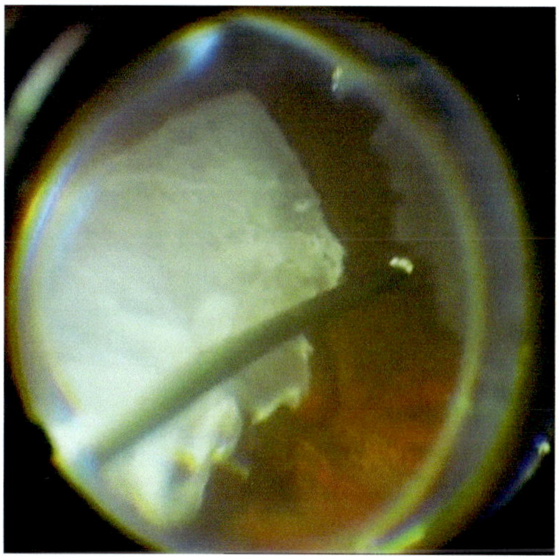

Fig. 22.7 A retinectomy of the anterior retina

PVR. *Remark*: In PVR stage D, a 180° retinotomy is usually not sufficient. In most cases, a 270°–360° retinotomy is required. If possible, avoid a 360° retinotomy because the risk for a macular rotation is increased. Prefer a 270° retinotomy which prevents a retinal/macular rotation.

7. **Retinectomy of anterior retina (Fig.** 22.6)

Remove the residual anterior retina with the vitreous cutter (Fig. 22.7).

8. **Removal of subretinal membranes**

Check if subretinal membranes are present and remove them. Check also if a napkin ring is present. A napkin ring is a fibrotic ring around the optic disc. It is located subretinally (Fig. 22.8). The annular membrane occurs after a chronic detachment. In order to remove the napkin ring, a 360° circumferential retinotomy is required.

9. **Instillation of PFCL**
10. **Flattening of retinal edges**
11. **Attachment test and rotation test**
12. **Laser treatment (Fig.** 22.9)

Inject now PFCL until the retinal edges are completely attached. If a retinal edge is rolled up,

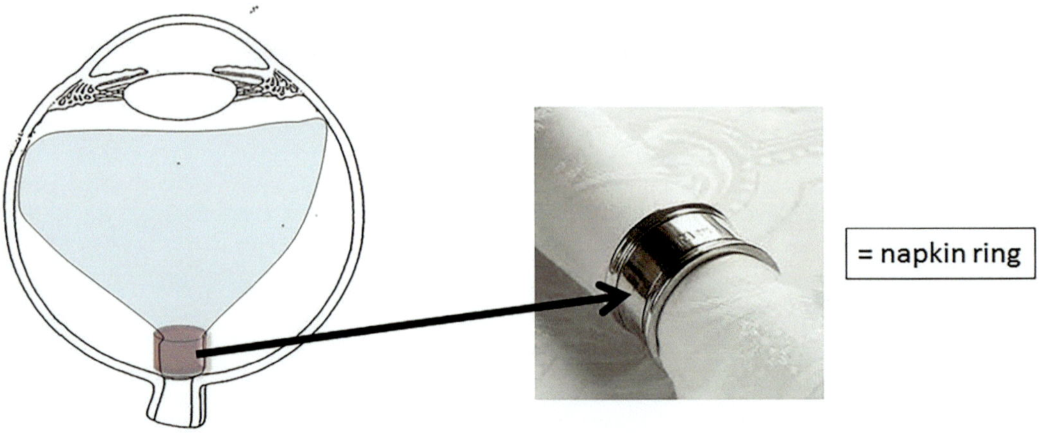

Fig. 22.8 A subretinal fibrotic ring around the retina located at the optic disc=napkin ring

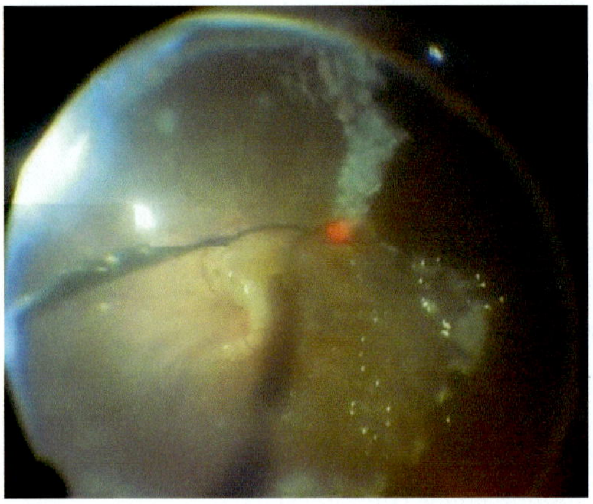

Fig. 22.9 Laser photocoagulation of retinal edges with increased laser power: 300 ms duration

then flatten it; if a fold in the retina is visible, then either massage it and if this does not help, then look for membranes and remove them. This manoeuvre can be carefully done under PFCL. If the retinal edges are 360° nicely attached, then observe if the macula is at the correct position. If not, rotate the retina with one or two vacuum cleaners. Continue with laser photocoagulation (Fig. 22.9). We need a high laser power for retinal edges to prevent a postoperative slippage. Choose laser settings of **300 ms** duration.

13. **PFCL against air and then against silicone oil exchange**

Finalize surgery with a PFCL against air exchange. When the PFCL reached the retinal edges, aspirate meticulously subretinal fluid at the retinal edges. Then remove the complete PFCL phase. Inject then 1300 or 5000 cSt silicone oil into the vitreous cavity.

22.3 Tips and Tricks

Lifted retinotomy edges during/after laser photocoagulation: Usually the retinotomy edges do not lift if you laser photocoagulate them; even if you use a high laser power. They will, however, lift when membranes are present. To prevent uplifting, all membranes must be removed. If the membranes cannot be removed because they are very attached and fibrotic, then perform a few radial cuts with the scissors at the retinotomy edge. This will result in an attachment of the retinotomy edges.

Tips and Tricks:
Laser photocoagulation for retinotomy: More laser power than usual: **300 ms** duration instead of 200 ms!!

23 Special Surgical Techniques for PVR Detachment

Ulrich Spandau and Zoran Tomic

23.1 Staining of Peripheral Membranes

The staining of central membranes is simple because the dye falls onto the posterior pole. The staining of peripheral membranes is, however, difficult because the dye cannot be applied on the peripheral retina. The trick is to stain under the air. The advantage is that you can drop the dye directly on the peripheral membrane and the contact between dye and retina is longer resulting in a good staining of the membranes. With this method, a higher concentration of the dye is achieved and therefore a better staining of the membranes.

The technique in detail:
We refill the dye into a regular 3 cc syringe because the dye can be ejected in a more controlled manner (Figs. 23.1 and 23.2).

Start with a complete fluid x air exchange. Then drop a few drops of the dye directly onto the membranes (Figs. 23.3 and 23.4). Wait approximately 30 s and aspirate the dye from the posterior pole. Place the tip of the Charles flute cannula at the optic disc. When the most dye is removed, continue with an air x fluid exchange.

23.2 Removal of Subretinal Membranes (See Video)

Instruments:
(1) 20G subretinal spatula DORC 1295-1 0995
(2) 20G subretinal forceps DORC 1286 01 1095
(3) 20G or 23G Serrated jaws forceps

The surgery step-by-step:
1. Identify the subretinal membranes which have to be removed and those which can be left: Instil PFCL and identify those subretinal membranes which lift the retina.
2. Create two 20G sclerotomies. Remove either both instrument trocars and enlarge the sclerotomy with a V-lance (Alcon) or create two new sclerotomies (Fig. 23.5).
3. Insert a chandelier light.
4. Plan a retinotomy in the middle of the subretinal membrane.
5. Insert the subretinal spatula, pierce the retina and dissect the subretinal membrane from the retina (Fig. 23.6).
6. Now work bimanual with serrated jaws forceps and subretinal forceps: Place the subretinal forceps through the retinotomy, grasp the subretinal membrane with the subretinal forceps and pull it through the retinotomy

U. Spandau
St. Eriks Hospital, University of Stockholm, Stockholm, Sweden

Z. Tomic (✉)
Milos Klinika, Belgrade, Serbia
e-mail: zorannos@yahoo.se

U. Spandau et al. (eds.), *Retinal Detachment Surgery and Proliferative Vitreoretinopathy*,
https://doi.org/10.1007/978-3-031-11946-0_23

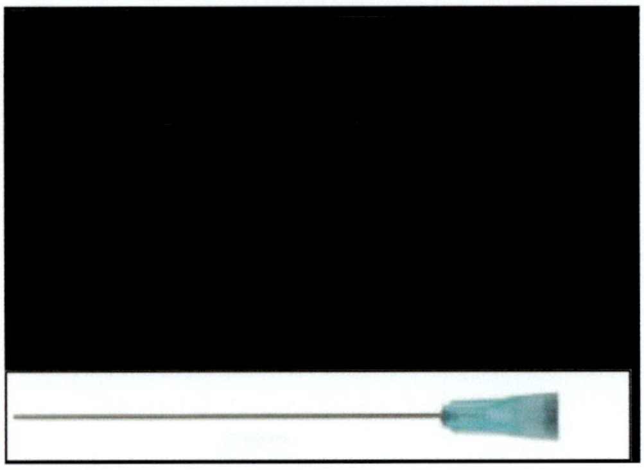

Fig. 23.1 A Charles flute needle

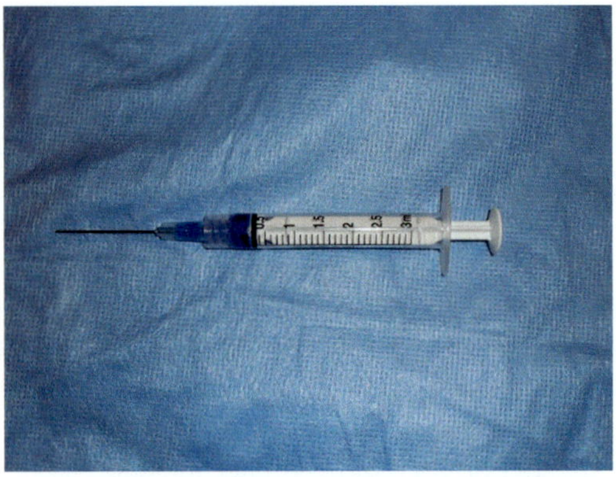

Fig. 23.2 A 3 cc syringe filled with trypane blue is easier to use than an original syringe

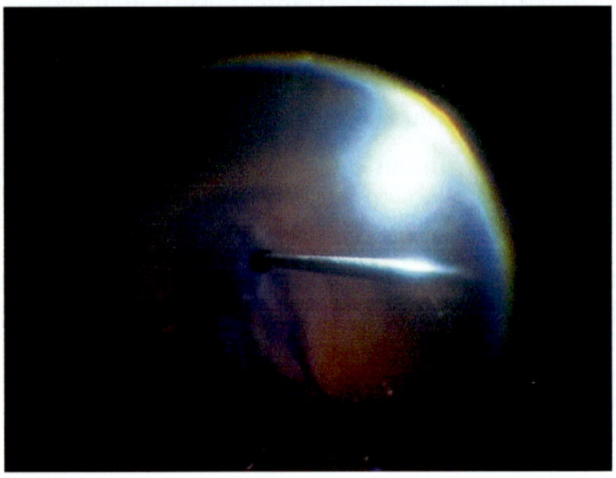

Fig. 23.3 The dye is dropped on the membrane

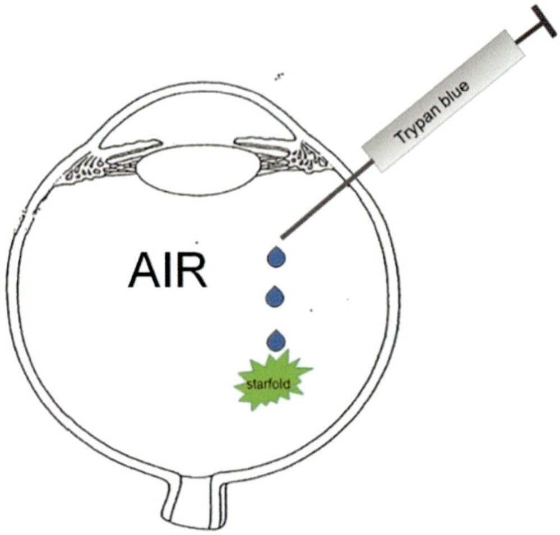

Fig. 23.4 The vitreous cavity is filled with air. This method increases the concentration of the dye and enables the staining of peripheral membranes

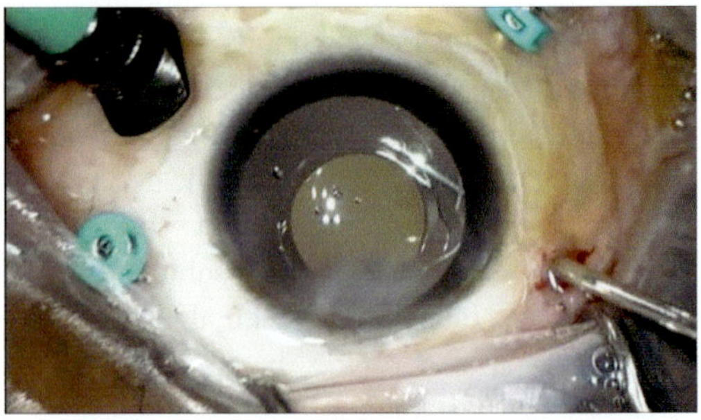

Fig. 23.5 Create first two 20G sclerotomies at 10 and 2 o'clock because the subretinal instruments are 20G

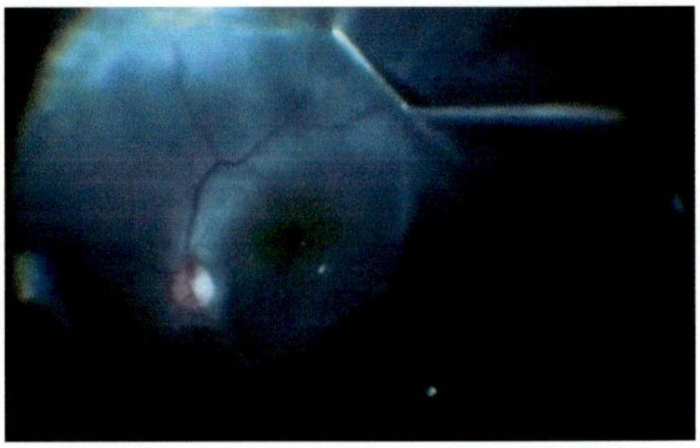

Fig. 23.6 Pierce the retina with the subretinal spatula and loosen the subretinal membranes

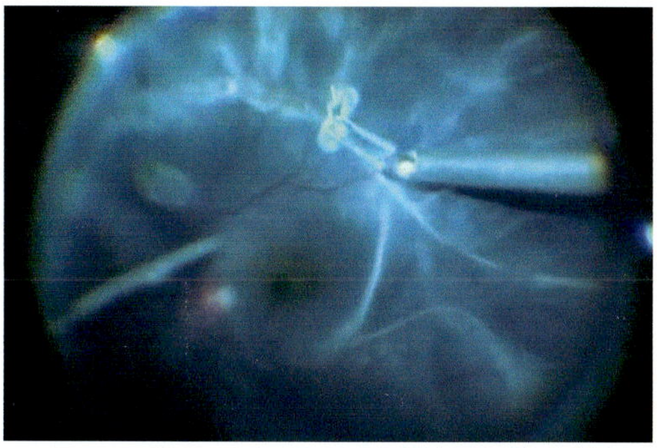

Fig. 23.7 Then grasp the membrane with the subretinal forceps and remove it together with a serrated jaws forceps

(Fig. 23.7). Then pull out the subretinal membrane with help of both forceps. If you do not work bimanual, then you will create a giant tear.

7. If the subretinal membrane breaks in small parts although it is not completely removed, then do not continue because the residual subretinal membrane creates no tension.
8. The manoeuvre 5–7 has to be performed from the nasal and temporal side for the same membrane.

23.3 180° Retinotomy

Introduction and definition: If despite meticulous transvitreal, epiretinal and subretinal dissection the retina remains foreshortened preventing an attachment of the retina with the retinal pigment epithelium, the surgeon should perform a retinotomy or retinectomy in order to relax the retina. **Retinotomy** involves incising the retina, whereas **retinectomy** involves excising the retina. The peripheral retina is cut parallel to the ora serrata (180, 270 or 360°) and the retinotomy edges are treated with laser photocoagulation in order to reattach the retina. See Diagram 23.1.

Retinotomy could be performed in a **radial** fashion, but most commonly it is done **circumferentially**, parallel to the ora serrata. The majority of PVR cases can be managed without retinotomy/retinectomy. We almost never use it in the first surgery, except for the penetrating injuries with PVR and incarceration of the retina in the penetrating wound. **The circumferential retinotomy** in repeated surgery for idiopathic PVR detachment is performed in the area with persistent contraction of the retina usually affecting the two lower quadrants, due to the

Diagram 23.1 The treatment algorithm regarding retinotomy

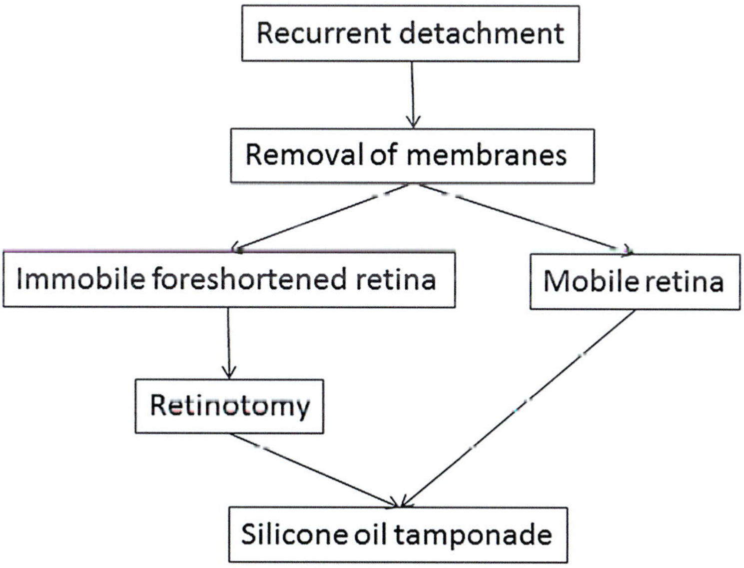

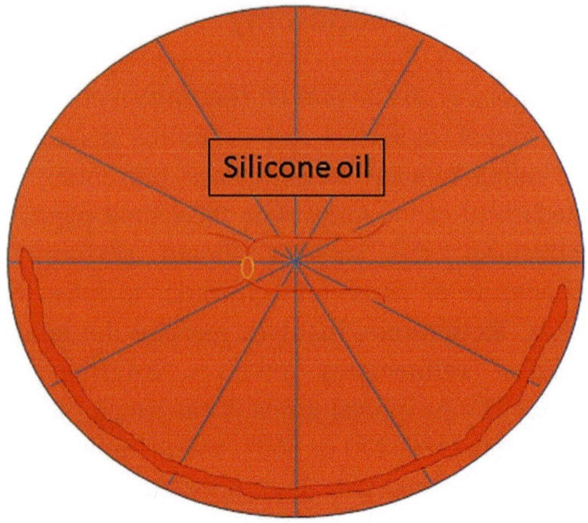

Fig. 23.8 A typical 180° retinotomy

physical property of the 1000 cSt silicone oil that is regularly used for the first surgery. This silicone oil is lighter than water and therefore is leaving some space filled with aqueous inferiorly thus tamponing better the upper two quadrants where recurrent detachment almost never occurs

Timing: A retinotomy (Figs. 23.8 and 23.9) should only be performed in the second (or later) surgery. You should avoid the retinotomy in the first surgery. Typically, it goes like this: PVR detachment and first surgery with silicone oil tamponade. Then inferior redetachment and second surgery with retinotomy and again silicone oil tamponade. Then 3 months later silicone oil removal.

Remark: Even if you perform a retinotomy, you need to remove all membranes up to the retinotomy edges. If you do not peel the membranes, then the retina will contract under silicone oil and the retinotomy edges will roll in.

Complications: The complication spectrum is big. Hypotony is a frequent side effect of retinotomy. The retina serves as a barrier between aqueous and choroid. A retinotomy and retinectomy remove this barrier partially and the IOP sinks. The consequences are hypotony and decompensated cornea which makes the removal of the silicone oil impossible. The redetachment rate after oil removal is reported to be 17–25%. In the silicone oil study, a redetachment rate of 20% after silicone oil removal has been observed. Around 40–50% of eyes with retinotomy are required to have a permanent silicone oil tamponade [1–10].

Remark: The technique of retinotomy is technically very difficult. Retinotomy does not mean: Circumferential cut in the retina with the vitreous cutter, then laser and finally injection of silicone oil. This eye will develop a PVR redetachment and the proliferating membranes did not develop after retinotomy but were present from the beginning. If you do a retinotomy, you must also remove all membranes; otherwise, you will fail. In my hands (US), retinotomy does not work well. I prefer to place a 90° circumferential buckle on the inferior equator and as the final technique I use retinotomy. In the hands of ZT, who masters the technique of macular translocation, retinotomy works well and the postoperative results are good.

Conclusion: Retinotomy and retinectomy are surgical procedures to attach foreshortened retina

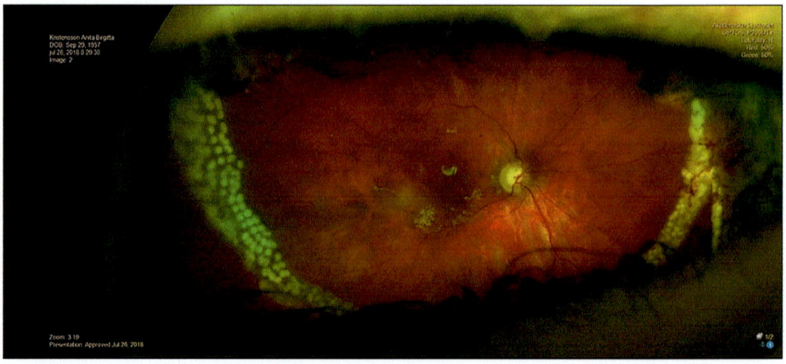

Fig. 23.9 Wide angle photo of a 180° retinotomy

secondary to intraretinal PVR. The procedure and the effect are traumatic for the eye and result in a huge complication spectrum in which hypotony dominates. A retinotomy is therefore the final step in our surgical repertoire to reattach the retina. An alternative is a 90° circumferential buckle giving the opportunity to perform a retinotomy at a later stage. If you perform a retinotomy in the first surgery, then you may regret your decision later on. You cannot bring back the retina which has been cut. In addition, if you did not remove the vitreous base completely and all epiretinal membranes, then a reproliferation will occur at the retinotomy edges. This will lead to a new, more centrally located retinotomy and this can trigger a vicious circle until you reach the temporal arcade. In addition, if you perform a retinotomy, you increase the risk of a permanent silicone oil tamponade. The larger the retinotomy, the bigger the risk for permanent tamponade.

The main surgical steps are as follows:

The relaxing retinotomy consists of three main surgical steps:

1. Ora parallel diathermy
2. Retinotomy
3. Removal of anterior retina (retinectomy).

The most common problem with retinotomy is the underestimation of the necessary size of the tissue to be removed so that contraction persists. The most common size of retinotomy is 180° tapered to the two lower quadrants and extending from 3 over 6 to 9 o'clock. A 360° retinotomy is seldom and may be required in penetrating injuries with the incarceration of the retina and PVR stage D. It is usually followed by some distortion of the retina after reattachment and requires relocation of the retina using the flute needle with a silicone tip in order to re-establish its normal anatomical position.

Instruments:

(1) 25G or 27G Vitreous cutter

or vertical scissors

(2) 23G or 25G knob spatula (Eye Tech, UK) **or** flute needle with silicone ti

(3) PFCL

(4) 1000 cSt or 5000 cSt silicone oil.

The surgery step-by step:

1. **Row of diathermy as anteriorly as possible within the contracted retina**
2. **Retinotomy**
3. **Retinectomy (Removal of remaining anterior retina)**
4. **Haemostasis of the retinotomy edge**
5. **Injection of PFCL**
6. **Flattening of retinotomy edges**
7. **Attachment test**
8. **Laser treatment**
9. **PFCL x air exchange**
10. **Air x silicone oil exchange**.

Every step in detail:

1. **Row of diathermy as anteriorly as possible within the contracted retina**

Retinotomy should be performed as anteriorly as possible in order to preserve the healthy retina. The area to be incised should be marked with a row of endodiathermy and incision should be tapered into the normal retina at both ends of the contracted retina. If endodiathermy is not possible, i.e. the retina does not become white during endodiathermy, then vitreous is left. Remove the residual vitreous with the vitreous cutter and continue with diathermy (Fig. 23.10). If you find a membrane at the edge, remove it at once; otherwise, it will continue to proliferate and cause a recurrent detachment.

2. **Retinotomy**
3. **Retinectomy (Removal of remaining anterior retina)**
4. **Haemostasis of the retinotomy edge**

The retinotomy is performed with the vitreous cutter at a low cut rate of 100–150 cuts/min or vertical scissors. A 27G vitreous cutter is due to its size very suitable for a retinotomy. The remaining anterior retina is then removed with

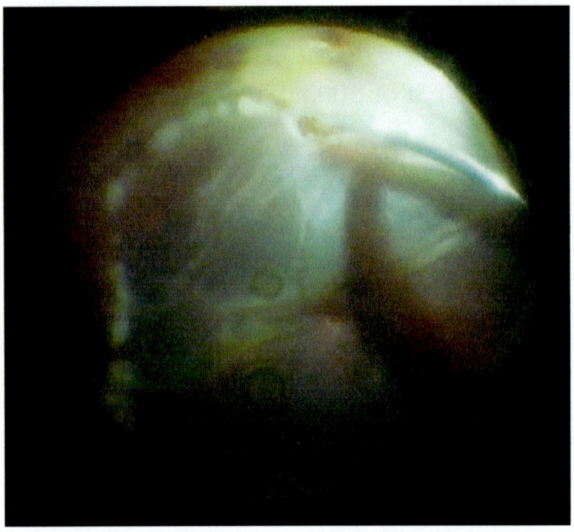

Fig. 23.10 Diathermy before retinotomy

the vitreous cutter at a higher cut rate of 5000–7500 cuts/min and is called **anterior retinectomy** (Fig. 23.11). Meticulous haemostasis of the retinotomy edge is essential, as any bleeding may lead to recurrent PVR.

5. **Injection of PFCL**
6. **Flatten the retinotomy edges**

The retina is then reattached using perfluorocarbon liquid (PFCL). Instil PFCL up to the retinal edge. Folds or areas of retinal distortion are adjusted with a retinal manipulator (knob spatula) or a flute needle with a silicone tip. In the case of residual membranes, dissect the membrane with a membrane pic or CRVO knife. The PFCL is not removed for this manoeuvre; it creates countertension. Grasp the membrane with forceps and remove it. You may need to work bimanual with the forceps in one hand and the dissection instrument in the other hand. If you lift the retina carefully, then the PFCL will not spill over the edges and flow subretinally.

7. **Attachment test**
8. **Laser treatment**

Before continuing with laser photocoagulation, check whether the retinotomy edges are

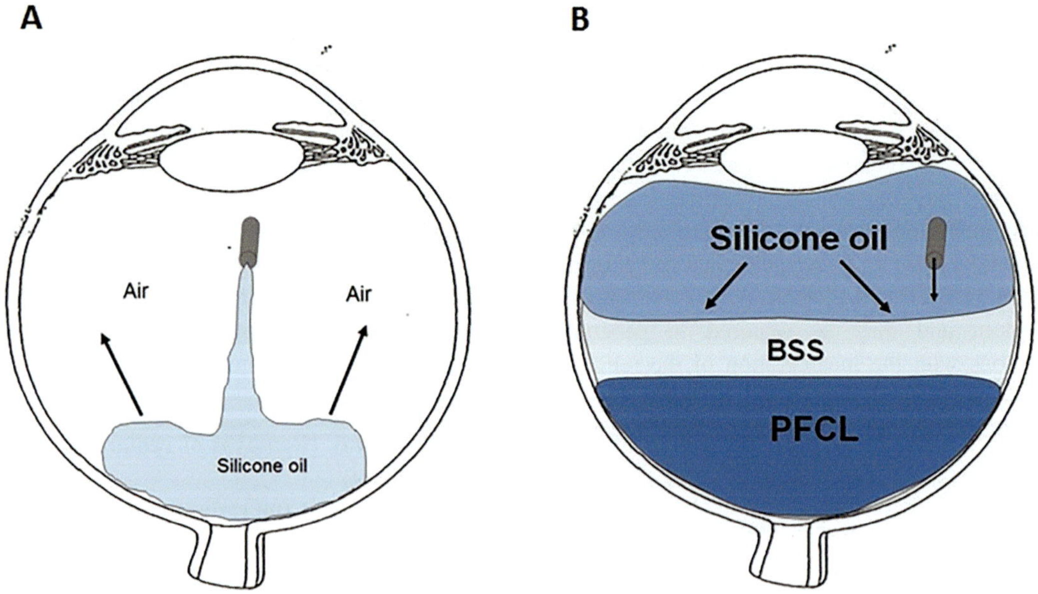

Fig. 23.11 Silicone oil injection in an air-filled eye (**A**) and in PFCL-filled eye (**B**). In an air-filled eye, the silicone oil fills the eye from posterior to anterior (**A**); in a PFCL-filled eye, the silicone oil fills the eye from anterior to posterior (**B**). In case of a retinotomy, it is advisable to use (**A**) instead of (**B**). Why? In (**A**), the retinotomy edges are attached under air and remain attached when the silicone oil is filled in. In (**B**), the retinotomy edges are attached under PFCL but detach as soon as the silicone oil comes

completely attached under PFCL). If not, then fix the problem: remove the membrane or enlarge the retinotomy. If the attachment test is positive, continue with laser treatment.

For laser photocoagulation of retinal edges, we recommend a higher laser power than usual. A higher laser power induces an immediate congealing of outer retinal proteins by heat resulting in a more immediate adhesion. Our laser power for retinotomy edges with an argon laser device (Iridex, CA) is Power: 100–300 mW; Duration: **300** ms; Interval: 300 ms. This is especially the case for laser treatment of retinotomy edges. For retinal holes and for a laser cerclage, a reduced laser power is recommended.

9. **PFCL x air exchange**
10. **Air x silicone oil exchange**

For this step, two methods are possible (Fig. 23.11): (1) First a PFCL x air exchange and then a silicone oil injection. (2) A direct PFCL x silicone oil exchange. We prefer the first method because the retinotomy edges detach and enrol with the second method.

Start with a PFCL x air exchange until the air reaches the retinal edges. It is important to aspirate thoroughly the fluid at the edges of the retinotomy to avoid slippage. Then continue to remove the residual PFCL. The whole procedure is finished with an injection of 1000 cSt silicone oil into the air-filled cavity. We use never gas in an eye with retinotomy because in case of recurrent detachment there will be a fast progression to PVR. Heavy silicone oil such as Densiron 68 can be used but is not necessary. If the retina is relieved, then 1000 cSt oil is sufficient.

FAQ's:

(1) How to avoid *slippage*? In the case of a large retinotomy (>180°), slippage is possible. Important is a strong laser treatment that creates immediate retinal adhesion and a meticulous aspiration of fluid at the retinotomy edges.
(2) *Too short retinotomy*: If the retinotomy is too short (if contracted retina remains), then the retina is under tension and silicone oil will flow subretinally. If this happens remove the silicone oil, enlarge the retinotomy and reinject the silicone oil.
(3) *Attachment test*. If the retinotomy edges are not attached under PFCL or air, then do not continue with a silicone oil tamponade. Silicone oil has a lower surface tension pressure than air. It is therefore likely that the retina detaches under silicone oil. Enlarge the retinotomy instead.
(4) *Is the retinotomy large enough*? In case of an inferior recurrent detachment with foreshortened retina, we recommend to do a 180° retinotomy from the beginning: from 3 o'clock over 6 o'clock to 9 o'clock.
(5) *PFCL x silicone oil tamponade* or PFCL x air x silicone oil tamponade? For silicone oil tamponades, two surgical techniques exist: (1) A PFCL against silicone oil exchange and (2) a PFCL against air and then an air against silicone oil exchange. We use a PFCL against silicone air exchange in giant tears and traumatic retinal detachments. Otherwise, we use always a PFCL against air exchange. Why? (1) Visualization of PFCL phase and silicone oil phase is difficult. (2) PFCL and air are very potent in attaching the retina. PFCL attaches the retina with its gravity and air with its high surface tension pressure. Silicone oil, however, has a low surface tension pressure. If you exchange from PFCL to silicone oil, then you remove a fluid with good attachment quality to a fluid with low attachment quality. If you do a PFCL against silicone oil exchange in an eye with 180° retinotomy, then the retinal edges lift up. This will not happen if you exchange from silicone oil to air. In an air-filled eye, the silicone oil falls on the posterior pole and fills the eye up from posterior to anterior.
(6) *Lifted retinotomy edges during/after laser photocoagulation*: Usually the retinotomy edges do not lift if you laser photocoagulate them; even if you use a high laser power. They will, however, lift when membranes are present. To prevent uplifting, all

membranes must be removed. If the membranes cannot be removed because they are very attached and fibrotic, then perform a few radial cuts with the scissors at the retinotomy edge. This will result in an attachment of the retinotomy edges.

References

1. Vitrectomy with silicone oil or sulfur hexafluoride gas in eyes with severe proliferative vitreoretinopathy: results of a randomized clinical trial. Silicone Study Report 1. Arch Ophthalmol. 1992;110(6):770–9.
2. Han DP, Lewis MT, Kuhn EM, et al. Relaxing retinotomies and retinectomies: surgical results and predictors of visual outcome. Arch Ophthalmol. 1990;108:694–7.
3. Federman JL, Eagle RC Jr. Extensive peripheral retinectomy combined with posterior 360° retinotomy for retinal reattachment in advanced proliferative vitreoretinopathy cases. Ophthalmology. 1990;97:1305–20.
4. Zivojnovic R. Silicone oil in vitreoretinal surgery. Dordrecht: Martinus Nijhoff/Dr W Junk;1987. p. 141–52.
5. Blumenkrantz MS, Azen SP, Aaberg T, et al. Relaxing retinotomy with silicone oil or long-acting gas in eyes with severe proliferative vitreoretinopathy. Silicone Study Report 5. The Silicone Oil Study Group. Am J Ophthalmol. 1993;116:557–64.
6. Bovey EH, De Ancos E, Gonvers M. Retinotomies of 180° or more. Retina. 1995;15:394–8.
7. Quiram PA, Gonzales CR, Hu W, et al. Outcomes of vitrectomy with inferior retinectomy in patients with recurrent rhegmatogenous retinal detachments and proliferative vitreoretinopathy. Ophthalmology. 2006;113:2041–7.
8. Grigoropoulos VG, Benson S, Bunce C, Charteris DG. Functional outcome and prognostic factors in 304 eyes managed by retinectomy. Graefes Arch Clin Exp Ophthalmol. 2007;245:641–9.
9. Shalaby KA. relaxing retinotomies and retinectomies in the management of retinal detachment with severe proliferative vitreoretinopathy (PVR). Clin Ophthalmol. 2010;4:1107–14.
10. Adelman RA, Parnes AJ, Sipperley JO, Ducournau D. Strategy for the management of complex retinal detachments: the European Vitreo-Retinal Society retinal detachment study report 2. Ophthalmology. 2013;120:1809–13.

Part V
Anterior and Intraretinal PVR Detachment

Intraretinal and anterior PVR come often together and are a major surgical challenge. This part describes first the pathophysiology of anterior PVR and then the surgical management. Then the pathology of intraretinal PVR is explained in detail followed by the surgical management.

All videos of this part are found in a playlist on my youTube channel:

https://youtube.com/playlist?list=PL0dKYclPD7yMn861X0g-aHCS6KZ5NcH1N

Chapter 24: **Vitreous Anatomy, Anterior PVR and Hypotony**

Anterior PVR Hypotony

PVR Prevention

Chapter 25: **Surgical Management of Anterior PVR**

Anterior retinal displacement

Anterior PVR secondary morning glory syndrome

Chapter 27: **Surgical Management of Intraretinal PVR**

27G vitrectomy and episcleral buckling

27G ppV and segmental buckle for primary RD with PVR at 9 o'clock

Inferior PVR detachment part 1

Inferior PVR detachment part 2

Inferior PVR detachment operated with scleral buckle

Failed RD surgery.

Vitreous Anatomy, Anterior PVR, and Hypotony

24

Diego Ruiz-Casas

24.1 Introduction

Chronic hypotony, defined as an intraocular pressure (IOP) lower than 5 mmHg for two consecutive measurements at least 1 month apart, is associated with poor visual outcomes, maculopathy, papillary edema, corneal opacification, membrane proliferation, retinal detachment (RD), and eventually phthisis bulbi [12, 26].

Chronic hypotony after vitrectomy to treat RD is associated with proliferative vitreoretinopathy (PVR) and ocular trauma in 18–24% of cases and 7–10% even with attached retina. Hypotony occurs twice as frequently with the use of C3F8 compared to silicone oil tamponade (31% versus 18%) [1, 3].

24.2 Hypotony Physiopathology

Many hypotheses have been forwarded to explain hypotony, i.e., cyclodialysis, intraocular inflammation, rerouting of aqueous outflow to the absorption compartment of the retinal pigment epithelium and choriocapillaris, or ciliary body damage [12, 26]. However, in cases of RD, if the retina is already attached, hypotony generally is related to ciliary body detachment due to anterior PVR, referred to as proliferative vitreociliopathy [7]. The contracted anterior hyaloid (AH) pulls the vitreous base (VB) anteriorly and detaches the ciliary body, leading to aqueous humor hyposecretion and increased outflow [1, 3, 8, 9, 18, 20, 21]. Coleman [7] reported that the IOP decreases when at least two clock hours of ciliary body detachment are present.

Meticulous removal of the AH during the initial surgery might prevent hypotony especially in eyes undergoing retinotomy or retinectomy [19]. The endoscopic examination has shown that despite the fact that retinectomy increases aqueous outflow, the main cause of hypotony in these cases is anterior PVR with AH contraction and ciliary body detachment. If the anterior retina was not removed completely, it was pulled anteriorly and integrated into a fibrotic tissue covering the ciliary body [3, 8, 11].

24.3 Chronic Hypotony Treatments

Several medical treatments are available to treat chronic hypotony: Ibopamine drops [13], monthly anterior chamber or pars plana viscoelastic injections [28], and intravitreous corticosteroids or laser trabecular meshwork sclerosis [24], but none is efficacious.

Surgical closure of cyclodialysis clefts is effective if they are present and no medical or laser treatment is effective [15].

D. Ruiz-Casas (✉)
Ramón y Cajal Hospital, University of Alcalá de Henares, Madrid, Spain
e-mail: drdiegoruizcasas@gmail.com

U. Spandau et al. (eds.), *Retinal Detachment Surgery and Proliferative Vitreoretinopathy*,
https://doi.org/10.1007/978-3-031-11946-0_24

Most cases of hypotony in RD result from anterior PVR, and different surgical techniques have been used to deal with anterior hyaloid (AH) scarring:

(a) Pars plana vitrectomy to remove lens remnants, intraocular lenses (IOLs), and anterior PVR membranes (covering the pars plana and pars plicata) resulted in resolution of the hypotony in 33–66% of cases [19, 22, 29]
(b) Endoscopic anterior membrane dissection that preserved the IOL resulted in resolution of the hypotony in 30% of patients [17].

24.4 Anterior Vitreous Base Anatomy

The vitreous base (VB), i.e., the retinal and pars plana area with intimate vitreoretinal and vitreo-pars plana epithelium adhesion, covers from 3 mm posterior to 2 mm anterior to the ora serrata. During vitreoretinal surgery, the posterior hyaloid (PH) is detached until it reaches its insertion point at the VB posterior edge, and then it is shaved at this area. Likewise, the anterior hyaloid (AH) is inserted at the anterior edge of the VB [10].

The AH is attached to several ocular structures through several ligaments:

- The posterior ciliary ligament (PCL) is the attachment of the AH to the anterior edge of the VB.
- The anterior ciliary ligament (ACL) is the strong attachment of the AH to the ciliary body and ciliary processes.
- Salzman's hiatus (SH) is the space between the epithelium of the pars plana and pars plicata and AH, limited posteriorly by the PCL and anteriorly by the ACL.
- The retrolental ligament or Wieger's ligament (RL) is the attachment of the AH to the posterior and peripheral lens capsule.
- Berger's space (BS) is the space between the posterior lens capsule and the AH medial to the RL and connected to Cloquet's canal.
- The canal of Petit (ChP) is the space between the posterior lens capsule and AH lateral to the RL and medial to the ACL and posterior zonular adhesions.

The VB ends anteriorly at the PCL; from this ligament, the AH is no longer intimately adherent to the epithelium of the pars plana and plicata. Thus, it is possible to detach and dissect the AH in this area [2] up to the ACL where there is strong adhesion between the AH and ACL and posterior zonules [2, 4, 6] (see Fig. 24.1).

24.5 Anterior Hyaloid Dissection

The AH is involved in accommodation by inducing VB traction when the ciliary body contracts. Therefore, unremoved AH between the ACL and PCL might be associated with anterior retinal traction and redetachment, [14]. Likewise, AH contraction in PVR causes anterior retinal loop and ciliary body detachment with subsequent hypotony [5]. Thus, AH removal might improve the success rate and reduce the recurrence rate of RD with and without PVR [23] (see Fig. 24.2).

AH detachment from RL is theoretically feasible [25]. The surgical techniques to detach the AH from RL are as follows:

(a) Hydrodissection by injecting fluid from the anterior and posterior chambers through the zonular area [16].
(b) Mechanical detachment of the AH: aspirating the AH at RL, Berger's space, or canal of Petit and then downward pulling in every quadrant [27].

AH detachment from RL was successful in up to 50% of cases, but it was still attached to the ciliary body and posterior zonule due to the strong adhesion of the AH at the ACL and posterior zonules [2, 4]. Thus, AH detachment did not allow vitreoretinal surgeons to remove the anterior vitreous traction from the ciliary body to the VB and it might damage the posterior zonular support.

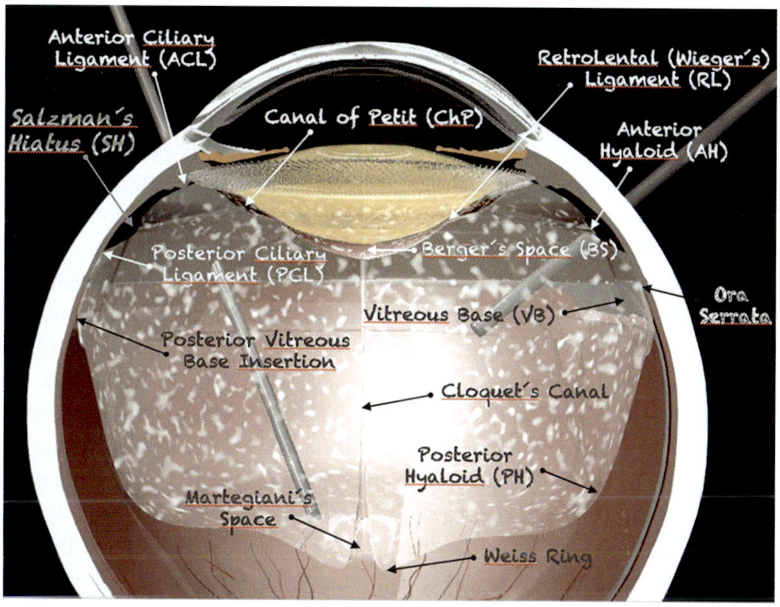

Fig. 24.1 Vitreous anatomy

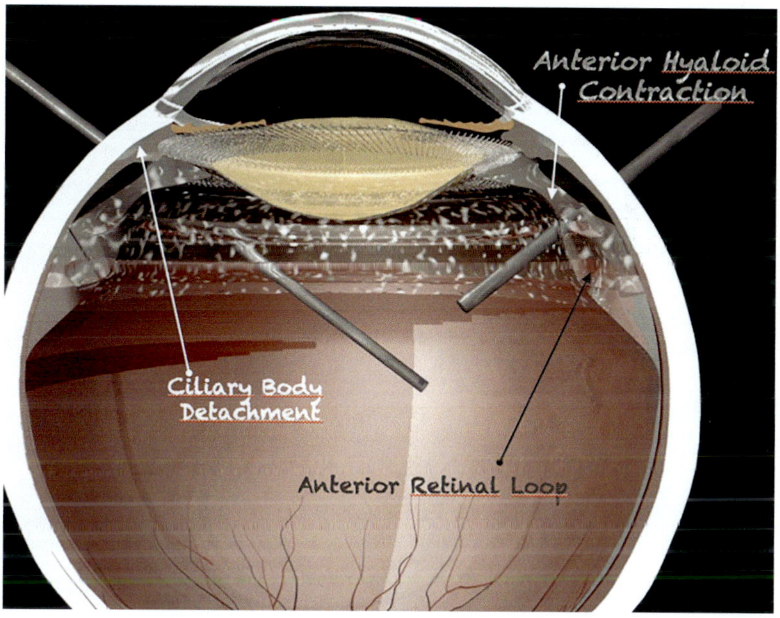

Fig. 24.2 Anterior PVR with anterior hyaloid contraction, ciliary body detachment, and anterior retinal loop due to unremoved anterior hyaloid

Nevertheless, there is an anatomic area between the ACL and PCL in which the AH is virtually detached from the epithelium of the pars plana and plicata, that is, Salzman's Hiatus (SH). In this area, the AH can be dissected by cutting with the vitrectome and removing any vitreous scaffold and traction from the ciliary body and zonular fibers to the VB [6].

Vitrectomy is performed first by inducing a posterior vitreous detachment (PVD), then removing the central vitreous without indentation (central vitrectomy), followed by shaving of the posterior hyaloid and VB with deep indentation (vitreous shaving), and finally dissecting the AH at SH (complete vitrectomy). AH dissection (AHD) is also referred to as hyaloido-zonulocapsulotomy [6].

Complete vitrectomy with AHD can be improved by detaching the AH from the RL and then removing the AH up to the posterior zonules and ACL attachments, but this maneuver does not relax the traction and might impair the stability of the posterior zonules and lens or IOL (see Fig. 24.3).

AHD is risky in phakic patients because of the anterior location of the SH. However, it is possible to perform AHD by placing scleral microcannulas 4–4.5 mm from the limbus and closer to 3 and 9 clock hours. Indentation is needed and it may be done from the opposite side by attempting to keep the vitrectome shaft parallel to the indented area or by indenting from the same side of the vitrectome at the superior, nasal, and temporal quadrants and moving the infusion line from the inferotemporal cannula to a superior one to dissect the AH at the inferior quadrant from the inferotemporal cannula without crossing the lens.

Since most phakic patients undergoing vitrectomy will develop significant cataracts in subsequent years, it is logical to perform combined phacovitrectomy in presbyopic cases with a RD. Phacovitrectomy allows complete vitreous removal and avoids future cataract surgery. In combined procedures, the anterior capsule should be polished thoroughly to improve intraoperative visualization and avoid capsular phimosis and opacification, and then a complete vitrectomy should be performed by dissecting the AH at SH. After complete vitrectomy with AHD, there are only two disconnected vitreous remnants at the VB and the ciliary body. If the AH also is detached from the RL, the ciliary body remnant is smaller but does not affect the VB traction (see Fig. 24.4).

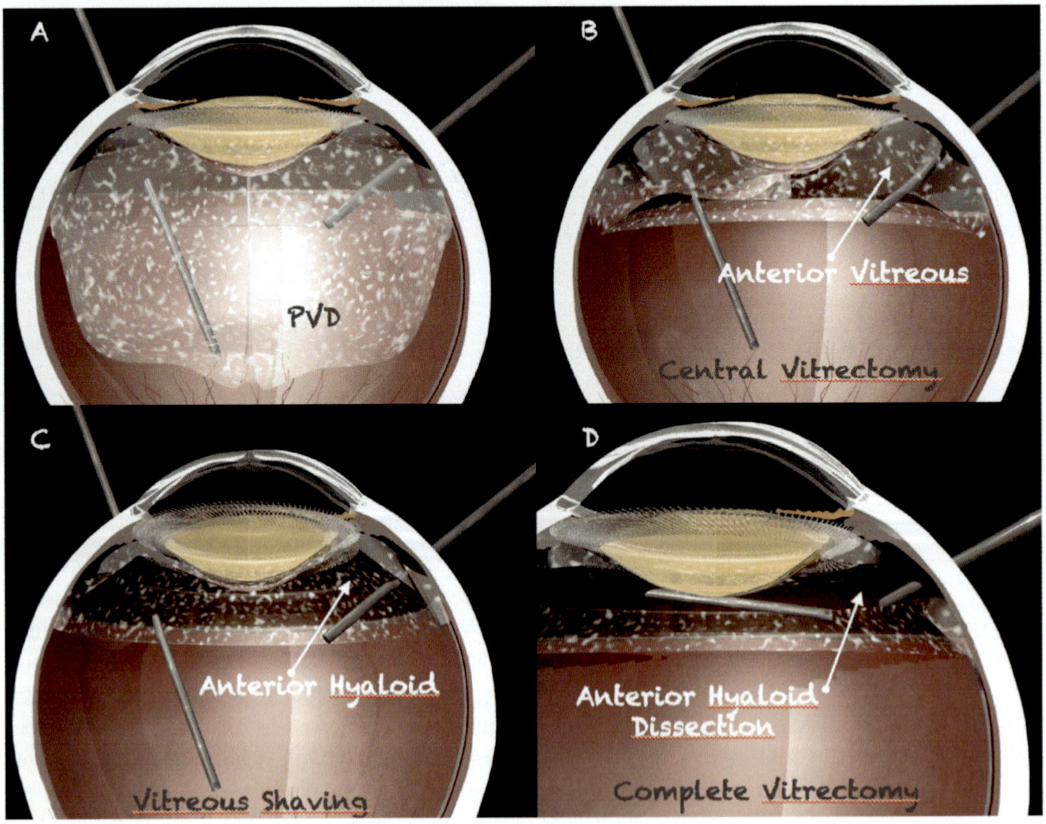

Fig. 24.3 Vitrectomy completeness in phakic patients. **A** PVD induction. **B** Central Vitrectomy. **C** Vitreous Shaving. **D** Complete vitrectomy with anterior hyaloid dissection (AHD)

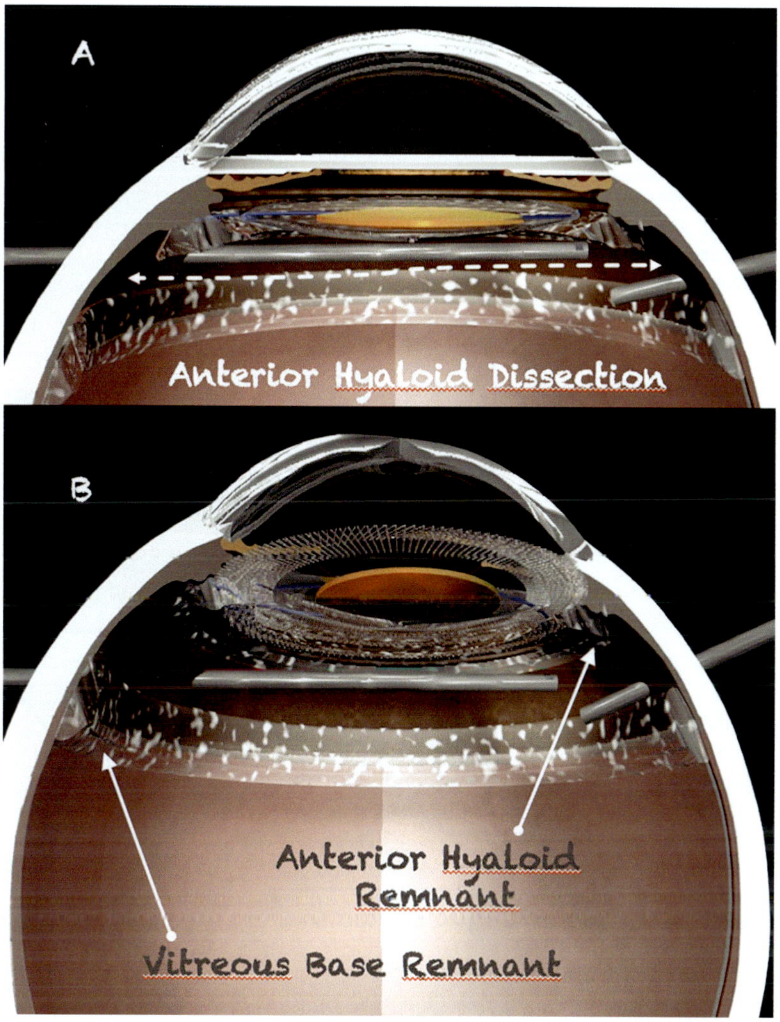

Fig. 24.4 Complete vitrectomy in pseudophakic eyes **A** Anterior Hyaloid Dissection (AHD), cutting of the anterior hyaloid connections between anterior and posterior ciliary ligaments through Salzman's space. **B** Complete vitrectomy with vitreous remnants at the vitreous base and ciliary body-zonular area

24.6 Anterior PVR

The development of PVR affects the retina with the formation of epiretinal and subretinal membranes, intraretinal shortening, and vitreous contraction. Vitreous contraction at the VB induces centripetal traction, which can be treated with encircling buckling and/or peripheral relaxing retinectomies. Retinectomies also relax anteroposterior traction (from the optic nerve to ora serrata) due to stiffening of the retina.

Likewise, AH contracts in PVR and pulls the ciliary body and VB together. This anteroposterior traction (from the ciliary body to VB) detaches the ciliary body inducing hypotony and displaces the peripheral retina anteriorly, creating an anterior retinal loop with or without retinal detachment. These complications occur even if an encircling buckle is used since the buckle relaxes centripetal traction but does not relieve anteroposterior traction. If a retinectomy is performed without AHD and complete retinal remnants/detached pars plana epithelium removal, these tissues are pulled anteriorly creating scar tissue over pars plana and pars plicata. In aphakic patients, the scar tissue also might involve lens capsular remnants and iris, pulling them posteriorly (see Fig. 24.5).

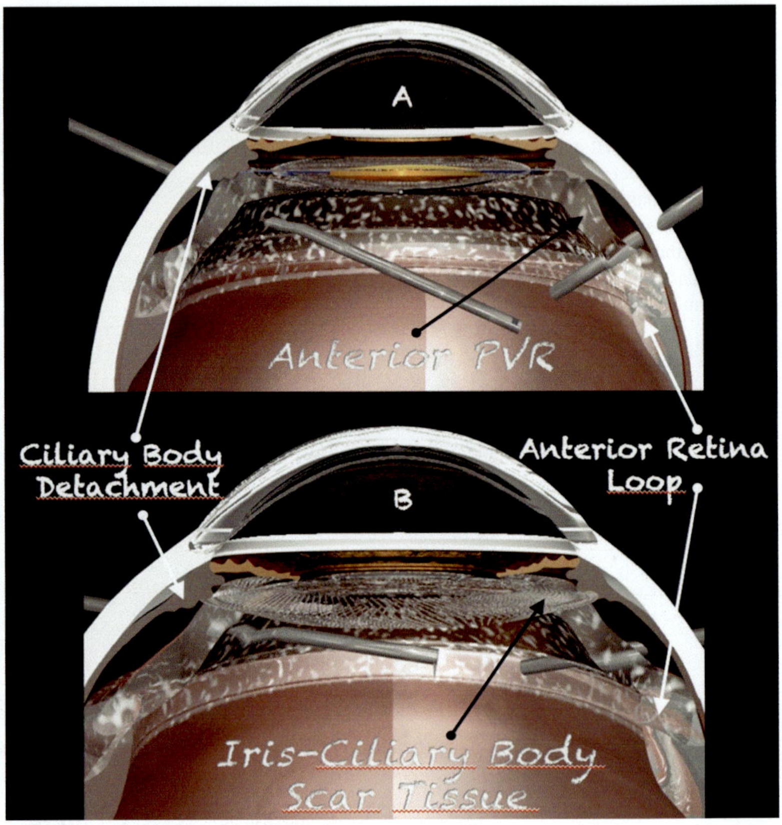

Fig. 24.5 **A** Anterior PVR in a pseudophakic eye. The AH contraction pulls on the VB and peripheral retina inducing an anterior retinal loop and on the ciliary body inducing ciliary body detachment. **B** Anterior PVR in an aphakic eye. The AH with zonular fibers and lens capsular remnants form scar tissue over the ciliary body. Scarring involves the iris, which is pulled posteriorly and becomes mydriatic. The AH contraction pulls on the VB and peripheral retina inducing an anterior retinal loop and on the ciliary body inducing ciliary body detachment

24.7 Surgical Technique to Remove Anterior PVR

Apart from dealing with RD and posterior PVR, vitreoretinal surgeons should look for anterior PVR and remove the AH traction on the VB and the ciliary body by detaching or dissecting the AH. Phakic patients with anterior PVR must be managed with a combination of phacovitrectomy or lensectomy to properly manage the anterior vitreous pathology.

AH detachment is easier to perform in PVR cases since collagen proliferation stiffens the AH. The AH can be aspirated using a vitreous cutter and then pulled downward until it detaches from the RL, posterior zonules, and ACL. If the AH adhesion is too strong to be aspirated, a retinal pick or forceps can be used to grasp it at the RL, Berger's space, or canal of Petit spaces and then pull it downward until it is completely detached. Finally, the AH is shaved up to the PCL and silicone oil is left in the eye to help ciliary body reattachment and hypotony recovery.

Frequently, detaching the AH can be unsuccessful or risky due to extreme AH adherence to the posterior zonules and ACL. In that case, anterior hyaloid dissection (AHD) at SH should be performed instead.

The AHD is harder in PVR cases because the vitreous cutter can barely penetrate the scarred AH. An MVR blade is used to incise the AH until SH is reached and opened. Vertical scissors also can be used to engage the AH, pull it from SH, and cut it. The AH gap then is widened to 360 degrees with the vitreous cutter or scissors (if too rigid). The AH then is shaved anteriorly up to the ACL and posteriorly up to the PCL leaving two remnant vitreous rings at the VB and ciliary body/posterior zonular area.

After the AHD, the AH anteroposterior traction is relaxed and the AH remnant at the ciliary body/posterior zonular area should not prevent the ciliary body from attaching, but aqueous secretion might decrease. However, stripping this AH remnant with forceps might damage the zonules, losing the iridozonular diaphragm and risking silicone oil migration into the anterior chamber. Since the hypotony recovery success rates range from 20 to 60%, leaving the AH remnant and IOL without risking zonular damage might be optimal (see Fig. 24.6).

In aphakic patients with PVR, the AH with capsular lens remnants and zonular fibers form scar tissue involving the iris, ciliary body, VB, and anterior retina. Aphakic patients have no irido-lens diaphragm to keep silicone oil in the vitreous cavity if aqueous secretion does not improve postoperatively. Thus, any scarred AH tissue from the ciliary body should be removed completely to eliminate all traction on the ciliary body and maximize the recovery of the ciliary body.

The AH is detached from the zonular remnants and ACL adhesions using a retinal pick or serrated forceps pulling the tissue downward in every quadrant. If remnants of the AH are found on the ciliary body, they are stripped with forceps to remove any traction. Once the strong ciliary body adhesion is relieved, some exudation from the ciliary processes and pigment dispersion from the iris and ciliary body usually occur. The detached scarred AH then is shaved up to the PCL. Finally, silicone oil (SO) is left in the eye to aid ciliary body reattachment and hypotony recovery. An inferior Ando iridotomy must be performed to keep silicone oil in the vitreous cavity and avoid anterior chamber silicone oil

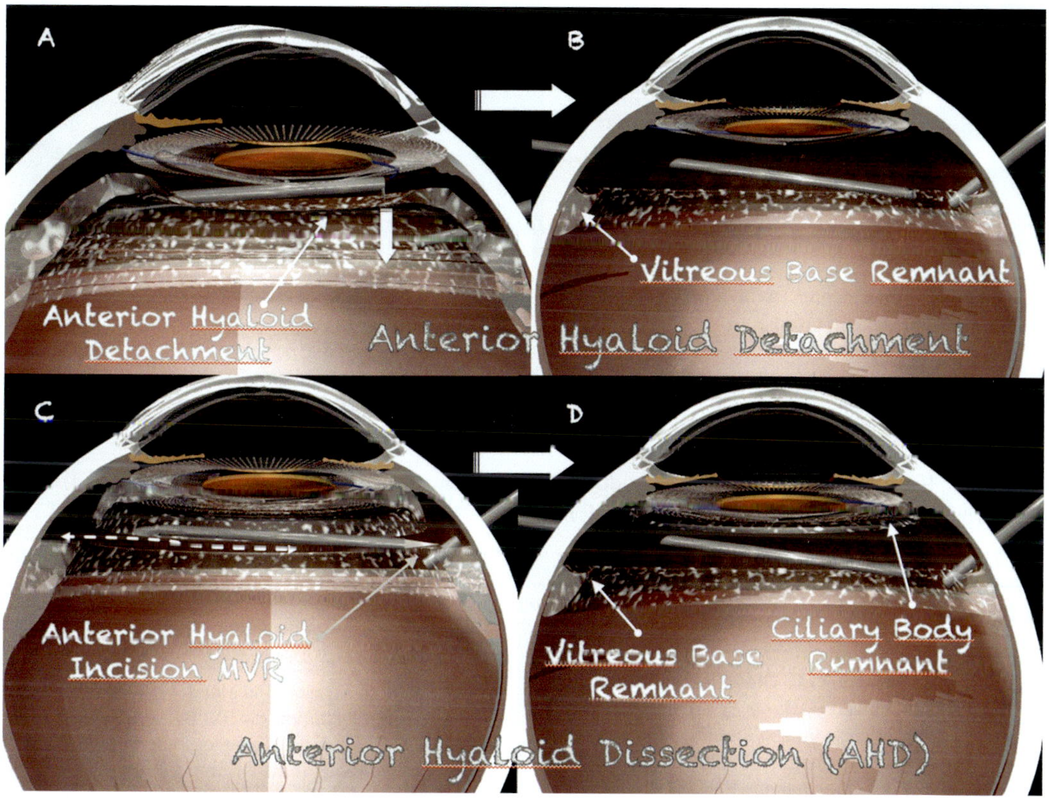

Fig. 24.6 Pseudophakic anterior PVR removal. **A**) Scarred AH detachment by downward pulling using a pick or forceps. **B** Complete traction removal from the ciliary body and the VB after removal of AH. **C** Incision of the scarred AH at SH with an MVR blade. **D** The final result after removing the AH with PVR leaving the VB and a scarred AH remnant at the ciliary body and zonular area

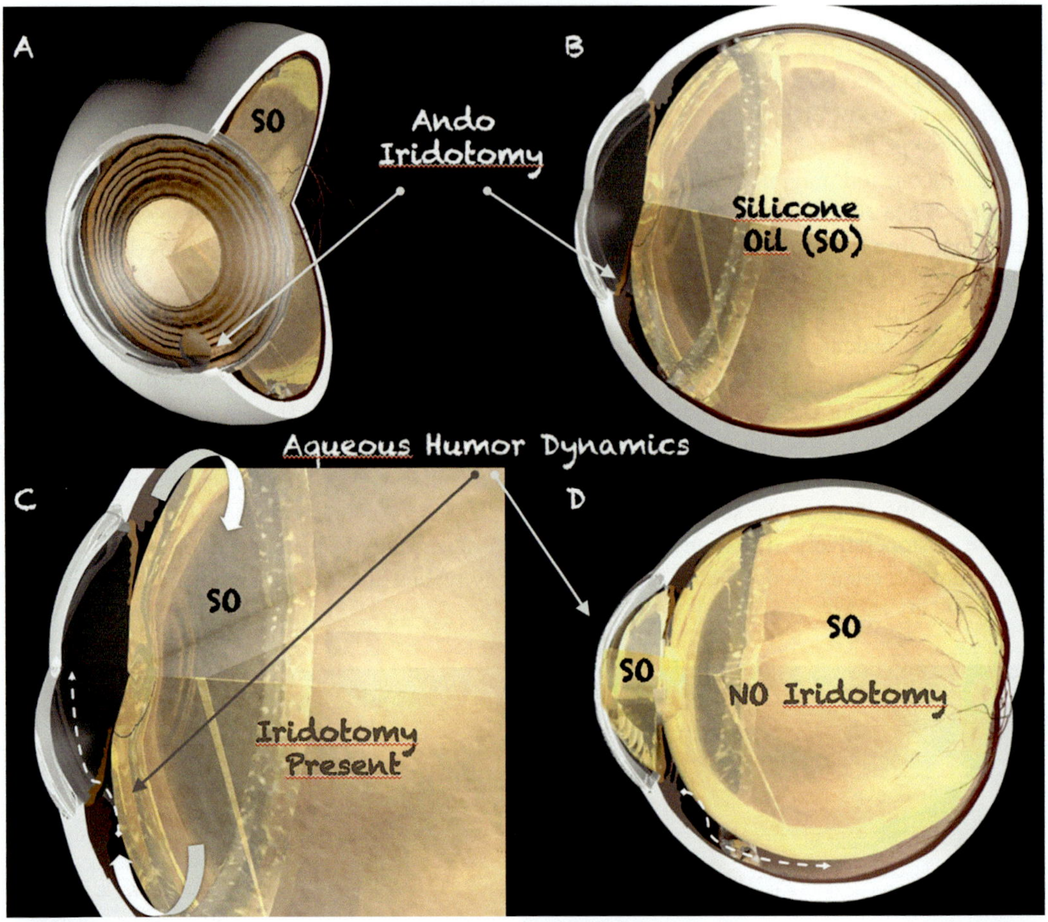

Fig. 24.7 Ando Iridotomy. **A** An inferolateral Ando iridotomy. **B** When an aphakic patient undergoes an inferior Ando iridotomy, aqueous moves into the anterior chamber and keeps the silicone oil in the vitreous cavity. **C** Aqueous humor dynamics with Ando iridotomy, aqueous moves around the ciliary body and into the anterior chamber through inferior iridotomy. **D** When an Ando iridotomy is not performed in an aphakic patient, the aqueous humor collects in the vitreous cavity and silicone oil is pushed into the anterior chamber

migration. If heavy oil was used, the iridotomy should be performed superiorly (see Fig. 24.7).

References

1. Adile SL, Peyman GA, Greve MD, Millsap CM, Verma LK, Wafapoor, H., & Soheilian, M. Postoperative chronic pressure abnormalities in the vitreon study. Ophthalmic Surg. 1994;25(9):584–9. http://www.ncbi.nlm.nih.gov/pubmed/7830998.
2. Albrecht M, Eisner G. The hyalo-capsular zonula. Graefe's Arch Clin Exp Ophthalmol. 1982;218 (2):88–92. http://www.ncbi.nlm.nih.gov/pubmed/7075966.
3. Barr CC, Lai MY, Lean JS, Linton KL, Trese M, Abrams G, Azen SP. Postoperative intraocular pressure abnormalities in the Silicone Study. Silicone Study Report 4. Ophthalmology. 1993;100 (11):1629–35. http://www.ncbi.nlm.nih.gov/pubmed/8233387.
4. Bernal A, Parel J-M, Manns F. Evidence for posterior zonular fiber attachment on the anterior hyaloid membrane. Invest Opthalmol Vis Sci. 2006;47 (11):4708. https://doi.org/10.1167/iovs.06-0441.
5. Boscher C, Kuhn F. An endoscopic overview of the anterior vitreous base in retinal detachment and anterior proliferative vitreoretinopathy. Acta Ophthalmol. 2014;92(4):e298–304. https://doi.org/10.1111/aos.12303.
6. Boscher C, Kuhn F. Endoscopic evaluation and dissection of the anterior vitreous base. Ophthalmic

Res. 2015;53(2):90–9. https://doi.org/10.1159/000370032.
7. Coleman DJ. Evaluation of ciliary body detachment in hypotony. Retina. 1995;15(4):312–8. http://www.ncbi.nlm.nih.gov/pubmed/8545577.
8. Diddie KR, Azen SP, Freeman HM, Boone DC, Aaberg TM, Lewis H, Ryan SJ. Anterior proliferative vitreoretinopathy in the silicone study. Silicone Study Report Number 10. Ophthalmology. 1996;103(7):1092–9. http://www.ncbi.nlm.nih.gov/pubmed/8684799.
9. Ding C, Zeng J. Clinical study on hypotony following blunt ocular trauma. Int J Ophthalmol. 2012;5(6):771–3. https://doi.org/10.3980/j.issn.2222-3959.2012.06.21.
10. Eisner G. [Gross anatomy of the vitreous body (author's transl)]. Graefes Arch for Clin Exp Ophthalmol. 1975;193(1):33–56. http://www.ncbi.nlm.nih.gov/pubmed/1078950.
11. Faude F, Wiedemann P. Vitreoretinal endoscope for the assessment of the peripheral retina and the ciliary body after large retinectomies in severe anterior PVR. Int Ophthalmol. 2004;25(1):53–6. http://www.ncbi.nlm.nih.gov/pubmed/15085977.
12. Fine HF, Biscette O, Chang S, Schiff WM. Ocular hypotony: a review. Compr Ophthalmol Update. 2007;8(1):29–37. http://www.ncbi.nlm.nih.gov/pubmed/17394757.
13. Ganteris-Gerritsen E, Ugahary LC, Jansen J, Mulder PGH, Cohen AF, van Meurs JC. Six months treatment with ibopamine in patients with hypotony after vitreoretinal surgery for retinal detachment, uveitis or penetrating trauma. Retina. 2012;32(4):742–7. https://doi.org/10.1097/IAE.0b013e3182265177.
14. Goldberg D. Computer-animated model of accommodation and theory of reciprocal zonular action. Clin Ophthalmol. 2011;5:1559. https://doi.org/10.2147/OPTH.S25983.
15. González-Martín-Moro J, Contreras-Martín I, Muñoz-Negrete FJ, Gómez-Sanz F, Zarallo-Gallardo J. Cyclodialysis: an update. Int Ophthalmol. 2017,37(2).441–457https://doi.org/10.1007/s10792-016-0282-8.
16. Ikeda T, Sato K, Katano T, Hayashi Y. Surgically induced detachment of the anterior hyaloid membrane from the posterior lens capsule. Arch Ophthalmol. 1999;117(3):408–9. http://www.ncbi.nlm.nih.gov/pubmed/10088827.
17. Lee GD, Goldberg RA, Heier JS. Endoscopy-assisted vitrectomy and membrane dissection of anterior proliferative vitreoretinopathy for chronic hypotony after previous retinal detachment repair. Retina. 2016;36(6):1058–63. https://doi.org/10.1097/IAE.0000000000000838.
18. Lewis H, Aaberg TM, Abrams GW. Causes of failure after initial vitreoretinal surgery for severe proliferative vitreoretinopathy. Am J Ophthalmol. 1991;111(1):8–14. http://www.ncbi.nlm.nih.gov/pubmed/1985496.
19. Lewis H, Verdaguer JI. Surgical treatment for chronic hypotony and anterior proliferative vitreoretinopathy. Am J Ophthalmol. 1996;122(2):228–35. http://www.ncbi.nlm.nih.gov/pubmed/8694091.
20. Lopez PF, Grossniklaus HE, Aaberg TM, Sternberg P, Capone A, Lambert HM. Pathogenetic mechanisms in anterior proliferative vitreoretinopathy. Am J Ophthalmol. 1992;114(3):257–79. http://www.ncbi.nlm.nih.gov/pubmed/1524114.
21. Nehemy MB, Zisman M, Marigo FA, Nehemy PG, Schachat AP. Ultrasound biomicroscopy after vitrectomy in eyes with normal intraocular pressure and in eyes with chronic hypotony. Eur J Ophthalmol. 2008;18(4):614–8. http://www.ncbi.nlm.nih.gov/pubmed/18609484.
22. O'Connell SR, Majji AB, Humayun MS, de Juan E. The surgical management of hypotony. Ophthalmology. 2000;107(2):318–23. http://www.ncbi.nlm.nih.gov/pubmed/10690833.
23. Pierro L, Azzolini C, Codenotti M, Locatelli C, Tremolada G, Brancato R. Ultrasound biomicroscopy of residual vitreous base after vitreoretinal surgery. Int J Ophthalmol. 2002;216(1):13–5. https://doi.org/10.1159/000048290.
24. Radius RL, Pederson JE. Laser-induced primate glaucoma. II. Histopathology. Arch Ophthalmol. 1984;102(11):1693–8. http://www.ncbi.nlm.nih.gov/pubmed/6541903.
25. Rosen E. Detachment of the anterior hyaloid membrane. Am J Ophthalmol. 1966;62(6):1185–94. http://www.ncbi.nlm.nih.gov/pubmed/5957895.
26. Schubert HD. Postsurgical hypotony: relationship to fistulization, inflammation, chorioretinal lesions, and the vitreous. Surv Ophthalmol. 1996;41(2):97–125.
27. Torii H, Takahashi K, Yoshitomi F, Miyata K, Ishii Y, Oshika T. Mechanical detachment of the anterior hyaloid membrane from the posterior lens capsule. Ophthalmology. 2001;108(12):2182–5. http://www.ncbi.nlm.nih.gov/pubmed/11733255.
28. Tosi GM, Schiff W, Barile G, Yoshida N, Chang S. Management of severe hypotony with intravitreal injection of viscoelastic. Am J Ophthalmol. 2005;140(5):952–4. https://doi.org/10.1016/j.ajo.2005.06.019.
29. Zarbin MA, Michels RG, Green WR. Dissection of epiciliary tissue to treat chronic hypotony after surgery for retinal detachment with proliferative vitreoretinopathy. Retina. 1991;11(2):208–13. http://www.ncbi.nlm.nih.gov/pubmed/1925084.

Surgical Management of Anterior PVR

25

Ulrich Spandau

25.1 Introduction

Anterior PVR is *the most common cause of failure to reattach the retina after vitrectomy for PVR.* Anterior PVR does usually not occur in primary detachment. It occurs typically in recurrent detachments after a vitrectomy surgery. Anterior PVR is PVR occurring at the height of the peripheral retina and the vitreous base. Three major tractional forces are present in anterior PVR. The first one is an *anteroposterior* tractional force, the second is a *circumferential* tractional force and the third minor force is a *perpendicular* tractional force.

A migration of proliferative cells into the vitreous base pulls the peripheral retina anteriorly (*anteroposterior* traction) resulting in a contraction of the vitreous base (Fig. 25.1). The contraction of the vitreous base is called a trough (Fig. 25.2) and results in an anterior traction of the retina (Fig. 25.3). The drawing in Fig. 25.4 shows the development of vitreous base contraction and anterior retinal traction (=anterior displacement) (Fig. 25.4).

A foreshortening and shrinkage of the vitreous base results in radial folds of the retina (like a hand fan; *circumferential* contraction).

U. Spandau (✉)
St. Eriks Hospital, University of Stockholm, Stockholm, Sweden
e-mail: ulrich_spandau@yahoo.de

Finally, a transvitreal proliferation results in a *perpendicular traction* and a funnel-shaped detachment.

The surgical aim is the removal of these tractional forces.

25.2 Surgical Treatment of Focal Anterior PVR

Stabilize first the anterior retina using perfluorocarbon liquids (PFCLs). In addition, PFCL pulls down the vitreous base.

(1) The anterior trough is incised and opened circumferentially with scissors or a 25G/27G cutter. The opened but still compressed vitreous base is then removed with the vitreous cutter.
(2) If radial retinal folds are present, then stain the circumferential membranes with trypan blue (air technique) and remove them with a delamination instrument and forceps.
(3) If all tractions are removed and the retina reattaches under PFCL, then continue with laser photocoagulation and silicone oil tamponade.
(4) If the retina does not reattach under PFCL, then a focal retinotomy is required (Figs. 25.5 and 25.6). The retinectomy is usually limited to 15–90°.

U. Spandau et al. (eds.), *Retinal Detachment Surgery and Proliferative Vitreoretinopathy*,
https://doi.org/10.1007/978-3-031-11946-0_25

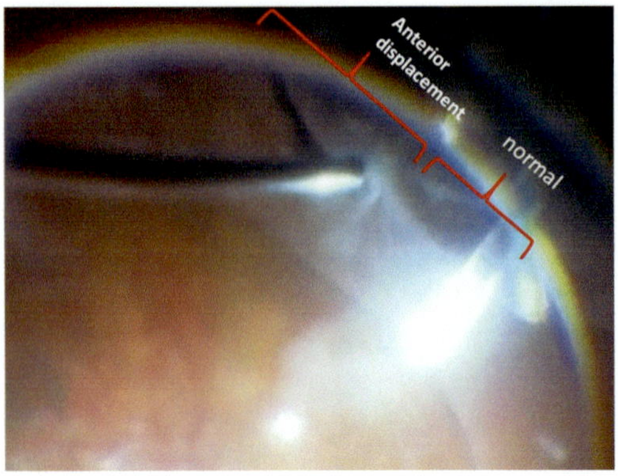

Fig. 25.1 Note the anterior displacement of the retina with a retinal band. The compressed vitreous base (trough) and then the retinal band must be opened with the vitreous cutter resulting in a mobilization of the retina

25.3 Surgical Treatment of Advanced Anterior PVR (3–4 Quadrants)

The two surgical options are an encircling band or a retinotomy. The problem is that a complete membrane removal at the height of the trough is not always possible. An encircling band may therefore lead to a recurrence. In the case of retinotomy, the trough and anterior retina can be completely removed and the recurrence risk is much lower.

If the anterior PVR extends to 3–4 quadrants, then we would choose a 270–360° retinotomy. The length depends on the extent of the anterior

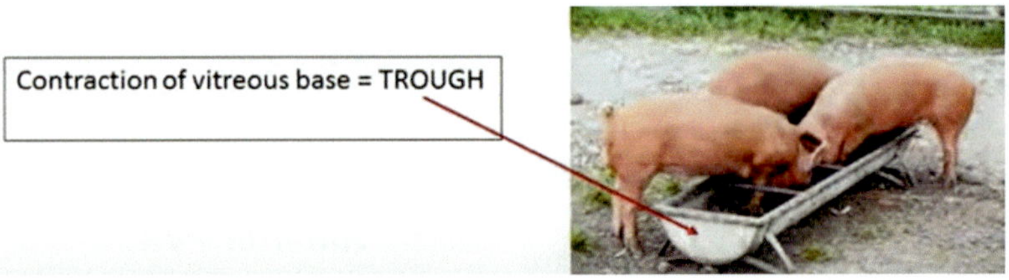

Fig. 25.2 A trough. The compressed vitreous base = trough

Fig. 25.3 The compressed vitreous base (trough) results in an anterior traction of the retina

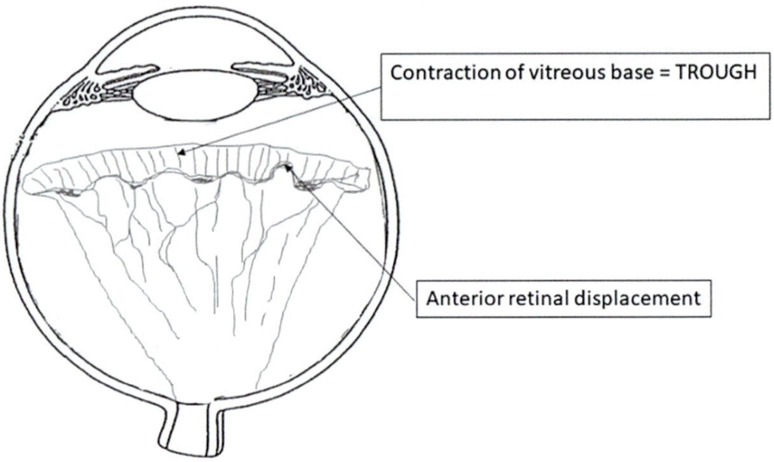

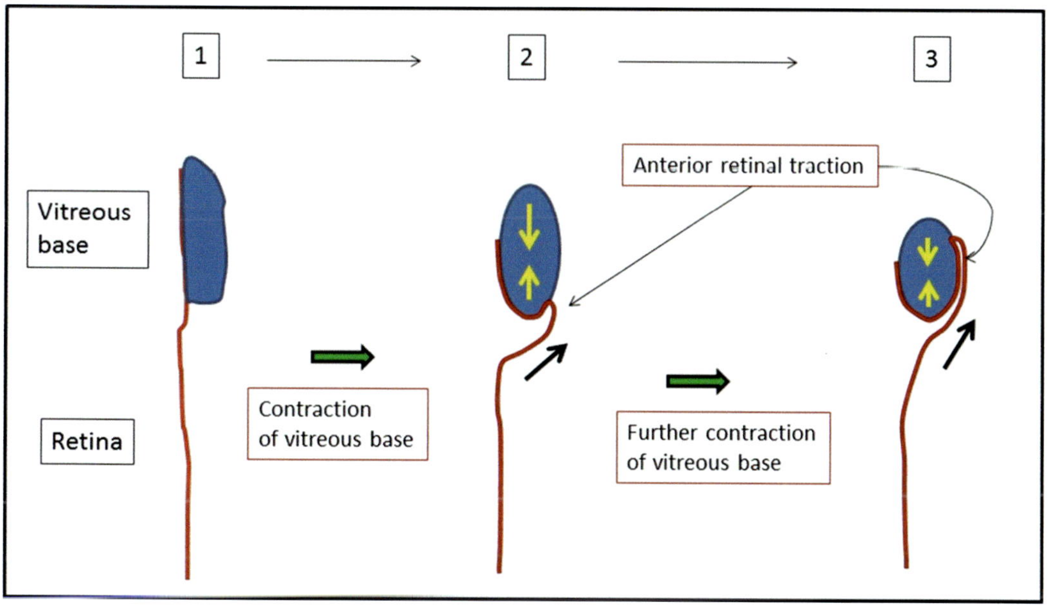

Fig. 25.4 Development of vitreous base contraction and anterior retinal traction. The vitreous base contracts and pulls up the retina. A vitreous trough is formed

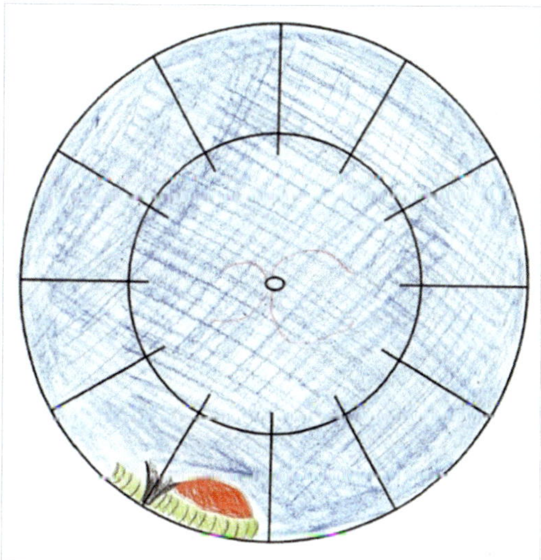

Fig. 25.5 An example of focal anterior PVR. A chronic and total detachment with an anterior PVR at 6–7 o'clock. The anterior PVR consisted of a trough formation and anterior retinal displacement

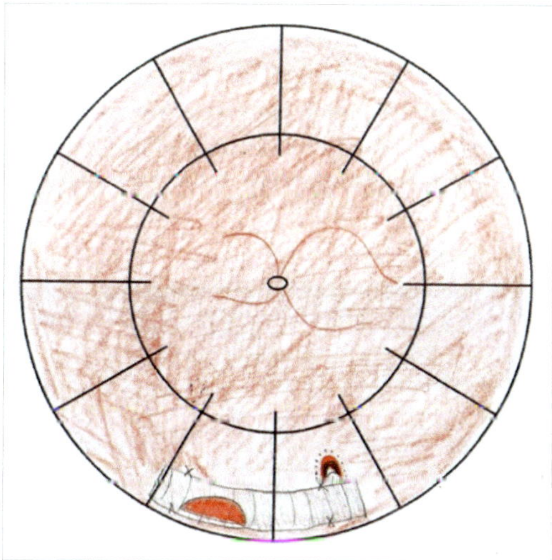

Fig. 25.6 After mobilizing the displaced retina, a circumferential buckle was placed from 5:00 to 7:00 The retinal break at 5:30 was caused by membrane peeling

PVR. Sometimes, it is not easy to perform an anterior retinectomy due to an anterior trough which is often present and may even cover the ciliary body. If you do not succeed in removing it completely, then the eye may get hypotonic which may result in a phthisis, a functional and anatomic loss of the eye.

Case report

A PVR stage D detachment *with anterior PVR* is the surgically most demanding case of all complicated retinal detachments. An encircling band does not solve the problem because the anterior retinal displacement persists. In most cases, the only surgical option is a 180–360° retinotomy, removal of all epiretinal and subretinal membranes and then a 1000 csts silicone oil tamponade.

Example: 17 y/o girl with a unilateral morning glory disc presented with total retinal detachment (Fig. 25.7) and PVR stage D. A combined vitrectomy with removal of epiretinal membranes and silicone oil tamponade was performed. A total PVR redetachment stage D under silicone oil occurred. In addition, a 360° anterior PVR with trough formation and anterior retinal displacement secondary to morning glory optic disc syndrome was present (Fig. 25.8). A surgery in

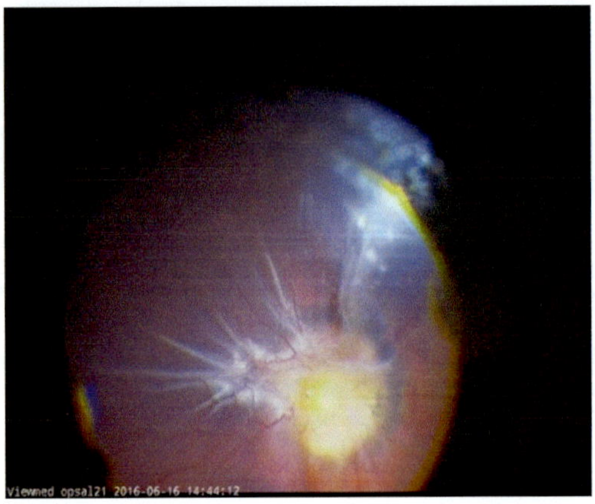

Fig. 25.7 Initial status. A total detachment with central and peripheral membranes. A retinal break is present at the edge of the optic disc. (morning glory syndrome)

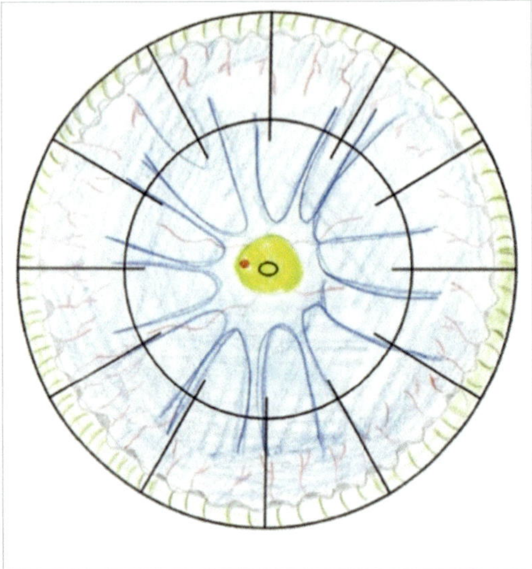

Fig. 25.8 Recurrent retinal detachment with PVR stage D and 360° anterior PVR. Note the break in the optic disc

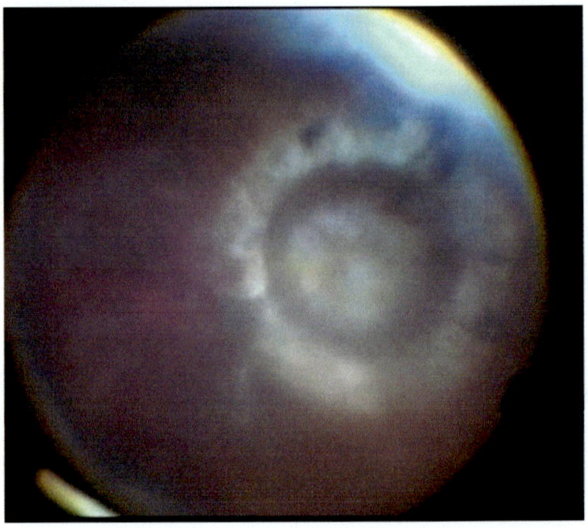

Fig. 25.9 Attached retina after 360° retinotomy and laser photocoagulation around the optic disc

general anaesthesia with a surgical time of 3 h was performed. 1000 cSt silicone oil was used as tamponade. In a final surgery, 1000 cSt silicone oil was removed, and preoperatively a redetachment at the posterior hole was observed and therefore 5000 cSt silicone oil was reinjected as permanent tamponade (Fig. 25.9).

26 Pathogenesis, Histopathology, and Classification of PVR

J. C. Pastor

26.1 Overview of the Disease. Pathogenesis

Proliferative vitreoretinopathy or PVR is a term adopted in 1983 for describing a complication occurring after some retinal detachments (RD) [1]. PVR develops in 5–10% of RD, and although it can occur spontaneously, before surgery, it is commonest after it [2]. Pathogenesis, in the original description, was focused on the formation of membranes on both surfaces of the retina, but more recently, the existence of intraretinal changes has been added as the more severe form of PVR [3].

Anyway, the initial mechanisms implicated in PVR are similar to any retinal injury repair process [2]. After separation of the neuroretina, photoreceptors started to die mainly by apoptosis (and also by other cell death mechanisms) very early, but also outer layers of the retina became ischemic, because of their separation from the choriocapillaris. Ischemia obviously produces the loss of neurons but also triggers several cell and molecular processes. This loss of neurons stimulates a reaction of retinal glial cells (Müller, astrocytes, and microglia) starting a new event directed to remodeling the retina and preserving the retinal structure [4]. Those changes lead to membrane formation, over and behind the retina, but above all, they induced intraretinal glial changes, which shorten the retina making it very difficult to reattach even by surgery, unless a retinectomy was performed [3].

Not all RD develop this severe complication, although all of them have many common facts: separation of retina layers, ischemia, breaks affecting the whole thickness of the retina, and a breakdown of the blood-retinal barriers allowing an intraocular inflammation and also facilitating the intraocular migration of cells which release more inflammatory products into the vitreous cavity [2]. Therefore, one of the current challenges is the appropriate identification of those patients with a high risk of developing this complication.

Initial approaches for detecting those patients at high risk of developing PVR were based on the identification of clinical factors [5], but since 2006 we have been working on elucidating the role of the genetic profile of each patient [6–8]. We are now convinced that genetics plays an important role in some crucial steps of this complication. For instance, cytokines production, which is a crucial element in retinal scarring, is a gene-regulated process [9, 10].

PVR still poses some challenges to the retina specialist, because, despite the efforts made over the past 40 years, we are still unable to prevent or treat it, and continues to be the most frequent and severe complication after RD surgery [2, 11].

J. C. Pastor (✉)
IOBA-Eye Institute, University of Valladolid, Paseo de Belen 17, Valladolid 47011, Spain
e-mail: pastor@ioba.med.uva.es

U. Spandau et al. (eds.), *Retinal Detachment Surgery and Proliferative Vitreoretinopathy*,
https://doi.org/10.1007/978-3-031-11946-0_26

For almost two decades, researchers have been focused on several steps of the disease: cell migration (giving a crucial role to RPE cells in PVR pathogenesis), epi and subretinal membrane formation, and further contraction of those membranes [11]. These events are essential parts of PVR but currently we know that there are more players in this story, and probably more relevant if our target is inhibiting this abnormal repairing process, and then getting an efficient prophylaxis. One, without any doubt, is the glial reactivity and hypertrophy which is a basic repair element in the retina as well as in any other part of the Central Nervous System [12]. And they are some others.

The lack of an appropriate classification is also a bottleneck that has prevented an adequate comparison of the proposed treatments for decades.

This problem has not yet been solved and seems an essential point to set the appropriate framework for an efficient clinical research, since now.

In fact, in a recent review of the literature [13], we found that only 74% of the revised papers related to treatments, published between 2000 and 2014, used a standardized classification, being in the 56,3% of cases the updated Retina Society classification of 1991 and in 33,9% the original one of 1983 [1] (Fig. 26.1). But when the updated Retina Society classification was used, only 10,4% of authors used a full C grade description (Fig. 26.2). It is clear that current classifications have a very limited value in clinical practice, but for clinical research purposes, we are convinced that a new one is needed.

We have pointed out some of the critical elements, which in our opinion must be part of this new classification [2]: type of morphologic changes, the extension of changes, signs of severity and progressiveness, and, for sure, some still unidentified signs.

Regarding the prophylactic measures or medical treatments, no one has been widely accepted for clinical use [2].

PVR is a complex process involving several risk factors. Over the last 25 years, and besides the spectacular evolution of vitreoretinal surgery techniques, which includes small gauge instrumentation, the emphasis has been placed on having a success in the primary surgery for RD repair, ignoring some other important factors. But the incidence of PVR remains unchanged, ranging from 4 to 34% in prospective studies [2].

Basic and clinical research has suggested that adjuvant agents could reduce that incidence. Pharmacological strategies have included anti-inflammatory drugs, anti-proliferative agents, anti-neoplastic, anti-growth factors, and antioxidants [2].

Clinical strategies would probably require a multimodal combinatorial approach, because, as mentioned, PVR is a complex and multifactorial disease. Surprisingly a few combined treatments have been reported in the literature. Last reports reiterate those approaches.

Resveratrol has been widely proposed for cardio protection, neuroprotection, chemotherapy, and antiaging therapy. And it seems to attenuate TGF-β2-induced wound closure and cell migration in ARPE-19 cells in a scratch wound test [14].

Also, dexamethasone-loaded polymer (Ozurdex®) has been evaluated for improving the outcomes of vitreoretinal surgery for established PVR. But results have failed in demonstrating this possible improvement [15].

To complete these examples, anti-VEGF (vascular endothelial growth factor) has been proposed as an adjuvant to inhibit PVR. But in a very recent meta-analysis [16], authors concluded that, based on the available evidence, intravitreal injection of bevacizumab in vitrectomy for patients with PVR-related RD did not decrease retinal re-detachment rate or improve visual function. Authors suggested better-designed studies with larger simple sizes and longer follow-up periods to reach valid conclusions. Moreover, they highlighted that evaluation of anti-VEGF therapy on surgical outcomes in eyes with milder subtypes of PVR or no PVR, but deemed at high risk of PVR, may be worthy of future consideration. This is a very interesting observation and emphasized the need for a more consistent classification useful for comparing different treatments [2, 13].

Fig. 26.1 Classification from the Retina Society Terminology Committee (1983). Modified from: The Retina Society Terminology Committee, "The classification of retinal detachment with proliferative vitreoretinopathy," Ophthalmology, vol. 90, no. 2, pp. 121–125, 1983

Retina Society Terminology Committee classification	
Grade	**Clinical Signs**
A (minimal)	vitreous haze and pigment clumps
B (moderate)	surface retinal wrinkling, rolled edges of the retinal, retinal stiffness and vessel tortuosity
C (marked)	full thickness fixed retinal folds in:
C-1	one quadrant
C-2	two quadrants
C-3	three quadrants
D (massive)	fixed retinal folds in four quadrants that result in:
D-1	a wide funnel shape;
D-2	a narrow funnel shape;
D-3	closed funnel without view of the optic disc

Nevertheless and besides those clear limitations, we have currently a more accurate and detailed understanding of its pathogenesis, and we are more than sure that in the near future its prevention could be possible, after a more accurate identification of high-risk patients and although surgery will be essential for managing it once it appears, some adjuvant measures will be adopted.

26.2 Histopathology

Because it is difficult to obtain human tissue samples, especially in the early stages of the disease, most of our current knowledge derives from experimental models. But we are very critical with these models because in our opinion, they do not mimic adequately the human disease [2]. Our group has proposed the use of organotypic cultures of the retina as potential tools for analyzing early changes in neuroretina structure [17–19].

In any RD, when neuroretina separates from the RPE, outer layers become ischemic. Neuroretina presents a high metabolic demand, but separation from the choriocapillaris does not lead to immediate neuron death, because intrinsic protective mechanisms are activated, specifically, stress-response genes and signaling pathways [20]. When these mechanisms failed, neurons died, mainly by apoptosis, but also by other cell death forms [21].

But ischemia is not the unique process involved in RD and in PVR. Inflammation and proliferation of several cell types as well as the production of local factors are also important events. Separation of the neuroretina from the RPE triggers the repairing response mediated by glial cells orientated to remodeling the retina which is losing neurons [22].

Very soon after RD, RPE cells de-differentiate into fibroblasts or macrophages-like cells. By this process, driven by factors not fully understood, contractile cellular or fibrocellular membranes are created. These membranes are considered a characteristic feature of PVR, but except for the peri-retinal membrane formation, the glial hyper-reactivity is quite similar to the one elicited by any RD not necessarily complicated with a PVR [22] (Fig. 26.3).

Therefore, a yet unidentified factor must be necessary to direct the above-mentioned events toward a PVR, which is currently interpreted as an exaggerated healing response [2].

The Retina Society updated classification	
Grade and Type	**Clinical Signs**
A	vitreous haze, pigment clumps, pigment clusters on inferior retina
B	Wrinkling of inner retinal surface, retinal stiffness, vessel tortuosity, rolled and irregular edge of retinal break, decreased mobility of vitreous
CP (posterior) - Type: I. Focal II. Diffuse III. Subretinal	Full-thickness retinal folds or subretinal strands posterior to equator (1-12 clock hours involvement) I. Starfolds posterior to vitreous base; II. Confluent starfolds posterior to vitreous base; optic disc may not be visible; III. Proliferation under the retina; annular strand near disc; linear strands; motheaten-appearing sheets
CA (anterior) - Type: I. Circumferential II. Anterior	Full-thickness retinal folds or subretinal strands anterior to equator (1-12 clock hours involvement), anterior displacement, condensed vitreous strands I. retina contraction inwards at the posterior edge of the vitreous base; with central displacement of the retina; peripheral retina stretched; posterior retina in radial folds; II. anterior contraction on the retina at the vitreous base; ciliary body detachment and epiciliary membrane; iris retraction

Fig. 26.2 The Retina Society updated classification (1991). Modified from: R. Machemer, T. M. Aaberg, H. M. Freeman, A. R. Irvine, J. S. Lean and R. M. Michels, "An updated classification of retinal detachment with proliferative vitreoretinopathy," Am J Ophthalmol, vol. 112, no. 2, pp. 159–165, 1991

As pointed out, many of the early changes have been obtained from animal models, due to the difficulties of getting human material. Therefore, findings should be extrapolated carefully to the humans.

In cats, photoreceptors degenerate within 24 h after detachment. Degeneration reaches a peak at 3 days and continues as long as the retina remains detached [23]. Müller cells become activated 15 min after RD [24]. RD also induces the proliferation of non-neuronal cells, such as astrocytes, endothelial cells, pericytes, and microglia [25]. Some of these changes are reversible with a prompt reattachment of the retina [26], but other changes are more consistent affecting photoreceptors and glial cells.

But once again, all these changes are also present in any RD even if they do not complicate with a PVR.

During the 1990s, RPE and glial cells were identified in epiretinal membranes [27] and they have been considered one of the main actors of PVR. In experimental models (cats), RPE cells initiate changes 24 h after RD [28]. They de-differentiate, lose their polarity, and migrate into the subretinal space. But in RD blood-retinal barriers are breakdown, allowing the passage of chemotactic and mitogenic factors into the

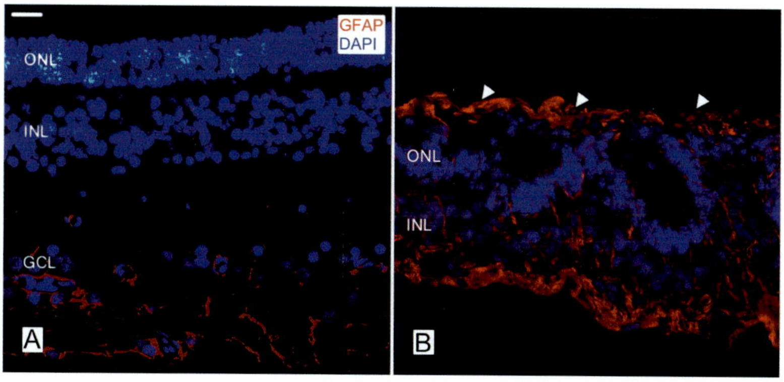

Fig. 26.3 Retinal distribution of glial fibrillary acidic protein (GFAP) in fresh neuroretina and 9-day culture samples. Freshly isolated retina explants (**A**) showed GFAP (red) staining at the end feet of Müller cells and in astrocytes. The outer nuclear layer (ONL), inner nuclear layer (INL), and ganglion cell layer (GCL) were identified with DAPI dye (blue; 4',6-diamino-2-phenylindole dihydrochloride). At 9 days of neuroretina culture (**B**), GFAP was markedly upregulated at the cytoplasm of glial cells, and GFAP-positive extensions formed a layered-like structure outside the retinal tissue (arrows). Cell modifications were also observed in the retinal structure. Scale bar: 20 μm (Courtesy of Dr. Ivan Fernandez-Bueno, IOBA, University of Valladolid, Spain)

vitreous cavity. These factors stimulate the migration and proliferation of both RPE and glial cells [28].

RPE cells migrate into the vitreous cavity through the retinal breaks and they participate in the formation of epiretinal membranes [29]. This process involves an epithelial-mesenchymal transition of the RPE cells which acquire a mesenchymal phenotype including the enhanced capacity of migration, invasiveness, more resistance to apoptosis, and above all the capacity of producing extracellular matrix, became RPE cells a fibroblast-like cells [29, 30].

The exact mechanism of RPE proliferation is not fully understood, but the presence of some growth factors seems necessary. Among them, platelet-derived growth factor (PDGF), fibroblast growth factor (FGF), epidermal growth factor (EGF), insulin-like growth factor (IGF), vascular endothelial growth factor (VEGF), hepatocyte growth factor (HGF), and transforming growth factor β (TGF-β) [29].

But also glial cells have a crucial role in PVR. As mentioned, PVR could be considered as an exaggerated response of the remodeling process of the retina, triggered by the retinal break [22]. Müller cells suffer changes visible 24 h after RD [31]. By the 3rd day, Müller cell bodies migrate to the outer layers (nuclear and plexiform) occupying the spaces left by dead photoreceptors and extending their processes into the subretinal space [30]. These cells, along with some others such as RPE cells, microglia and macrophages contribute to form the subretinal membranes, which are relatively uncommon in PVR, but more often after ocular trauma.

In some cases, the reactivity of Müller cells and microglial cells are not confined in the detached areas but have been also observed in intact attached areas of the retina. This finding could be important in explaining the loss of vision detected in a significant percentage of patients with macula-on and successful RD surgery [32].

Macrophages are also important players in PVR development [27]. Any RD has a breakdown of the blood-retinal barriers allowing the passage of these cells into the subretinal space and into the vitreous cavity. The presence of a high number of these cells in the vitreous fluid has been considered a fact associated with a high risk of developing PVR after rhegmatogenous RD [33]. These cells have been also found inside the retinal tissue and around retinal vessels in human PVR samples [3]. (Figs. 26.4 and 26.5).

In summary, three major cell types are implicated in RD and in PVR: RPE, glial, and

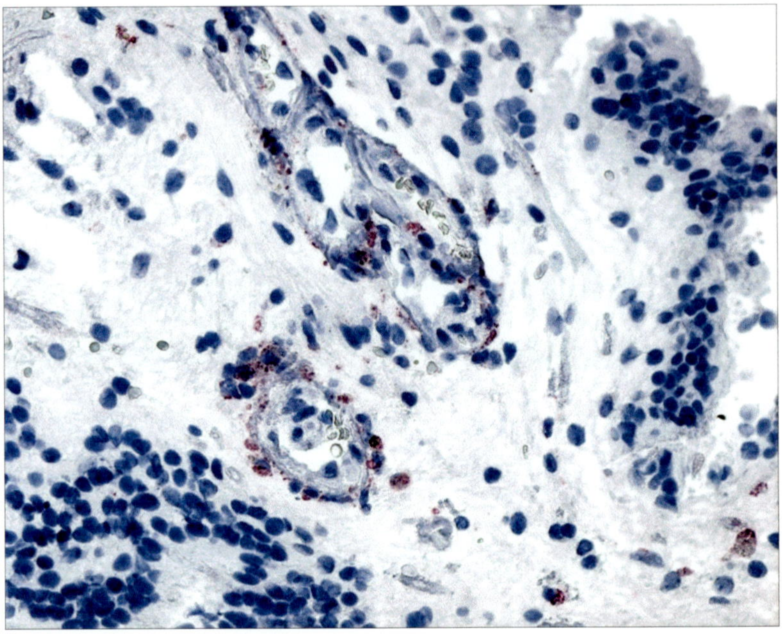

Fig. 26.4 Human retina in an eye with proliferative vitreoretinopathy (PVR). Sample obtained by retinectomy due to retina shortening. Immunostained with CD68 particularly useful as a marker for the various cells of the macrophage lineage, including monocytes, histiocytes, and others. The image shows CD68 positive cells and macrophages (red stained) located around blood vessels at the top and bottom center of the figure (Magnification 40x)

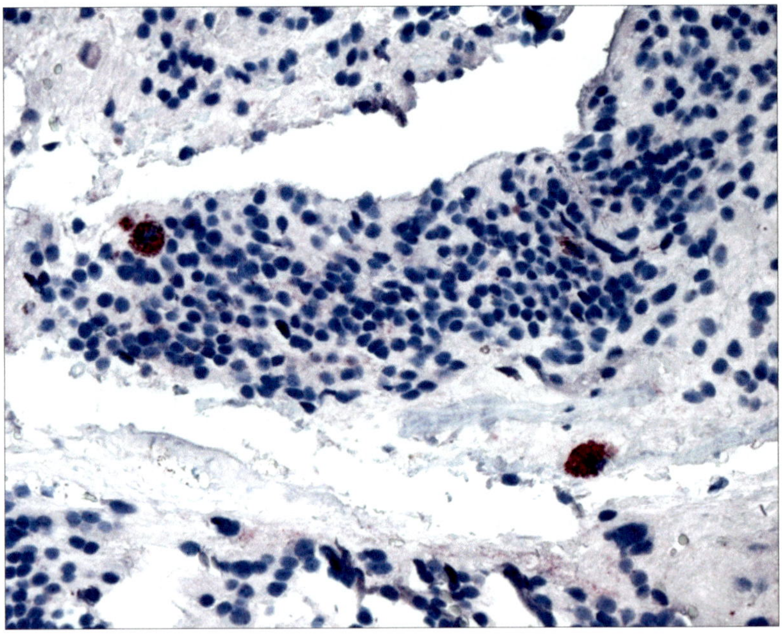

Fig. 26.5 Human retina in an eye with proliferative vitreoretinopathy (PVR). Sample obtained by retinectomy due to retina shortening. Immunostained with CD68 (marker of macrophages/histiocytes). Two CD68 positive macrophages (red stained) are identified inside of the retina (Magnification 40x)

macrophages, whose major role is remodeling of the retinal structure after neuron death caused by RD. And three major histological changes can be observed in PVR-affected retinas: subretinal membranes, which are rare, epiretinal membranes, considered for many years the most specific finding of PVR, and retinal gliosis and shortening which is now recognized as the most severe form [2] (Figs. 26.6, 26.7 and 26.8a, b).

Finally, and very briefly, these are our ideas on the pathogenesis of PVR (Fig. 26.9).

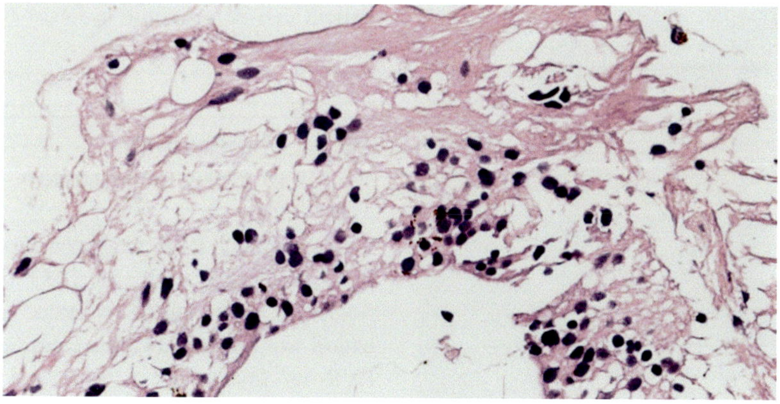

Fig. 26.6 Human retina obtained after retinectomy in a case of retinal shortening by PVR after RD. Picture shows diffuse architectural disorganization and loss of neurons. (H&E) (Magnification 40x)

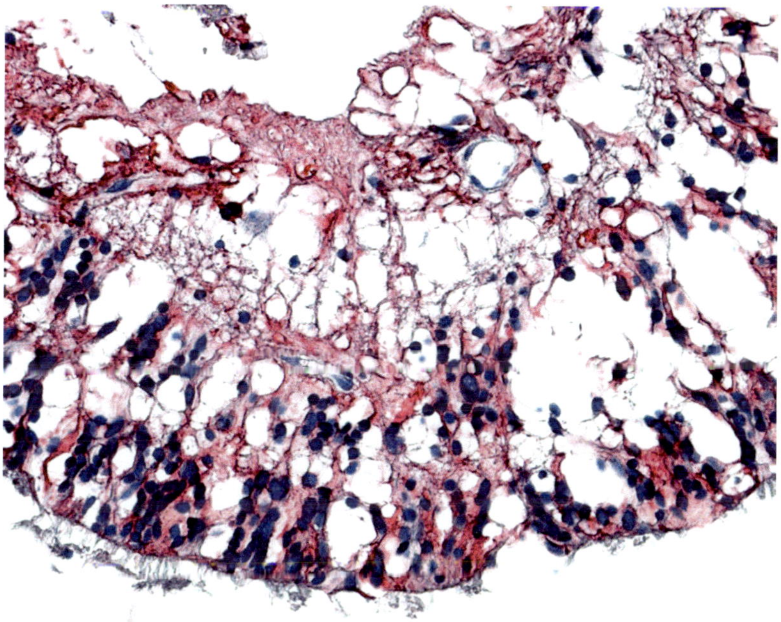

Fig. 26.7 Human retina sample obtained by retinectomy in a case of retinal shortening by PVR. Immunostained with glial fibrillary acidic protein (GFAP) an intermediate filament protein that is expressed by numerous cell types of the central nervous system (CNS) including astrocytes. The image shows widespread positivity of the retina stained in red; therefore, the reactivity of Müller cells and astrocytes, which are replacing the neurons. This causes a shortening of the retinal tissue preventing its reattachment to the eyeball. We named this form as "intraretinal PVR" (Magnification 40x)

Initial mechanisms are not different between PVR and any RD. After RD, outer retinal layers become ischemic and photoreceptors start to die. This loss of neurons stimulates a remodeling process directed to maintain the retinal structure, where Müller cells, astrocytes, and microglia play an important role.

At the same time, and due to the blood-retinal barriers breakdown, microglia and macrophages migrate into the subretinal space and the vitreous

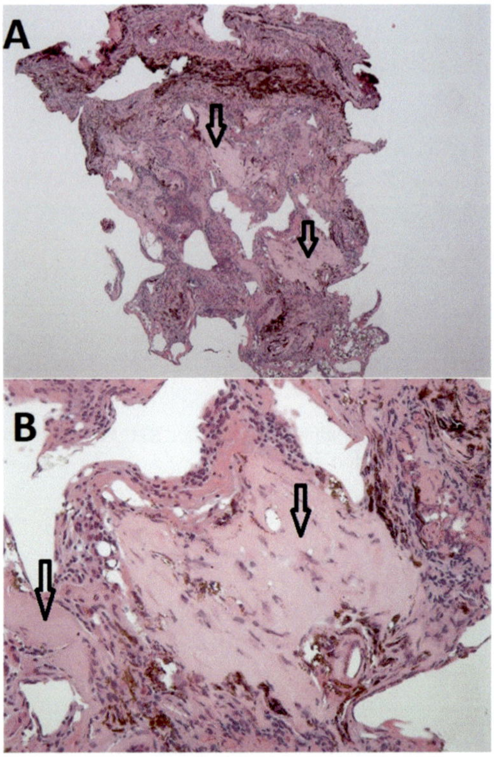

Fig. 26.8 **A** Human retina in an eye with proliferative vitreoretinopathy (PVR) in its more severe form: intraretinal PVR. Intraretinal fibrous tissue: light pink areas (arrows). (H&E Magnification 5x). **B** Detail of an area with collagen fiber deposits: Collagen bundles stain light pink with H&E. Retinal tissue and neurons have been replaced by fibrous tissue arrows. Fibroblasts are also seen as the spindle-shaped nuclei stained in purple (H&E Magnification 20x)

cavity where they release inflammatory products. Then, some cells, mainly RPE enter in a mesenchymal transformation, deriving into fibroblast-like cells able to synthesize extracellular matrix, and therefore producing peri-retinal membranes.

Our hypothesis is that when inflammation reaches a certain level, the remodeling mechanisms elicited in any RD are exaggerated and amplify entering in the PVR process. It is possible that, according to the clinical experience, this critical inflammatory level may be caused by the accumulation of clinical and surgical factors, such as extensive RD, presence of blood in the vitreous, excessive retinopexy, and others [5]. But in some other cases, the genetic profile of the patient can be a definitive factor in PVR development [6–8, 34–36].

26.3 The Problem of the Classification

As mentioned, PVR was identified as an independent clinical entity in 1983 by the Retina Society Terminology Committee and a classification was created [1]. This classification divided PVR into four stages, A, B, C, and D, apparently by increasing its severity, from minimal to massive PVR (Fig. 26.1). As mentioned, PVR was considered only a problem related to cellular proliferation, at that time. This classification is simple to use but does not provide clinically relevant information in terms of medical or surgical decisions. Unfortunately, this classification had numerous limitations. It did not consider the location of the vitreoretinal traction and the magnitude of the contraction. In addition, some of the stages provide a false idea of severity; for instance, D3 caused by a localized epiretinal membrane could be more easily treated by surgery than a C1 caused by intraretinal changes.

Even more, grade A was defined as the presence of vitreous haze and pigment clumps, but these findings are not specific to PVR. They are present, for instance, in many posterior uveitis and in some long-lasting RD without any additional sign of PVR [37].

A more specific sign is the presence of rolled edges of the retinal break, with or without retinal stiffness, and vessel tortuosity, which was considered by the Retina Society as Grade B. But these signs can be present in RD which does not further develop a more extensive PVR, and some surgeons treated them successfully with scleral techniques, which usually failed in established PVR [38].

In 1989, the Silicone Study Group introduced a new classification [39] adding new characteristics, such as the location, anterior or posterior, and the type of contraction. The most important contribution of this classification was the inclusion of proliferative phenomenon in the pre-equatorial zone of the retina and vitreous base, which is relatively frequent after previous

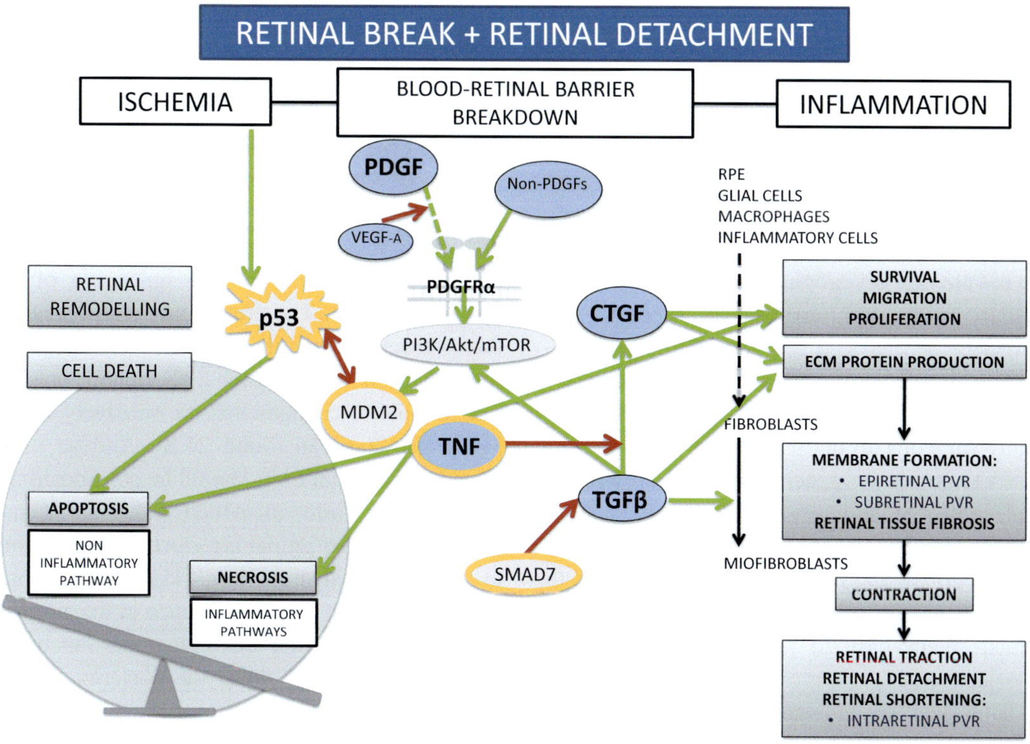

Fig. 26.9 Pathogenesis of PVR: our conception. Adapted from: Pastor JC, Rojas J, Pastor-Idoate S, Di Lauro S, Gonzalez-Buendia L, Delgado-Tirado S. Proliferative vitreoretinopathy: A new concept of disease pathogenesis and practical consequences. Prog Retin Eye Res. 2016 Mar;51:125–55. Reproduced by permission of the Editor and Publisher

attempts to reattach the retina, named anterior PVR. Nevertheless, the authors stated that they do not attempt to predict the PVR severity which is a crucial point from the clinical point of view.

The classification was then updated in 1991[40] according to modifications proposed by the Silicone Study Group and also by other authors (Fig. 26.2). But this classification appears to be difficult to use in clinical practice and may not offer any special advantage for decision-making in relation to the treatment of the disease. Thus, this relative new classification has been rarely used in clinical work.

As mentioned, papers dealing with PVR treatment evaluation made between 2000 and 2014 were analyzed in 2016 [13]. We localized 138 publications and we found that only in 103 of them, authors used standardized classifications. The most used one was the updated Retina Society classification [40] (Fig. 26.2), followed by the first classification of 1983 [1] (Fig. 26.1), and only four used the Silicone Study grading system [39]. In addition, four papers used "customized" classifications, and four publications showed serious mistakes in the application of the mentioned classifications.

It seems clear that this lack of uniformity reflects the uselessness of the existent classifications and made difficult the comparison between series and proposed treatments. Current classifications are purely descriptive and do not provide any information on the pathobiology of this complex disease. They do not provide information on the stage of activity of the process, which is crucial for estimating the risk of re-proliferation after surgery or when surgeons decided to remove the long-lasting endo-tamponade. Furthermore, current classifications do not provide any prognostic information neither visual results nor anatomical success, after surgery.

Results of our review suggested that current classifications have a limited value, and in fact, many surgeons do not use any of them referring to PVR grades by generic names such as minimal, moderate, and severe [41, 42]. Even more, grades A and B present in each classification are often ignored, and most authors refer only to the most advanced stages of PVR, basically grade C, which seems easy to identify from a clinical perspective [13].

This lack of an appropriate classification might have prevented advances in the understanding the pathogenesis of the disease and then the search for a more adequate treatment or prophylaxis.

For instance, because the Retina Society Committee defined PVR as a "proliferative disease," many treatments based on the inhibition of cell proliferation were developed for more than 20 years, none of which appears to have produced a significant clinical advance. Therefore, a review of both the classification and the pathogenesis of PVR appears to be appropriate to aid the development of new treatments [2, 43, 44]. This use of different and non-normalized classifications creates severe communication problems between clinicians and comparison of different studies became problematic or even impossible. Thus, it is clear that over the last 20 years clinicians have progressively abandoned PVR classifications [13].

Considering these facts, we believe that a new classification is needed, paying attention not only to the type of morphologic changes and their extension, but also to the presence of signs of severity and progressiveness, including the amount of intraocular inflammation and the pro-inflammatory genetic profile of each patient.

26.4 The Problem of the Intraretinal Changes

One of the most important absences in any of the existing classifications is the ignorance of the intraretinal PVR. The crucial fact is that besides the peri-retinal membranes, in PVR the neuroretina itself might suffer a shortening process due to cellular changes that are relatively recent [3] (Figs. 26.6, 26.7 and 26.8). And as mentioned, intraretinal PVR should be considered the most severe form in which there are major changes affecting retinal architecture and leading to significant dysfunction [45]. Furthermore, these forms have a huge influence in the surgical complexity and in the anatomical and functional outcomes, especially when the posterior pole is involved. Epiretinal or subretinal membranes can be relatively easily removed by surgery, and therefore, the prognosis of an epiretinal membrane is better than an intraretinal change [2, 3, 11]. As explained in the pathogenesis section, glial cells, including Müller and astrocytes, not only become reactive but also do replicate inside of the retina in PVR and it is thought that this gliosis, as well as the loss of neurons, contributes to retinal shortening [3]. RPE cells are also involved in this process, although their numbers appear to be small compared to their relevant role in peri-retinal membranes formation. But in this form of PVR, gliosis, with or without epiretinal and/or subretinal membranes, can cause marked retinal distortion and localized retinal thickening that can lead to the formation of a focal mass. However, until now, intraretinal changes have been detectable only during surgery when the surgeon could not reattach the retina to the eye wall by pushing it back by air or PFCL. Also, little attention has been paid to the identification of these changes before surgery or in the post-operative period. Even in some recent papers, these retinal changes have not been fully recognized [37], although they are evident for any

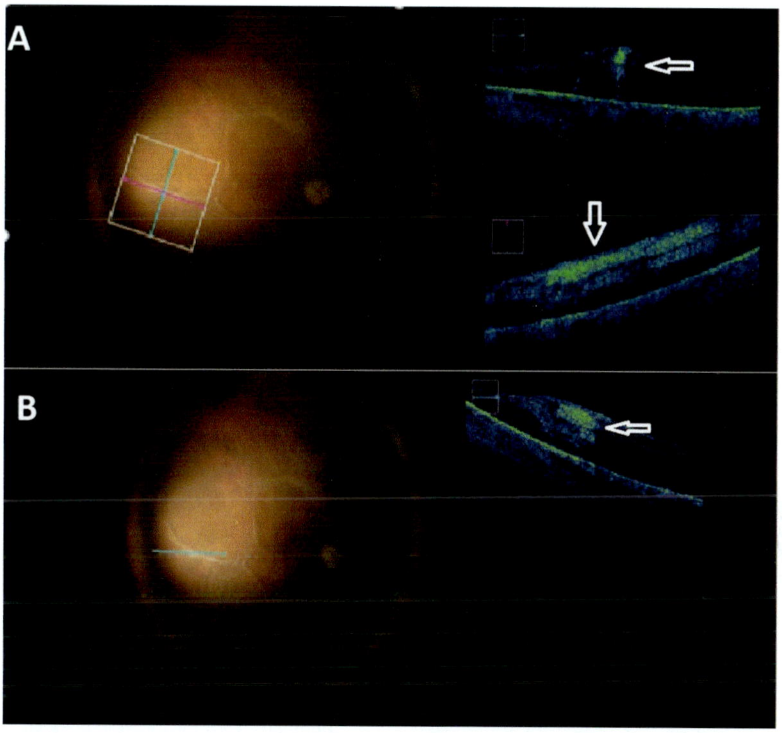

Fig. 26.10 **A** and **B** Intraoperative OCT (iOCT) application in PVR management. In this case with established PVR, iOCT allows intraretinal changes identification (arrows). These changes are neither epiretinal nor subretinal membranes and cannot be surgically removed. Thus, a retinectomy is mandatory to reattach the retina. Image obtained with the Zeiss Rescan® 700 iOCT (Carl Zeiss Meditech, Oberkochen, Germany)

experienced surgeon, probably because they are not easy to identify by routine clinical examination.

Nevertheless, there is hope that the use of new imaging technologies could add relevant information regarding the intraretinal changes [46, 47]. Considering these facts, we believe that attention should be focused on changes in the retinal tissue rather than membrane extensions [2].

26.5 OCT Imaging

One of the crucial points in PVR management should be the clear identification of epiretinal, subretinal, and above all intraretinal changes. Recent advances in Optic Coherence Tomography (OCT) and the development of intraoperative OCT (iOCT) may be extremely useful in clinical practice allowing intraoperative assessment of retinal status. The iOCT may be useful to identify intraretinal changes and/or subretinal PVR membranes which cannot be easily peeled as the epiretinal membranes [2] (Fig. 26.10a, b). Intraretinal forms are especially difficult to identify pre-operatively but their presence may be crucial in surgical management because the attempt to remove the presumed membrane may result in severe retinal tissue damage and iatrogenic tears. Therefore, surgical technique and even tamponade choice may be seriously affected by OCT imaging results.

We expect that in the near future, prospective clinical studies can be developed with the aim of establishing the advantages of this intraoperative evaluation in the current management of PVR.

References

1. Committee TRST. The classification of retinal detachment with proliferative vitreoretinopathy. Ophthalmology. 1983 Feb;90(2):121–5. PubMed PMID: 6856248. Epub 1983/02/01. eng.
2. Pastor JC, Rojas J, Pastor-Idoate S, Di Lauro S, Gonzalez-Buendia L, Delgado-Tirado S. Proliferative vitreoretinopathy: a new concept of disease pathogenesis and practical consequences. Prog Retinal Eye Res. 2016 Mar;51:125–55. PubMed PMID: 26209346. Epub 2015/07/26. eng.
3. Pastor JC, Mendez MC, de la Fuente MA, Coco RM, Garcia-Arumi J, Rodriguez de la Rua E, et al. Intraretinal immunohistochemistry findings in proliferative vitreoretinopathy with retinal shortening. Ophthalmic Res. 2006;38(4):193–200. PubMed PMID: 16679807.
4. de Souza CF, Kalloniatis M, Polkinghorne PJ, McGhee CN, Acosta ML. Functional and anatomical remodeling in human retinal detachment. Exp Eye Res. 2012 Apr;97(1):73–89. PubMed PMID: 22406310. Epub 2012/03/13. eng.
5. Rodriguez de la Rua E, Pastor JC, Aragon J, Mayo-Iscar A, Martinez V, Garcia-Arumi J, et al. Interaction between surgical procedure for repairing retinal detachment and clinical risk factors for proliferative vitreoretinopathy. Current Eye Res. 2005 Feb;30 (2):147–53. PubMed PMID: 15814473. Epub 2005/04/09. eng.
6. Rojas J, Fernandez I, Pastor JC, Garcia-Gutierrez MT, Sanabria RM, Brion M, et al. Development of predictive models of proliferative vitreoretinopathy based on genetic variables: the Retina 4 project. Investig Ophthalmol Visual Sci. 2009 May;50 (5):2384–90. PubMed PMID: 19098314. Epub 2008/12/23. eng.
7. Pastor-Idoate S, Rodriguez-Hernandez I, Rojas J, Fernandez I, Garcia-Gutierrez MT, Ruiz-Moreno JM, et al. The p53 codon 72 polymorphism (rs1042522) is associated with proliferative vitreoretinopathy: the Retina 4 Project. Ophthalmology. 2013 Mar;120 (3):623–8. PubMed PMID: 23207172. Epub 2012/12/05. eng.
8. Sanabria Ruiz-Colmenares MR, Pastor Jimeno JC, Garrote Adrados JA, Telleria Orriols JJ, Yugueros Fernandez MI. Cytokine gene polymorphisms in retinal detachment patients with and without proliferative vitreoretinopathy: a preliminary study. Acta Ophthalmologica Scandinavica. 2006 Jun;84(3):309–13. PubMed PMID: 16704689. Epub 2006/05/18. eng.
9. Murakami Y, Notomi S, Hisatomi T, Nakazawa T, Ishibashi T, Miller JW, et al. Photoreceptor cell death and rescue in retinal detachment and degenerations. Prog Retinal Eye Res. 2013 Nov;37:114–40. PubMed PMID: 23994436. Pubmed Central PMCID: PMC3871865. Epub 2013/09/03. eng.
10. Saika S, Yamanaka O, Sumioka T, Miyamoto T, Miyazaki K, Okada Y, et al. Fibrotic disorders in the eye: targets of gene therapy. Prog Retinal Eye Res. 2008 Mar;27(2):177–96. PubMed PMID: 18243038. Epub 2008/02/05. eng.
11. Pastor JC, de la Rua ER, Martin F. Proliferative vitreoretinopathy: risk factors and pathobiology. Prog Retinal Eye Res. 2002 Jan;21(1):127–44. PubMed PMID: 11906814. Epub 2002/03/22. eng.
12. Luna G, Keeley PW, Reese BE, Linberg KA, Lewis GP, Fisher SK. Astrocyte structural reactivity and plasticity in models of retinal detachment. Exp Eye Res. 2016 Sep;150:4–21. PubMed PMID: 27060374. Pubmed Central PMCID: PMC5031520. Epub 2016/04/10. eng.
13. Di Lauro S, Kadhim MR, Charteris DG, Pastor JC. Classifications for proliferative vitreoretinopathy (PVR): an analysis of their use in publications over the last 15 years. J Ophthalmol. 2016;2016:7807596. PubMed PMID: 27429798. Pubmed Central PMCID: PMC4939352. Epub 2016/07/19. eng.
14. Chen CL, Chen YH, Tai MC, Liang CM, Lu DW, Chen JT. Resveratrol inhibits transforming growth factor-beta2-induced epithelial-to-mesenchymal transition in human retinal pigment epithelial cells by suppressing the Smad pathway. Drug Des Dev Ther. 2017;11:163–73. PubMed PMID: 28138219. Pubmed Central PMCID: PMC5241127. Epub 2017/02/01. eng.
15. Banerjee PJ, Quartilho A, Bunce C, Xing W, Zvobgo TM, Harris N, et al. Slow-release dexamethasone in proliferative vitreoretinopathy: a prospective, randomized controlled clinical trial. Ophthalmology. 2017 Jun;124(6):757–67. PubMed PMID: 28237428. Epub 2017/02/27. eng.
16. Zhao XY, Xia S, Wang EQ, Chen YX. Efficacy of intravitreal injection of bevacizumab in vitrectomy for patients with proliferative vitreoretinopathy retinal detachment: a meta-analysis of prospective studies. Retina (Philadelphia, PA). 2017. PubMed PMID: 28272285. Epub 2017/03/09. eng.
17. Fernandez-Bueno I, Fernandez-Sanchez L, Gayoso MJ, Garcia-Gutierrez MT, Pastor JC, Cuenca N. Time course modifications in organotypic culture of human neuroretina. Exp Eye Res. 2012 Nov;104:26–38. PubMed PMID: 23022403. Epub 2012/10/02. eng.
18. Di Lauro S, Rodriguez-Crespo D, Gayoso MJ, Garcia-Gutierrez MT, Pastor JC, Srivastava GK, et al. A novel coculture model of porcine central neuroretina explants and retinal pigment epithelium cells. Mol Vis. 2016;22:243–53. PubMed PMID: 27081295. Pubmed Central PMCID: PMC4812504. Epub 2016/04/16. eng.
19. Rodriguez-Crespo D, Di Lauro S, Singh AK, Garcia-Gutierrez MT, Garrosa M, Pastor JC, et al. Triple-layered mixed co-culture model of RPE cells with neuroretina for evaluating the neuroprotective effects of adipose-MSCs. Cell Tissue Res. 2014 Dec;358

(3):705–16. PubMed PMID: 25213807. Epub 2014/09/13. eng.
20. Zacks DN, Han Y, Zeng Y, Swaroop A. Activation of signaling pathways and stress-response genes in an experimental model of retinal detachment. Investig Ophthalmol Vis Sci. 2006 Apr;47(4):1691–5. PubMed PMID: 16565410. Epub 2006/03/28. eng.
21. Murakami Y, Miller JW, Vavvas DG. RIP kinase-mediated necrosis as an alternative mechanisms of photoreceptor death. Oncotarget. 2011 Jun;2(6):497–509. PubMed PMID: 21670490. Pubmed Central PMCID: PMC3248194. Epub 2011/06/15. eng.
22. Garweg JG, Tappeiner C, Halberstadt M. Pathophysiology of proliferative vitreoretinopathy in retinal detachment. Surv Ophthalmol. 2013 Jul–Aug;58 (4):321–9. PubMed PMID: 23642514. Epub 2013/05/07. eng.
23. Sakai T, Calderone JB, Lewis GP, Linberg KA, Fisher SK, Jacobs GH. Cone photoreceptor recovery after experimental detachment and reattachment: an immunocytochemical, morphological, and electrophysiological study. Investig Ophthalmol Vis Sci. 2003 Jan;44(1):416–25. PubMed PMID. 12506104. Epub 2002/12/31. eng.
24. Lewis GP, Fisher SK. Up-regulation of glial fibrillary acidic protein in response to retinal injury: its potential role in glial remodeling and a comparison to vimentin expression. Int Rev Cytol. 2003;230:263–90. PubMed PMID: 14692684. Epub 2003/12/25. eng.
25. Geller SF, Lewis GP, Anderson DH, Fisher SK. Use of the MIB-1 antibody for detecting proliferating cells in the retina. Investig Ophthalmol Vis Sci. 1995 Mar;36(3):737–44. PubMed PMID: 7890504. Epub 1995/03/01. eng.
26. Lewis GP, Charteris DG, Sethi CS, Leitner WP, Linberg KA, Fisher SK. The ability of rapid retinal reattachment to stop or reverse the cellular and molecular events initiated by detachment. Investig Ophthalmol Vis Sci. 2002 Jul;43(7):2412–20. PubMed PMID: 12091445. Epub 2002/07/02. eng.
27. Campochiaro PA. Pathogenic mechanisms in proliferative vitreoretinopathy. Arch Ophthalmol (Chicago, IL: 1960). 1997 Feb;115(2):237–41. PubMed PMID. 9046259. Epub 1997/02/01. eng.
28. Anderson DH, Stern WH, Fisher SK, Erickson PA, Borgula GA. The onset of pigment epithelial proliferation after retinal detachment. Investig Ophthalmol Vis Sci. 1981 Jul;21(1 Pt 1):10–6. PubMed PMID: 7251293. Epub 1981/07/01. eng.
29. Chiba C. The retinal pigment epithelium: an important player of retinal disorders and regeneration. Exp Eye Res. 2014 Jun;123:107–14. PubMed PMID: 23880527. Epub 2013/07/25. eng.
30. Tamiya S, Kaplan HJ. Role of epithelial-mesenchymal transition in proliferative vitreoretinopathy. Exp Eye Res. 2016 Jan;142:26–31. PubMed PMID: 26675400. Epub 2015/12/18. eng.
31. Wickham L, Charteris DG. Glial cell changes of the human retina in proliferative vitreoretinopathy. Dev Ophthalmol. 2009;44:37–45. PubMed PMID: 19494651. Epub 2009/06/06. eng.
32. Di Lauro S, Castrejon M, Fernandez I, Rojas J, Coco RM, Sanabria MR, et al. Loss of visual acuity after successful surgery for macula-on rhegmatogenous retinal detachment in a prospective multicentre study. J Ophthalmol. 2015;2015:821864. PubMed PMID: 26640704. Pubmed Central PMCID: PMC4660023. Epub 2015/12/08. eng.
33. Martin F, Pastor JC, De La Rua ER, Mayo-Iscar A, Garcia-Arumi J, Martinez V, et al. Proliferative vitreoretinopathy: cytologic findings in vitreous samples. Ophthalmic Res. 2003 Jul–Aug;35 (4):232–8. PubMed PMID: 12815199. Epub 2003/06/20. eng.
34. Pastor-Idoate S, Rodriguez-Hernandez I, Rojas J, Fernandez I, Garcia-Gutierrez MT, Ruiz-Moreno JM, et al. The T309G MDM2 gene polymorphism is a novel risk factor for proliferative vitreoretinopathy. PLoS One. 2013;8(12):e82283. PubMed PMID: 24349246. Pubmed Central PMCID: PMC3857251. Epub 2013/12/19. eng.
35. Pastor-Idoate S, Rodriguez-Hernandez I, Rojas J, Fernandez I, Garcia-Gutierrez MT, Ruiz-Moreno JM, et al. BAX and BCL-2 polymorphisms, as predictors of proliferative vitreoretinopathy development in patients suffering retinal detachment: the Retina 4 project. Acta Ophthalmologica. 2015 Nov;93(7): e541–9. PubMed PMID: 25991504. Epub 2015/05/21. eng.
36. Pastor-Idoate S, Rodriguez-Hernandez I, Rojas J, Gonzalez-Buendia L, Delgado-Tirado S, Lopez JC, et al. Functional characterization of rs2229094 (T > C) polymorphism in the tumor necrosis factor locus and lymphotoxin alpha expression in human retina: the Retina 4 project. Clin Ophthalmol (Auckland, NZ). 2017;11:973–81. PubMed PMID: 28579748. Pubmed Central PMCID: PMC5449105. Epub 2017/06/06. eng.
37. Rouberol F, Chiquet C. [Proliferative vitreoretinopathy: pathophysiology and clinical diagnosis]. J francais d'ophtalmologie. 2014 Sep;37(7):557 65. PubMed PMID: 24997864. Epub 2014/07/07. Proliferation vitreo-retinienne: physiopathologie et diagnostic clinique. fre.
38. Afrashi F, Akkin C, Egrilmez S, Erakgun T, Mentes J. Anatomic outcome of scleral buckling surgery in primary rhegmatogenous retinal detachment. Int Ophthalmol. 2005 Jun;26(3):77–81. PubMed PMID: 16957875. Epub 2006/09/08. eng.
39. Lean JS, Stern WH, Irvine AR, Azen SP. Classification of proliferative vitreoretinopathy used in the silicone study. The Silicone Study Group. Ophthalmology. 1989 Jun;96(6):765–71. PubMed PMID: 2662099. Epub 1989/06/01. eng.
40. Machemer R, Aaberg TM, Freeman HM, Irvine AR, Lean JS, Michels RM. An updated classification of retinal detachment with proliferative vitreoretinopathy. Am J Ophthalmol. 1991 Aug 15;112(2):159–65. PubMed PMID: 1867299. Epub 1991/08/15. eng.

41. Lai MM, Ruby AJ, Sarrafizadeh R, Urban KE, Hassan TS, Drenser KA, et al. Repair of primary rhegmatogenous retinal detachment using 25-gauge transconjunctival sutureless vitrectomy. Retina (Philadelphia, PA). 2008 May;28(5):729–34. PubMed PMID: 18463517. Epub 2008/05/09. eng.
42. Oliveira LB, Reis PA. Silicone oil tamponade in 23-gauge transconjunctival sutureless vitrectomy. Retina (Philadelphia, PA). 2007 Oct;27(8):1054–8. PubMed PMID: 18040244. Epub 2007/11/28. eng.
43. Pastor JC. Proliferative vitreoretinopathy: an overview. Surv Ophthalmol. 1998 Jul–Aug;43(1):3–18. PubMed PMID: 9716190. Epub 1998/08/26. eng.
44. Sadaka A, Giuliari GP. Proliferative vitreoretinopathy: current and emerging treatments. Clin Ophthalmol (Auckland, NZ). 2012;6:1325–33. PubMed PMID: 22942638. Pubmed Central PMCID: PMC3429288. Epub 2012/09/04. eng.
45. Pastor JC, Rodriguez de la Rua E, Martin F, Mayo-Iscar A, de la Fuente MA, Coco R, et al. [Retinal shortening: the most severe form of proliferative vitreoretinopathy (PVR)]. Archivos de la Sociedad Espanola de Oftalmologia. 2003 Dec;78(12):653–7. PubMed PMID: 14689321. Epub 2003/12/23. Acortamiento retiniano: la forma mas grave de la vitreorretinopatia proliferante (VRP). spa.
46. Toygar O, Riemann CD. Intraoperative optical coherence tomography in macula involving rhegmatogenous retinal detachment repair with pars plana vitrectomy and perfluoron. Eye (London, England). 2016 Jan;30(1):23–30. PubMed PMID: 26656086. Pubmed Central PMCID: PMC4709554. Epub 2015/12/15. eng.
47. Junker B, Maier M, Agostini H, Hattenbach LO, Pielen A, Framme C. [Intraoperative optical coherence tomography in retinal detachment]. Der Ophthalmologe: Zeitschrift der Deutschen Ophthalmologischen Gesellschaft. 2016 Aug;113 (8):663–7. PubMed PMID: 27378449. Epub 2016/07/06. Intraoperative optische Koharenztomographie bei Ablatio retinae. ger.

Surgical Management of Intraretinal PVR

27

Zoran Tomic and Ulrich Spandau

27.1 Introduction

A foreshortened retina may be caused by epiretinal, intraretinal and anterior PVR. Remove first all epiretinal membranes. If the retina does not mobilize, then an anterior and/or intraretinal PVR must be present (Fig. 27.1). Remove next the anterior PVR and examine whether the retina is mobile and attached. If the retina does not reattach, then an intraretinal PVR must be present. Depending on the extent of the intraretinal PVR, different surgical approaches are required [1–7].

27.2 Inferior Detachment with PVR

Intraretinal PVR occurs most often at the inferior pole. Inferior PVR detachments occur often and especially after silicone oil removal. According to the silicone oil study, a recurrent retinal detachment occurs in 20% of cases after silicone oil removal [1], and in other studies with 17–25% [2–7]. Reasons for a recurrent detachment may be an undetected hole (rhegmatogenous retinal detachment) or a tractive detachment. The inferior recurrent detachment occurs more often than a superior recurrent detachment. The reason for this is that all proliferative cells accumulate due to gravity at the inferior pole and cause a PVR reaction resulting in a PVR detachment (Fig. 27.2). After removal of epiretinal and subretinal PVR, intraretinal PVR persists and causes a foreshortened retina.

The possible surgical techniques are shown in Diagram 27.1. The most popular surgical technique is an encircling band with C_3F_8; other possibilities are a retinotomy and an inferior circumferential buckle. The easiest technique is, however, a tamponade with a heavy silicone oil (Densiron Xtra) which tamponades the inferior pole.

The correct choice of these techniques depends on the *extent of intraretinal PVR*, i.e. how much the inferior retina is foreshortened.

If an inferior **mildly** foreshortened retina is present, then the following surgical techniques can be used:

(1) Encircling band
(2) Densiron Xtra tamponade

If an inferior **severely** foreshortened retina is present, then the following surgical techniques are possible:

(1) Retinotomy with silicone oil
(2) Inferior circumferential buckle with silicone oil

Z. Tomic
Milos Klinika, Belgrade, Serbia

U. Spandau (✉)
St. Eriks Hospital, University of Stockholm, Stockholm, Sweden
e-mail: ulrich_spandau@yahoo.de

U. Spandau et al. (eds.), *Retinal Detachment Surgery and Proliferative Vitreoretinopathy*,
https://doi.org/10.1007/978-3-031-11946-0_27

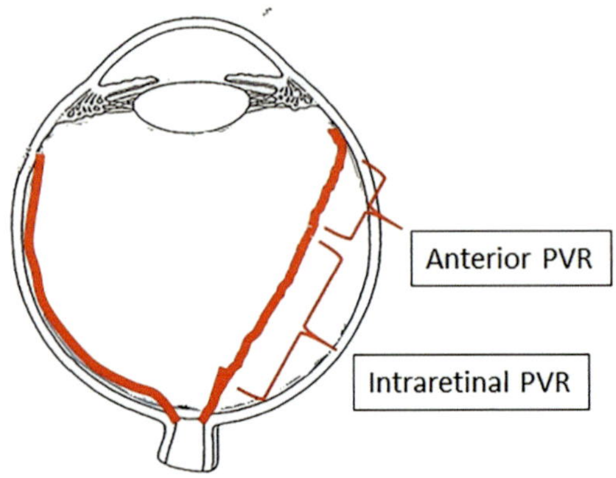

Fig. 27.1 A foreshortened retina may be caused by epiretinal, intraretinal and anterior PVR. Remove first all epiretinal membranes. If the retina does not mobilizes, then an anterior and/or intraretinal PVR must be present

The surgical management of a ***mildly*** *foreshortened inferior retina*

Cerclage and C_3F_8 (Figs. 27.2 and 27.3).

The advantage of a gas compared to silicone oil is the higher surface tension pressure. In addition, C_3F_8 maintains a good gas filling of the vitreous cavity for 2 months. The disadvantage of gas is a poor tamponade of the inferior pole. This disadvantage of a gas tamponade for inferior detachments can be encountered with an encircling band (Figs. 27.2 and 27.3).

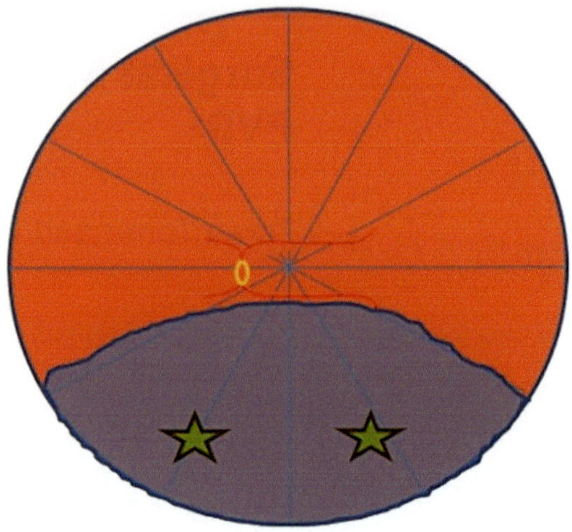

Fig. 27.2 A recurrent inferior detachment is present. Epiretinal PVR with a mild intraretinal PVR is present

Densiron Xtra (Fig. 27.4).

Densiron Xtra is a wonderful tamponade for inferior detachments. The surgery is simple and fast. Depending on how much the inferior retina is shortened, an encircling band is required.

Inferior circumferential segmental buckle (Fig. 27.5)

An alternative is an inferior segmental buckle. In this technique, a segmental circumferential

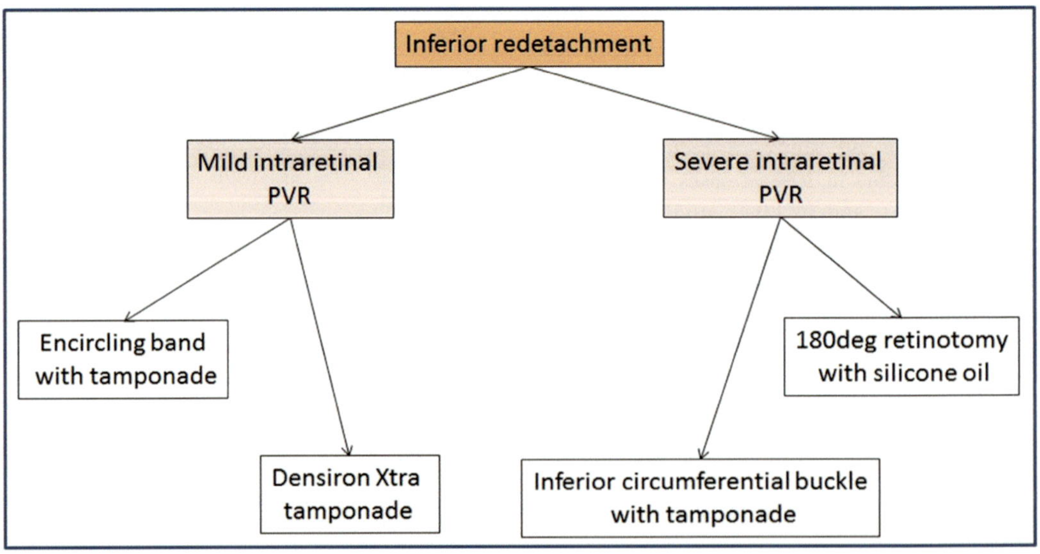

Diagram 27.1 Surgical options for inferior recurrent detachment

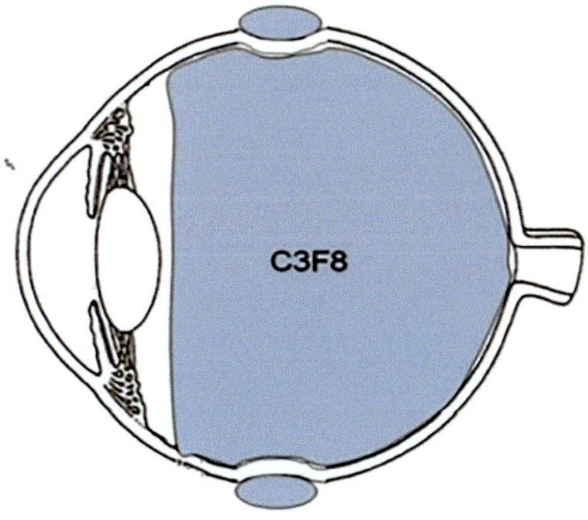

Fig. 27.3 The indenting effect of an encircling band and the high surface tension pressure of C_3F_8 may reattach a mild foreshortened retina

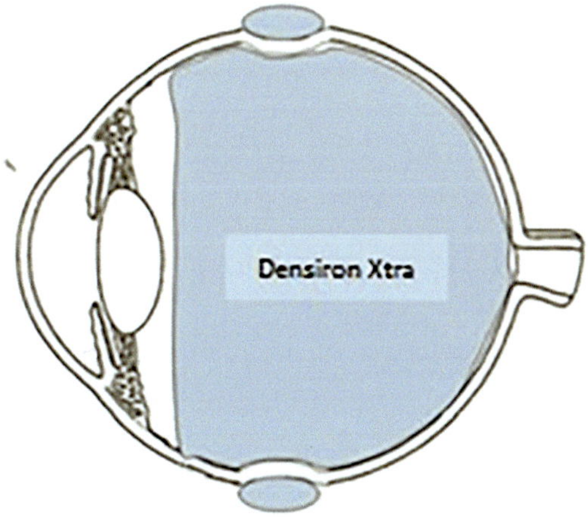

Fig. 27.4 An encircling band with a Densiron Xtra tamponade reattaches an inferior retina with mild intraretinal PVR

buckle is placed on the inferiorly detached retina approximately from 4 o'clock to 8 o'clock. In the case of a foreshortened retina, an inferior buckle on the height of the equator reattaches the retina. If the retina is severely foreshortened, we add a Densiron Xtra tamponade. If the inferior retina is less foreshortened, a C_3F_8 or 1300 cSt silicone oil tamponade may be sufficient.

C_3F_8 versus Densiron Xtra

In the case of inferior PVR, we prefer an encircling band with Densiron Xtra and not C_3F_8. Our rationale for this is as follows: The best silicone oil for inferior detachments is Densiron Xtra. In the case of an inferior PVR, we prefer Densiron Xtra because a redetachment under C_3F_8 progresses fast to an advanced PVR detachment and requires immediate surgery. In contrast, a redetachment under Densiron Xtra progresses slowly and does not require immediate surgery.

The surgical management of a severely foreshortened inferior retina

The most popular surgical procedure for an inferior foreshortened retina is an inferior 180° retinotomy (Figs. 27.6 and 27.7). This technique is surgically difficult because all preretinal membranes must be removed meticulously. Otherwise, the retina will reattach (Fig. 27.8). The complication spectrum of this technique is therefore high and a high amount of eyes require a permanent silicone oil tamponade.

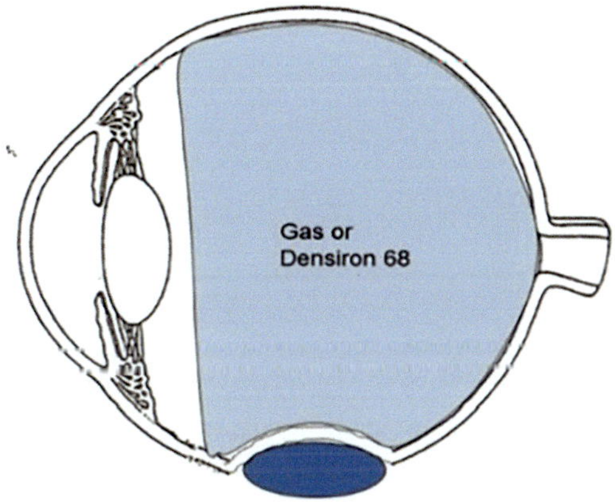

Fig. 27.5 The inferior segmental buckle indents the sclera much more than an encircling band. If you add a tamponade with Densiron Xtra, then you have a second help to attach the inferior retina

Treatment algorithm for inferior PVR detachment at the University of Uppsala

The easiest surgical option is a tamponade of the inferior pole and available on the market is Densiron Xtra (Fluoron, Germany). If this technique fails or if the inferior retina is severely foreshortened, then two surgical options are available: Retinotomy OR segmental buckle on the inferior equator. See Diagram 27.2.

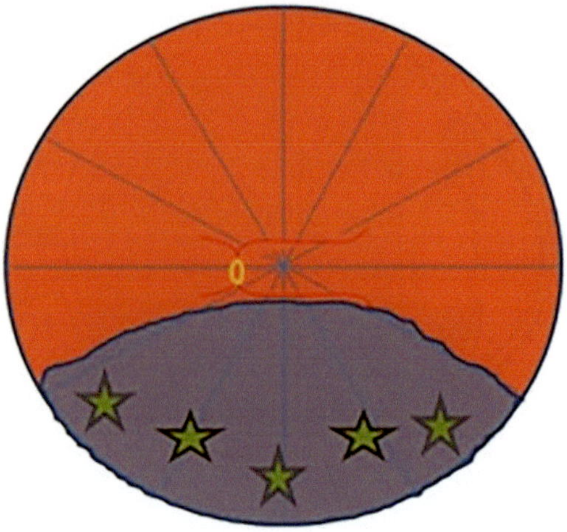

Fig. 27.6 A recurrent inferior detachment with severe intraretinal PVR

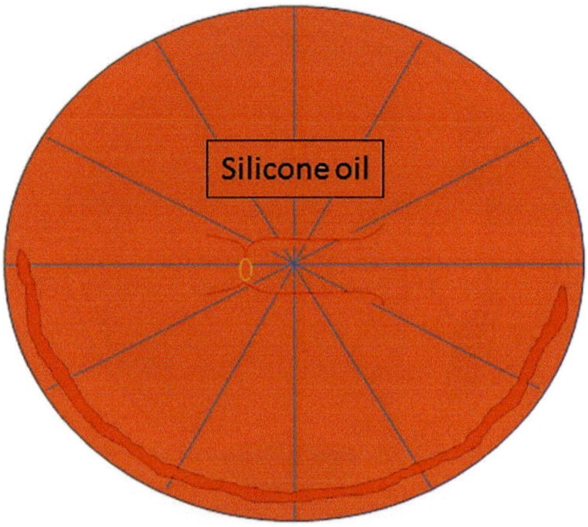

Fig. 27.7 A 180° retinotomy

Retinotomy versus inferior segmental buckle

A retinotomy requires a *complete membrane removal*. An inferior circumferential buckle does *not* require a complete membrane removal. In the hands of ZT, a retinotomy is the best option. He masters this technique in perfection from the macular translocation surgery. In the hands of the US a combination of episcleral buckling with Densiron Xtra is the best method. He would try to treat with an episcleral buckle and Densiron

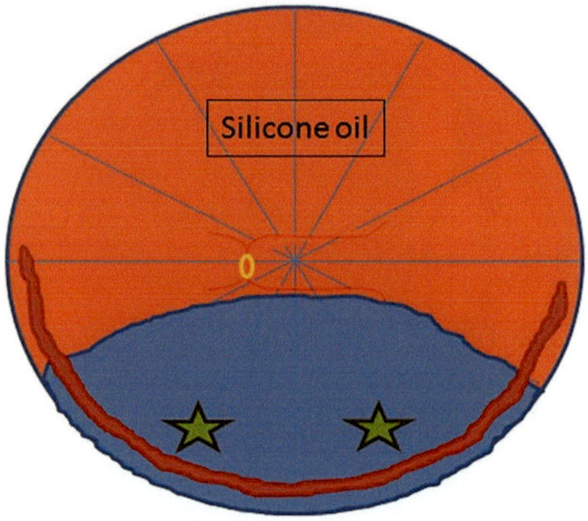

Fig. 27.8 If the preretinal membranes are not removed, then the inferior retina will redetach. After the removal of silicone oil, the detachment risk is 20%

Xtra. In case of a failure, US would perform a retinotomy. The big disadvantage of retinotomy is its large late complication spectrum: Approximately 20% hypotony, approximately 20% decompensated cornea, approximately 40% permanent silicone oil tamponade and approximately 20% retinal detachment after silicone oil removal (1–6). The advantages and disadvantages of the different techniques are listed in Table 27.1. The surgical technique is demonstrated in the chapter "Special surgical techniques for PVR detachment".

Tips and tricks

Timing of surgical procedure: You can use Densiron Xtra for first and second surgery; you can perform an inferior buckle at the (first and) second surgery; avoid retinotomy in the first surgery; perform a retinotomy only in a second surgery; an exception is a PVR stage D.

Conclusion

In case of an inferior detachment intraretinal PVR, we prefer a Densiron Xtra tamponade with an encircling band. An alternative is a segmental buckling with Densiron Xtra. In case of a severe intraretinal PVR, a 180° retinotomy is recommended.

Diagram 27.2 Our treatment algorithm for inferior recurrent detachment with foreshortened retina

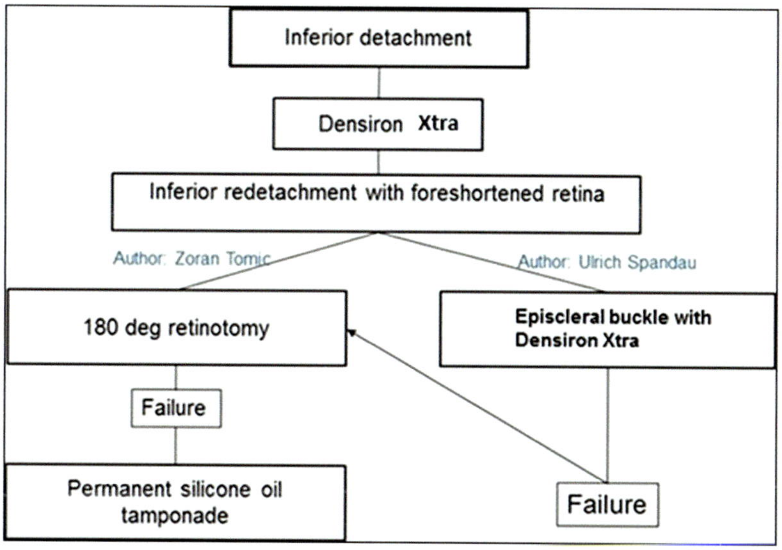

Table 27.1 This 180 retinotomy vs segmental buckling (inferior and circumferential (=ora parallel) from 4 o'clock to 8 o'clock)

	Advantages	Disadvantages
Encircling band (cerclage)	Moderate impression, good for mild foreshortened retina	Not sufficient impression for severe foreshortened retina
	Technically easy	Causes ametropia
	Relaxes the vitreous base in PVR	
Segmental buckling	Excellent impression	
	Technically easy	Causes ametropia
Retinotomy	Good method for severe foreshortened retina	Technically difficult, **complete removal of preretinal membranes required**
	No ametropia	Retinal slippage
		Proliferations at the retinotomy edges
		Many late complications: Hypotony (25%), decompensated cornea (25%), permanent silicone oil tamponade (40%), recurrent retinal detachment after silicone oil removal (20%) (1–9)

27.3 Combined Buckle/Vitrectomy

If despite thorough removal of epiretinal membranes the inferior retina remains immobile, i.e. the retina does not reattach under PFCL or air, then a retinotomy or an episcleral buckling procedure is required in order to reattach the retina onto the underlying retinal pigment epithelium. US usually places a 90° segmental circumferential buckle onto the inferior equator. Why a 90° segmental buckle and not a 360° encircling buckle? A segmental buckle creates a stronger impression than a 360° encircling band because the segmental buckle has no counter pressure (Figs. 27.9 and 27.10) **(see videos)**.

In the hands of the US this is the safest and easiest procedure for inferior recurrent

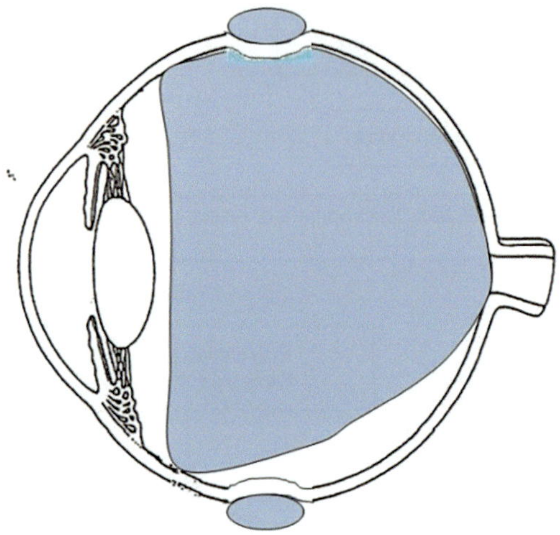

Fig. 27.9 An encircliing band creates a minor indentation of the sclera than a segmental buckle. The inferior retina may not attach

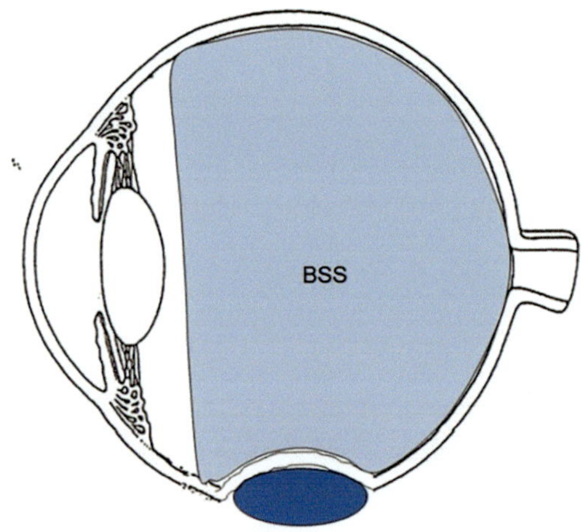

Fig. 27.10 A segmental buckle creates a stronger indentation of the sclera because the sponge is wider and no counterpressure is present. The inferior retina attaches in the most cases

detachment. If the inferior retina is foreshortened and if you do not have Densiron Xtra available, then this is a wonderful surgical option with excellent postoperative results. The surgery is already presented in a previous chapter. In this chapter, we will only demonstrate the placement of an inferior segmental circumferential buckle. Usually, the buckle is placed under the inferior muscle and sutured at 4 and 8 o'clock. But this might vary according to the location of the pathology.

Instruments and material

Silicone sponge 5 × 3.77 (Labtician, Canada) (Fig. 27.11).

Sponge suture: Mersilene 5–0 (Alcon) or Supramid 4–0 (Serag-Wiessner, Germany).

The surgery step-by-step

(1) **Inferior peritomy**
(2) **3 holding sutures**
(3) **3-port vitrectomy**
(4) **Identification of holes or PVR**
(5) **Marking of left and right end of the buckle at the limbus or sclera**
(6) **Marking of sutures**
(7) **Placing of two sutures**
(8) **Place the silicone sponge first under the inferior rectus**
(9) **Fasten the suture on the right side of the inferior rectus**
(10) **Fasten the suture on the left side of the inferior rectus**
(11) **Fluid x air exchange**
(12) **Laser treatment**
(13) **Tamponade**

Every step in detail

(1) **Inferior peritomy**
(2) **3 holding sutures**
(3) **3-port vitrectomy**

Start with an inferior peritomy and dissect the tenon capsule from the sclera. Place 3 holding sutures at the medial, inferior and temporal rectus. Then insert three trocars. The setup is a 3-port vitrectomy. If peripheral vitreous is present, then perform a meticulous removal of the residual vitreous. Staining with triamcinolone helps to visualize the vitreous.

(4) **Identification of holes or PVR**
(5) **Marking of left and right end of the buckle at the limbus** (Figs. 27.12 and 27.13)
(6) **Marking of sutures** (Fig. 27.14)

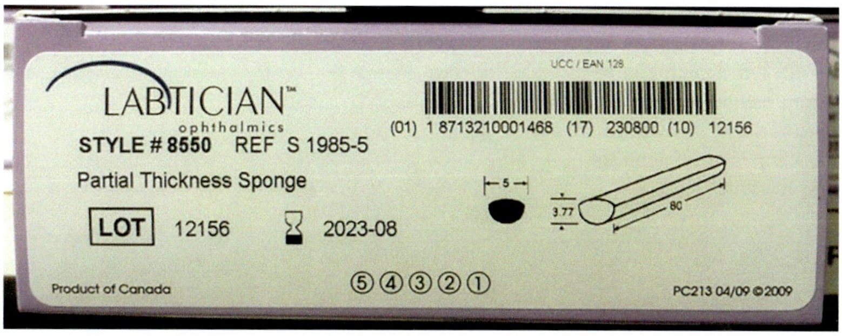

Fig. 27.11 Our favorite silicone sponge for inferior retinal detachments for combined buckle/vitrectomy

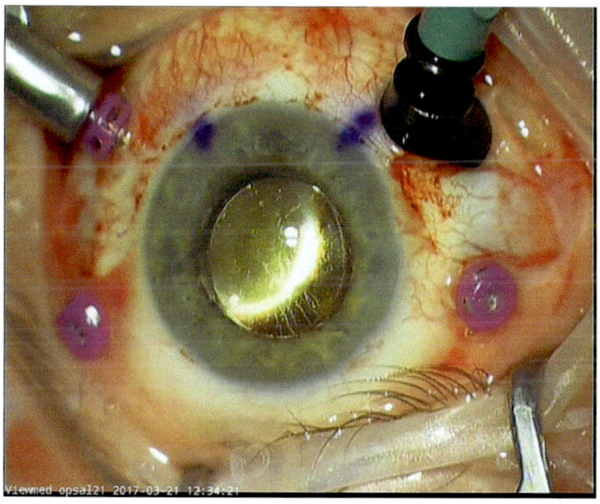

Fig. 27.12 Mark the cornea at both ends of the planned sponge. Note the scleral depressor at 4 o'clock

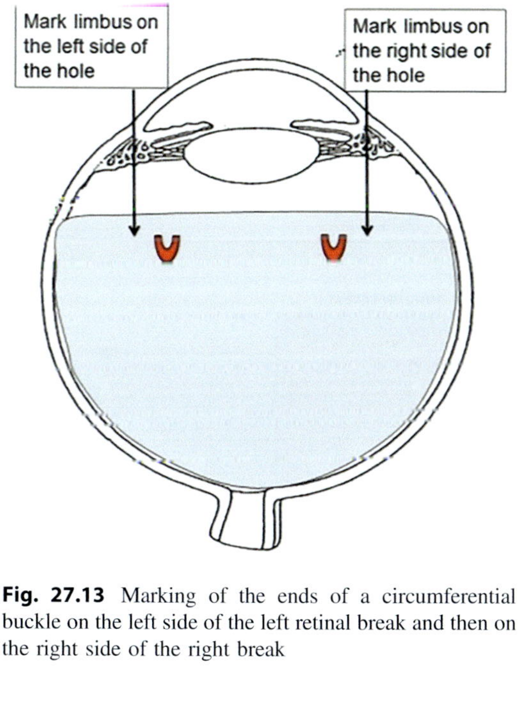

Fig. 27.13 Marking of the ends of a circumferential buckle on the left side of the left retinal break and then on the right side of the right break

The first important step is the localization of the PVR pathology and the retinal breaks. If holes are present, then cauterize the hole edges. If no holes are present, then place the buckle under the PVR pathology, i.e. star folds.

Examine the inferior pathology with a hand hold light fiber in one hand and the scleral depressor in the other hand. First you localize the left end of the pathology with the scleral depressor or cotton wool swab, remove the light fiber, flick out the BIOM and then mark the limbus on the height of the depressor. Then the same maneuver for the right hand of the buckle. Now you have two limbal or scleral markings.

The buckle is placed circumferential (ora parallel) on the height of the equator. If you suture as posterior as possible, then you have the correct height. I use always the standard buckle from Labtician, Canada (5 × 3.77). The caliper is set at 7 mm. Posterior to the first limbal marking place the first suture marking 1–2 mm behind the muscle insertion. The second suture marking is located 7 mm posterior to the first suture marking; now the same maneuver with the second limbal marking. Mark the sclera 1–2 mm behind the muscle insertion and 7 mm more posterior. Remark: Dry the sclera with a cotton swab before marking.

(7) **Placing of two sutures** (Fig. 27.16)
(8) **Place the silicone sponge first under the inferior rectus**
(9) **Fasten the suture on the right side of the inferior rectus**
(10) **Fasten the suture on the left side of the inferior rectus**

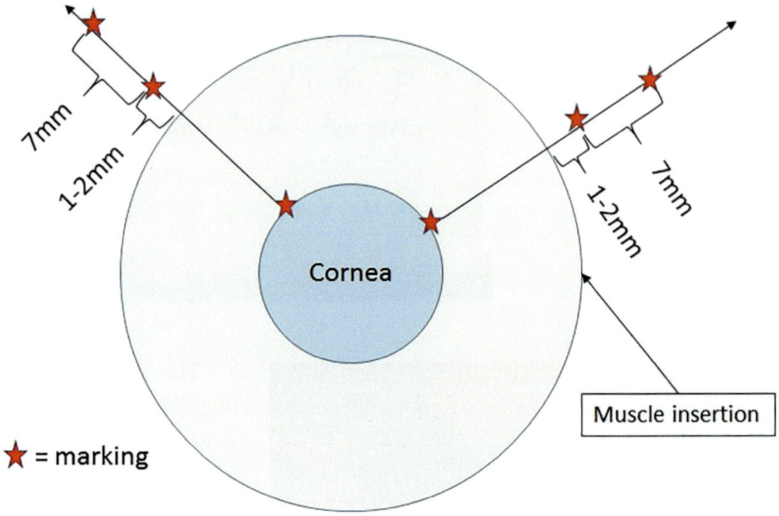

Fig. 27.14 After marking of the limbus, the sutures must be marked. One marking 1-2 mm behind the muscle insertion and the second marking 7 mm behind the first marking

Remove now the infusion line. You need two sutures (Supramid or Mersilene) with one needle each. The assistant pulls two holding sutures and holds the orbita spatula. Work now under microscope view. Place the first suture on the anterior scleral marking. Move the needle a long bite slightly under the sclera; approximately 3–4 mm. The posterior suture is difficult due to the lack of space. The suture is easier if you indent the sclera with anatomic forceps. Then repeat the maneuver on the other side.

Place the sponge first under the inferior rectus using two surgical forceps (Fig. 27.15). Then place one end of the sponge under one suture. Before fastening the suture, check the tension of the globe. If the tension is over 10 mmHg, then release some BSS with a flute needle. If the tension is lower than 6 mmHg, then continue to fasten the sponge. The globe impresses very much during this maneuver. Don't worry. Later when the globe is normotensive, it will look perfect. Then the same maneuver on the other side.

(11) **Fluid x air exchange**
(12) **Laser treatment**
(13) **Tamponade**

Reinsert the infusion line. Continue with a fluid x air exchange. The next step is a laser

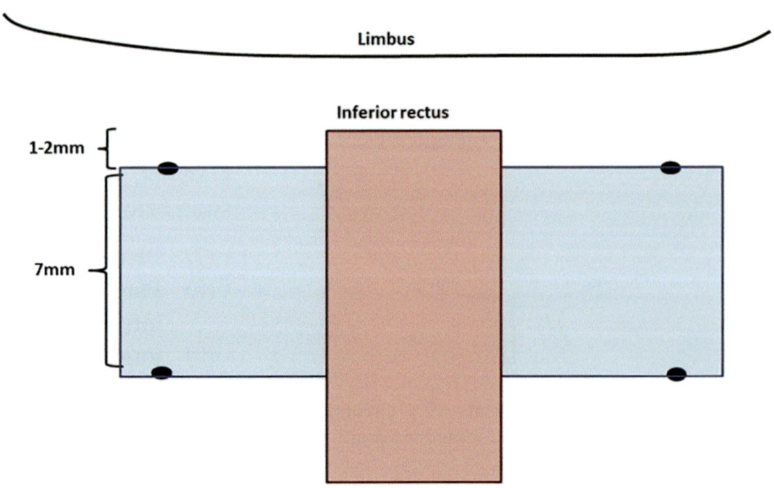

Fig. 27.15 Place the silicone sponge under the rectus muscle and sutures and then tie the sutures

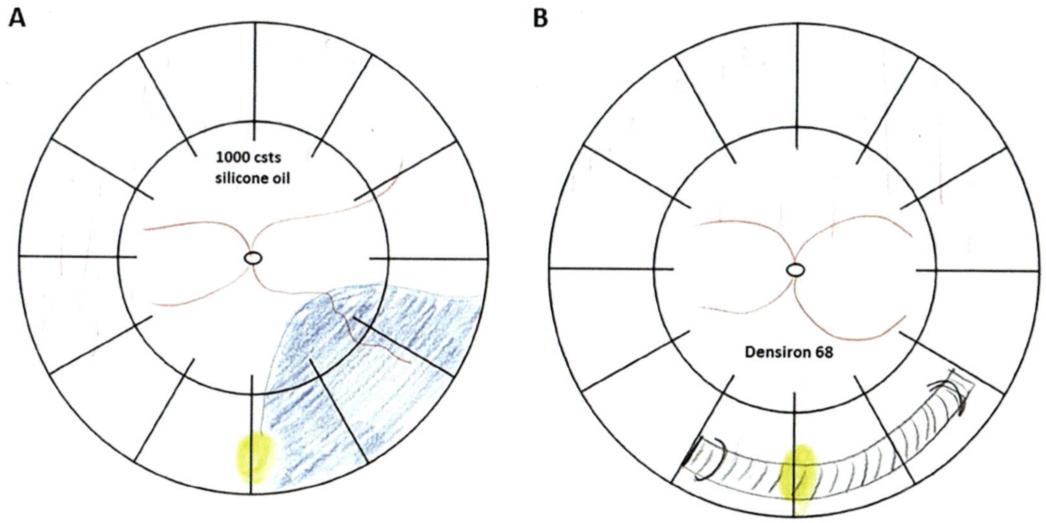

Fig. 27.16 A focal recurrent detachment under silicone oil. **A** The silicone oil was removed and a circumferential buckle was placed from 4:00 to 7:00 and Densiron Xtra was injected. **B** Two months later, the silicone oil was removed and the retina remained attached

photocoagulation. If the inferior retina has much PVR changes and much subretinal fluid, we recommend Densiron Xtra. If the retina is dry, then use gas or 1000 cSt silicone oil as tamponade.

Case report

A 74 y/o male patient was operated with vitrectomy and silicone oil. Four weeks postoperative a focal recurrent detachment under silicone oil was observed (Fig. 27.16A). The silicone oil was removed and a circumferential buckle was placed from 4:00 to 7:00 and Densiron Xtra was injected (Fig. 27.16B). Two months later, the silicone oil was removed and the retina remained attached.

27.4 Retinotomy and Retinectomy

If despite meticulous transvitreal, epiretinal and subretinal dissection the retina remains foreshortened preventing an attachment of the retina with the retinal pigment epithelium, the surgeon should perform a retinotomy or retinectomy in order to relax the retina. **Retinotomy** involves incising the retina, whereas **retinectomy** involves excising the retina. The peripheral retina is cut parallel to the ora serrata and the retinotomy edges are treated with laser photocoagulation in order to reattach the retina (Figs. 27.17).

Retinotomy could be performed in a **radial** fashion, but most commonly it is done **circumferentially**, parallel to the ora serrata. Most PVR cases can be managed without retinotomy/retinectomy. We almost never use it in the first surgery, except for the penetrating injuries with PVR and incarceration of the retina in the penetrating wound. **The circumferential**

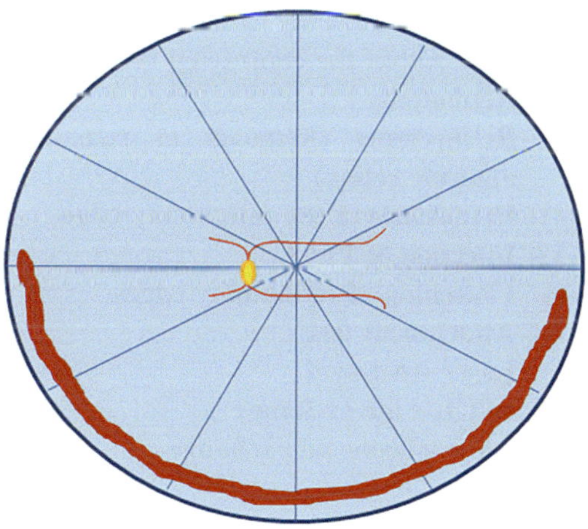

Fig. 27.17 A 180° retinotomy at the inferior pole

retinotomy in repeated surgery for idiopathic PVR detachment is performed in the area with persistent contraction of the retina usually affecting the two lower quadrants, due to the physical property of the 1000 csts silicone oil that is regularly used for the first surgery. This silicone oil is lighter than water and therefore is leaving some space filled with aqueous inferiorly thus tamponing better the upper two quadrants where recurrent detachment almost never occurs.

The most common problem with retinotomy is the underestimation of the necessary size of the tissue to be removed so that contraction persists. The most common size of retinotomy is 180° tapered to the two lower quadrants and extending from 3 over 6 to 9 o'clock. A 360° retinotomy is seldom and may be required in penetrating injuries with the incarceration of the retina and PVR stage D. It is usually followed by some distortion of the retina after reattachment and requires relocation of the retina using the flute needle with a silicone tip in order to re-establish its normal anatomical position. See video.

Instruments

(1) 25G or 27G Vitreous cutter
or vertical scissors.
(2) 23G or 25G knob spatula (Eye Tech, UK)
or flute needle with silicone tip.
(3) PFCL
(4) 1000 csts or 5000 csts silicone oil

The surgery step-by step

(1) **Row of diathermy as anteriorly as possible within the contracted retina**
(2) **Retinotomy**
(3) **Retinectomy (Removal of remaining anterior retina)**
(4) **Hemostasis of the retinotomy edge**
(5) **Injection of PFCL**
(6) **Flattening of retinotomy edges**
(7) **Attachment test**
(8) **Laser treatment**
(9) **PFCL x air exchange**
(10) **Air x silicone oil exchange**

Every step in detail

1. **Row of diathermy as anteriorly as possible within the contracted retina**

   Retinotomy should be performed as anteriorly as possible in order to preserve the healthy retina. The area to be incised should be marked with a row of endodiathermy and the incision should be tapered into the normal retina at both ends of the contracted retina. If endodiathermy is not possible, i.e. the retina does not become white during endodiathermy, then vitreous is left. Remove the residual vitreous with the vitreous cutter and continue with diathermy. If you find a membrane at the edge, remove it at once; otherwise, it will continue to proliferate and cause a recurrent detachment.

2. **Retinotomy**
3. **Retinectomy (Removal of remaining anterior retina)**
4. **Hemostasis of the retinotomy edge**

   The retinotomy is performed with the vitreous cutter at a low cut rate of 100–150 cuts/min or vertical scissors. A 27G vitreous cutter is due to its size very suitable for a retinotomy. The remaining anterior retina is then removed with the vitreous cutter at a higher cut rate of 5000–7500 cuts/min and is called **anterior retinectomy**. Meticulous hemostasis of the retinotomy edge is essential, as any bleeding may lead to recurrent PVR.

5. **Injection of PFCL**
6. **Flatten the retinotomy edges**

   The retina is then reattached using perfluorocarbon liquid (PFCL). Instill PFCL up to the retinal edge. Folds or areas of retinal distortion are adjusted with a retinal manipulator (knob spatula) or a flute needle with a silicone tip. In the case of residual membranes, dissect the membrane with a membrane pic (27G membrane pic, DORC).

The PFCL is not removed for this maneuver; it creates counter tension. Grasp the membrane with forceps and remove it. You may need to work bimanual with the forceps in one hand and the dissection instrument in the other hand. If you lift the retina carefully, then the PFCL will not spill over the edges and flow subretinal.

7. **Attachment test**
8. **Laser treatment**

Before continuing with laser photocoagulation, check whether the retinotomy edges are completely attached under PFCL). If not, then fix the problem: remove the membrane or enlarge the retinotomy. If the attachment test is positive, continue with laser treatment. For laser photocoagulation of retinal edges, we recommend a higher laser power than usual. A higher laser power induces an immediate congealing of outer retinal proteins by heat resulting in a more immediate adhesion. Our laser power for retinotomy edges with an argon laser device (Iridex, CA) is Power: 100–300 mW; Duration: **300** ms; Interval: 300 ms. This is especially the case for laser treatment of retinotomy edges. For retinal holes and for a laser cerclage, a reduced laser power is recommended.

Surgical pearls no. 94

Laser photocoagulation for retinotomy: More laser power than usual: **300 ms** duration instead of 200 ms!!

9. **PFCL x air exchange**
10. **Air x silicone oil exchange**

For this step, two methods are possible: (1) First a PFCL x air exchange and then a silicone oil injection. (2) A direct PFCL x silicone oil exchange. We prefer the first method because the retinotomy edges detach and enroll with the second method.

Start with a PFCL x air exchange until the air reaches the retinal edges. It is important to aspirate thoroughly the fluid at the edges of the retinotomy to avoid slippage. Then continue to remove the residual PFCL. The whole procedure is finished with an injection of 1000 csts silicone oil into the air-filled cavity. We use never gas in an eye with retinotomy because in case of recurrent detachment there will be a fast progression to PVR. Heavy silicone oil such as Densiron Xtra can be used but is not necessary. If the retina is relieved, then 5000 csts silicone oil is sufficient.

References

1. Vitrectomy with silicone oil or sulfur hexafluoride gas in eyes with severe proliferative vitreoretinopathy: results of a randomized clinical trial. Silicone Study Report 1. Arch Ophthalmol. 1992 Jun;110(6):770–9.
2. Han DP, Lewis MT, Kuhn EM, et al. Relaxing retinotomies and retinectomies: surgical results and predictors of visual outcome. Arch Ophthalmol. 1990;108:694–7.
3. Federman JL, Eagle RC Jr. Extensive peripheral retinectomy combined with posterior 360° retinotomy for retinal reattachment in advanced proliferative vitreoretinopathy cases. Ophthalmology. 1990;97:1305–20.
4. Zivojnovic R. Silicone oil in vitreoretinal surgery. Dordrecht: Martinus Nijhoff/Dr W Junk; 1987. p. 141–52.
5. Blumenkrantz MS, Azen SP, Aaberg T, et al. Relaxing retinotomy with silicone oil or long-acting gas in eyes with severe proliferative vitreoretinopathy. Silicone Study Report 5. The Silicone Oil Study Group. Am J Ophthalmol 1993;116:557–64.
6. Bovey EH, De Ancos E, Gonvers M. Retinotomies of 180 degrees or more. Retina. 1995;15:394–8.
7. Quiram PA, Gonzales CR, Hu W, et al. Outcomes of vitrectomy with inferior retinectomy in patients with recurrent rhegmatogenous retinal detachments and proliferative vitreoretinopathy. Ophthalmology 2006;113:2041–7.

Part VI
Difficult Cases

All videos of this part are found in a playlist on my youtube channel:
https://youtube.com/playlist?list=PL0dKYclPD7yMn861X0g-aHCS6KZ5NcH1N

Chapter 28: **Traumatic Retinal Detachment Secondary to Open Globe**

Surgical management of a corneal and scleral perforation

Implantation of an iris-IOL (Ophtec) for traumatic aniridia and aphakia

Napkin ring

Trauma with kick scooter with Napkin ring

Trauma with snowblower

PVR detachment secondary to trauma

Chapter 29: **Choroidal Detachment: Surgical Management of a Serous Choroidal Detachment**

Choroidal detachment for dummies

Chapter 30: **Suprachoroidal Haemorrhage**

Suprachoroidal haemorrhage after dry vitrectomy

Chapter 31: **Surgical Techniques for Silicone Oil and PFCL**

27G silicone oil removal

Densiron 68 removal with 25G.

28 Traumatic Retinal Detachment Secondary to Open Globe

Zoran Tomic and Ulrich Spandau

28.1 General Introduction

Trauma presents with a huge variety of pathology. Not one traumatic case can be compared with the other. This makes trauma surgery exciting and demanding but makes also recommendations for the surgical procedure rather difficult. Generally, a globe injury is divided up into an open globe injury and a closed globe injury [1]. Here, we will only talk about open globe injuries. For open globe injury, two major traumas are possible: (1) An ocular injury with intraocular foreign body (IOFB) and (2) globe injuries affecting the sclera (= scleral injury) or the cornea (=corneal injury). Remark: A corneal injury is often called a perforation and a scleral rupture is also named a globe rupture. See Fig. 28.1.

The IOFB causes in most cases only a small defect in the cornea or sclera which is good for the prognosis of the globe. But if the IOFB is of organic material such as wood, then the risk for endophthalmitis is high and the prognosis is poor. If the IOFB is of metal, then the prognosis is better. An endophthalmitis is seldom.

In case of a globe injury affecting the cornea, the prognosis is good because the endophthalmitis risk is low and the posterior segment is not affected. In the case of a scleral injury, the prognosis is poor because the retina may be incarcerated and a subchoroidal, subretinal or intravitreal haemorrhage may be present. Many eyes get lost in a hypotony.

Indication of vitrectomy: The indication for surgery is a retinal detachment. Not every eye with an open globe has a retinal detachment. If the scleral defect is located at the height of the limbus, then the retina is not involved. If you are insecure, then measure the distance between the limbus and scleral rupture with the calliper. If the distance is shorter than 4 mm (pars plana), then a retinal engagement is unlikely. It is helpful to perform a preoperative ultrasound. In addition, control if light perception in all directions exists.

Why not perform a prophylactic vitrectomy? An eye that suffered trauma is very inflamed. A vitrectomy in an inflamed tissue (vitreous and retina) increases the risk of a retinal detachment. Example: Vitreous haemorrhage after open globe injury. A wound at the limbus from 12 o'clock to 3 o'clock is sutured successfully. Two days later you perform an ultrasound and suspect a retinal detachment. You perform a vitrectomy and find an attached retina. One week later, the eye has with big likelihood a PVR retinal detachment.

Timing of surgery: In an initial surgery we close the globe and 2 weeks later we perform a

Z. Tomic
Milos Klinika, Belgrade, Serbia

U. Spandau (✉)
St. Eriks Hospital, University of Stockholm, Stockholm, Sweden
e-mail: ulrich_spandau@yahoo.de

U. Spandau et al. (eds.), *Retinal Detachment Surgery and Proliferative Vitreoretinopathy*,
https://doi.org/10.1007/978-3-031-11946-0_28

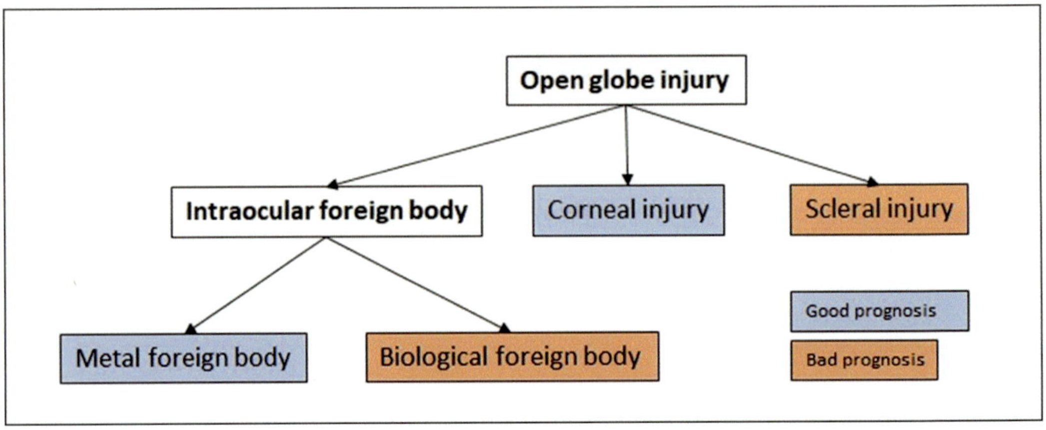

Fig. 28.1 Open globe injury and different prognosis

vitrectomy. See our treatment algorithm in Fig. 28.2. Other authors recommend to operate after 5–7 days (1). Even eyes with minimal or no light perception can be operated because visual acuity often increases after surgery. Perform an ultrasound: Is a subchoroidal haemorrhage (SCH) present? Is a vitreous haemorrhage present? Is a retinal detachment present? This information will help you to find your way during vitrectomy (Kuhn 2014).

But the prognosis is often poor. The main reason for failure in the long run is hypotony and corneal decompensation. But the spectrum of trauma is very large which makes it very difficult to generalize. We use to inform the patient that the prognosis is very poor but that in the majority of cases the outcome is better than without surgery. In our experience, patients with open globe rupture are postoperatively much more satisfied than patients with chronic and total retinal detachment.

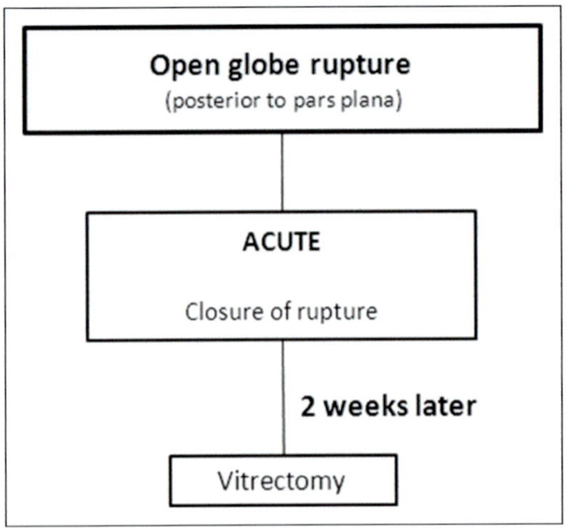

Fig. 28.2 Our treatment algorithm for open globe injuries

Anatomical characteristics of the posterior segment in open globe injuries are an *attached posterior hyaloid*, an *incarcerated retina* and a *napkin ring* (subretinal annular ring around the optic disc) (Figs. 28.3, 28.4 and 28.5)

Planning of surgery: The main indication for surgery is a retinal detachment. Silicone oil is the most common tamponade. The situation of the anterior chamber, therefore, is very important for surgery. Assess whether a cataract surgery has been performed or not. In many cases, aphakia

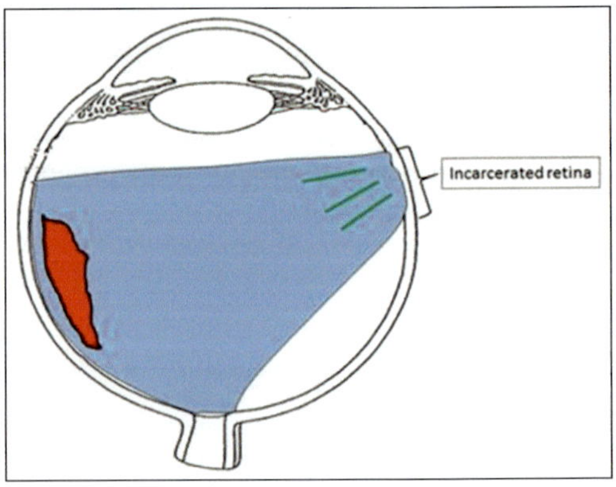

Fig. 28.3 The retina is incarcerated in the scleral wound on the right side and a large break is present on the left side

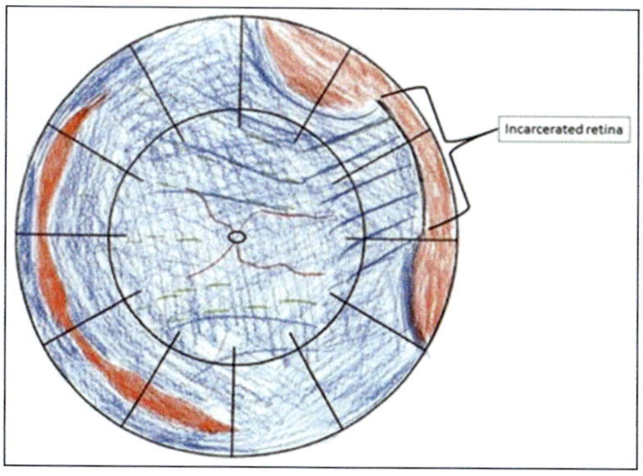

Fig. 28.4 A large retinal break on the left side and a retinal incarceration on the right side

due to a luxated lens/IOL and sometimes even aniridia are present. Aniridia and aphakia, however, are a big hinder to silicone oil tamponade. In the case of aphakia, an Artisan IOL can prevent a silicone oil prolapse. In the case of aphakia and aniridia, an iris IOL prosthesis (Opthec, NL) or a suture net is a good option.

Characteristics of surgery: The surgery is difficult due to poor visualization secondary to cloudy media and blood. Due to the extensive intravitreal, subretinal and subchoroidal haemorrhage, it is very difficult to see the difference between blood, vitreous, retina and choroid. The retina may be incarcerated in the wound and has to be relieved from the wound through a retinotomy. A PVD is usually not present.

A napkin ring may form subretinally at the optic disc. It has the shape of a ring and constricts the retina (Fig. 28.5). The annular membrane occurs after a chronic detachment. In order to remove the napkin ring, a 360° circumferential retinotomy is required. The surgery should be performed in general anaesthesia and the surgical time is 2–4 h.

The surgical management of an open globe with scleral injury

Material and instruments

1. 23G or 25G trauma trocars (Alcon)
2. Chandelier light
3. Maybe: Artisan IOL
4. PFCL
5. Silicone oil

The surgery step-by-step

1. **Insertion of anterior chamber maintainer**
2. **Removal of hyphema**
3. **Inspection of posterior segment**
4. **Core vitrectomy**
5. **Insertion of trauma trocars**
6. **Peripheral vitrectomy and PVD**
7. **Endodiathermy of traumatic retinal edges**
8. **Retinotomy of incarcerated retina**
9. **Removal of subretinal membranes**
10. **Removal of napkin ring**
11. **Instillation of PFCL**
12. **Attachment test and rotation test**

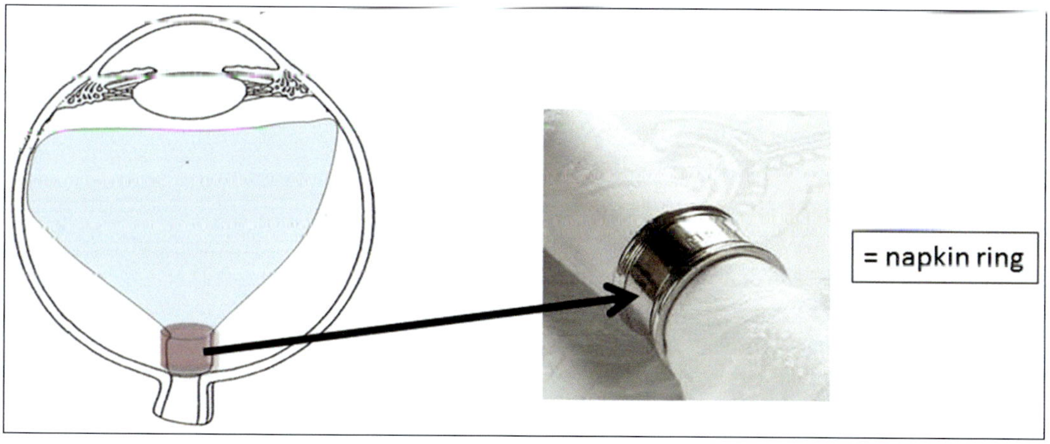

Fig. 28.5 A subretinal fibrotic ring around the retina located at the optic disc = napkin ring

13. **Laser treatment**
14. **Preparation of anterior chamber before silicone oil tamponade**
15. **PFCL against air and exchange**
16. **1000 cSt silicone oil tamponade**

Every step in detail

1. **Insertion of anterior chamber maintainer**
2. **Removal of hyphema**

   In many trauma cases, a hyphema is present. Remove the hyphema with irrigation and aspiration. If the cornea is cloudy, perform a corneal abrasion. If the view does not improve, then a haemorrhagic cornea is likely. The only solution is now a corneal transplantation. Examine the iris and the lens status. If the iris is haemorrhagic, do not insist to remove the blood but cut only a central pupil with the vitreous cutter.

3. **Inspection of posterior segment**
4. **Core vitrectomy**

   Insert the light fibre through a side incision and examine the retina, i.e. try to examine the retina. If you do not see anything, then work carefully because the retina may be totally detached. Start to cut centrally on the height of the pars plana. Try to identify retina, choroid and haemorrhagic vitreous from each other. If you cannot identify any structures in the centre behind the pars plane, then continue to work in the periphery. Even if you cut the retina in the periphery, this is not a problem because a large retinotomy is required in the end.

5. **Insertion of trauma trocars**
6. **Peripheral vitrectomy with PVD**
7. **Endodiathermy of traumatic retinal edges**

   Assess the periphery for a suitable area to insert the trocars. Try to insert at least two instrument trocars so that you can work easier in the posterior segment. As trocars we use 23G or 25G trauma trocars from Alcon. Then continue with a vitrectomy. In many cases, a PVD is absent. Induce a PVD and then instil PFCL to flatten the central retina. Perform a thorough peripheral vitrectomy as possible. If you leave the peripheral vitreous and use silicone oil as tamponade, then the silicone oil will press the peripheral vitreous against the ciliary body causing ciliary body insufficiency and hypotony. Perform a meticulous diathermy of bleeding retinotomy edges in order to prevent recurrent PVR.

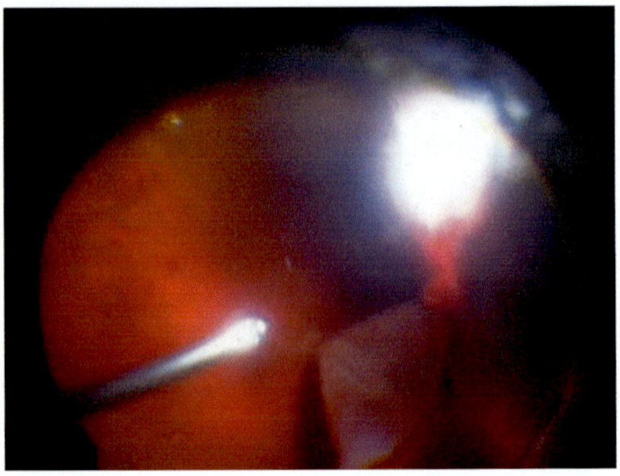

Fig. 28.6 The retina is incarcerated on the right side into the scleral wound

8. **Retinotomy of incarcerated retina** (Figs. 28.6 and 28.7)
9. **Removal of subretinal membranes**
10. **Removal of napkin ring** (Fig. 28.8)
11. **Instillation of PFCL**

    If the retina is incarcerated into the scleral wound, then perform a retinotomy at the scleral wound in order to mobilize the incarcerated retina (Figs. 28.6 and 28.7).

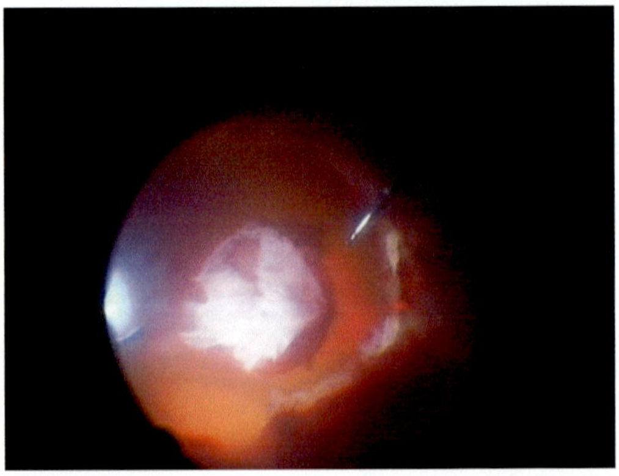

Fig. 28.7 After retinotomy: Note the residual retina in the scleral wound on the right side

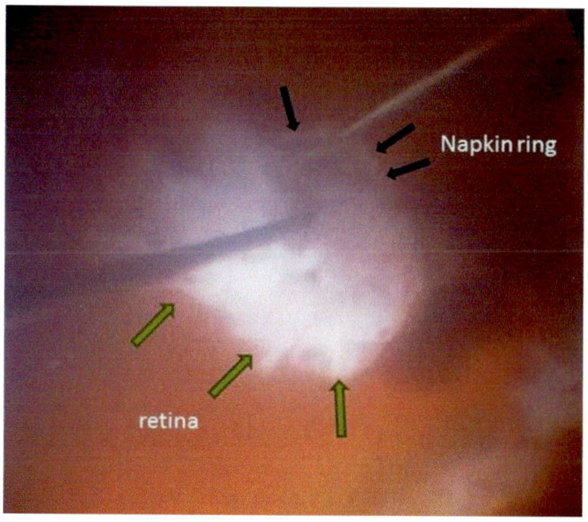

Fig. 28.8 Note the napkin ring which is located subretinally around the optic disc

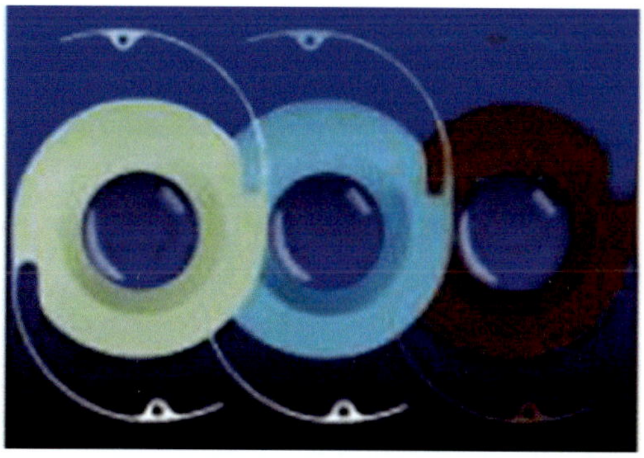

Fig. 28.10 An IOL-iris prosthesis from Opthec, Netherlands. The diameter is 9 mm. A large incision is therefore required. The colour of the prosthesis turns out brighter when inserted in the eye. We use only the brown iris. The prize is approximately 400 Euros

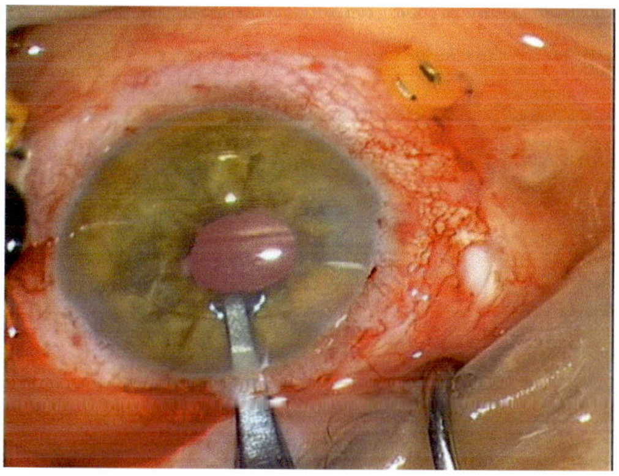

Fig. 28.9 In case of aphakia insert an IOL, in this case an Artisan IOL with retropupilar fixation. It will prevent a silicone oil prolapse

Continue with the removal of subretinal membranes. Finally, remove the fibrous ring around the optic disc. Then reattach the retina through instillation of PFCL over the retinotomy edges. Check if the retina is completely attached to the optic disc. If not, then you did not remove the complete napkin ring (Fig. 28.8). This procedure is difficult because the retina is mobile. Check also the retinal edges. Are they attached or enrolled? Flatten the distorted retina with a Charles flute needle with a silicone tip or a knob spatula. If a membrane causes a radial retinal distortion, then remove the membrane.

12. **Attachment test and rotation test**
13. **Laser treatment**

    Check now if the macula is correctly located or if a rotation is present. If you observe a rotation, then rotate the retina with the vacuum cleaner or a knob spatula. Continue with three rows of the laser along the retinotomy edges. For retinal edges, a laser duration of 300 ms is required. Remark: The usual laser duration for retinal breaks is 200 ms.

14. **Preparation of anterior chamber before silicone oil tamponade** (Figs. 28.9, 28.10 and 28.11)
15. **PFCL against air and exchange**
16. **1000 cSt silicone oil tamponade** (Fig. 28.12)

Before continuing with a tamponade, the anterior chamber must be prepared for the tamponade. Is an aphakia present? If aphakia is present and you plan to use silicone oil, then an iridectomy is required to prevent a pupillary block. If possible insert an Artisan iris-claw IOL with a retropupillary implantation (Fig. 28.9). If aniridia is present, then implant an iris-IOL prosthesis (Opthec, NL) (Fig. 28.10). An alternative is a suture net (Fig. 28.11). If you plan a silicone oil tamponade, then fill the anterior chamber with

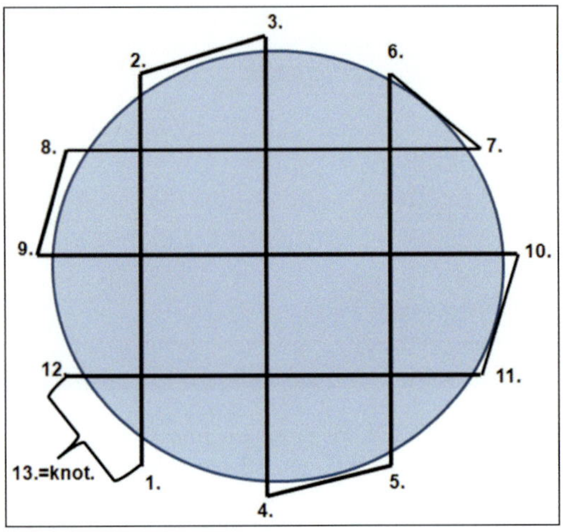

Fig. 28.11 A drawing of the suture. Start with 1 and end with 12 Number 13 is the knot. One continuous suture

methylcellulose to prevent a intraoperative prolapse of silicone oil into the anterior chamber. The next step is a PFCL against silicone oil exchange. If you prefer first a PFCL against air exchange, then perform a meticulous fluid aspiration at the retinotomy edges. Close the case with a 1300 St or 5000 cSt silicone oil tamponade (Fig. 28.12).

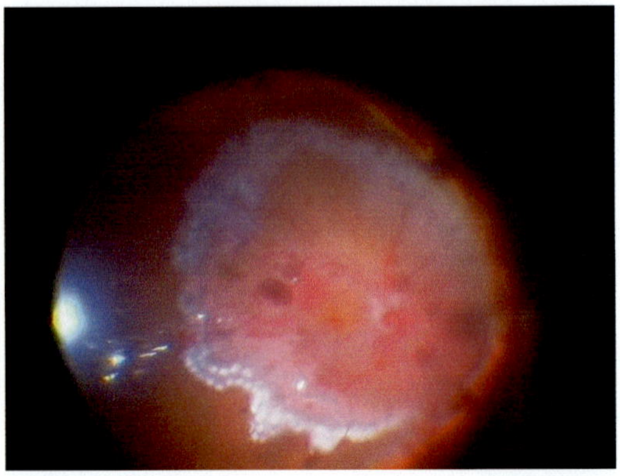

Fig. 28.12 The final view to retina. Visual acuity is 0,1, the globe is normotensive and the patient is satisfied. The minority of these cases have such a good outcome

Reference

1. Kuhn F. The timing of reconstruction in severe mechanical trauma. Ophthalmic Res. 2014;51(2):67–72.

29 Choroidal Detachment: Surgical Management of a Serous Choroidal Detachment

Zoran Tomic and Ulrich Spandau

A choroidal detachment occurs if the IOP drops below 6 mmHg. A choroidal detachment may be caused by hypotony for example after a trabeculectomy. Another typical example is a ciliary body insufficiency secondary to uveitis. Clear fluid is present between sclera and choroid. A so-called "choroidal effusion" or serous choroidal detachment has developed (Table 29.1). The surgery of a choroidal effusion has a low complication profile because the serous fluid can be removed easily and complete. As a basic rule, the subchoroidal fluid is removed from the scleral side, and not transretinal. But the surgery can become difficult if a combined choroidal effusion and rhegmatogeneous retinal detachment develop.

Indication for surgery: A surgery is recommended when kissing choroids are present. This is however only necessary in an avitreal eye. In an avitreal eye the retina of both sides stick to each other. In case of an eye with vitreous this risk is very much reduced. If kissing choroids occur after a trabulectomy then the first surgical approach is to close the scleral flap with extra sutures. If the IOP improves and increases over 8 mmHg then the choroidal detachment will disappear.

Timing for surgery: In case of a ciliary body insufficiency we would treat first with oral and topical steroids for approximately 1–2 weeks. If the IOP does not improve, we inject 0,1 ml intravitreal triamcinolone. In our experience a triamcinolone injection is more effective than topical or oral medication. If the IOP does not improve after 2 weeks, we would perform surgery because the risk for a PVR detachment increases.

Instruments

1. 23 or 25-Gauge 4-port trocar system
2. Anterior chamber maintainer
3. 6 mm trocar cannulas (23G and 25G from Alcon)

An *anterior chamber maintainer* is an infusion, which is inserted in the limbus and injects BSS into the anterior chamber.

Tamponade

PFCL, 1000 or 5000 csts silicone oil.

Individual steps

1. Limbal peritomy.

2. Place traction sutures beneath all four rectus muscles.

3. Insert an anterior chamber maintainer.

4. Drainage sclerotomies.

5. Drainage of serous fluid.

5. Insertion of trocars.

6. Core vitrectomy.

Z. Tomic
Milos Klinika, Belgrade, Serbia

U. Spandau (✉)
St. Eriks Hospital, University of Stockholm, Stockholm, Sweden
e-mail: ulrich_spandau@yahoo.de

U. Spandau et al. (eds.), *Retinal Detachment Surgery and Proliferative Vitreoretinopathy*,
https://doi.org/10.1007/978-3-031-11946-0_29

Table 29.1 Diagram of the anatomy of a choroidal detachment. Remark to the pars plana anatomy: The retina ends at the ora serrata and goes over to the pars plana epithelium. The choroid is contiguous with the ciliary body. If the choroid is detached, then the pars plana epithelium detaches too

Sclera
Serous fluid in the suprachoroidal space
Choroid
Retina
Vitreous

7. **Injection of PFCL.**
8. **Trimming of vitreous base.**
9. **Exchange of PFCL against silicone oil.**

1. Limbal peritomy

2. Place traction sutures beneath all four rectus muscles

Perform a 360° peritomy and place traction sutures underneath all horizontal muscles.

3. Insert an anterior chamber maintainer

An inferotemporal paracentesis is performed, the anterior chamber maintainer is inserted, and the infusion line is opened (Fig. 29.1). Now the eyeball becomes normotensive. An infusion of the anterior chamber works particularly well when there is a pseudophakia.

4. Drainage sclerotomies

5. Drainage and expression of subchoroidal blood

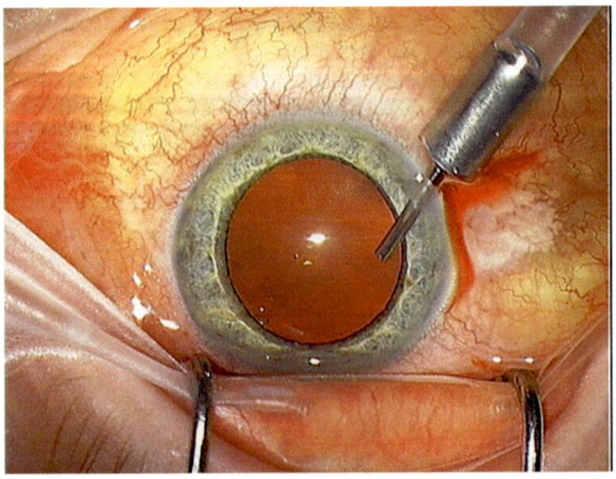

Fig. 29.1 Insert an anterior chamber maintainer to increase IOP

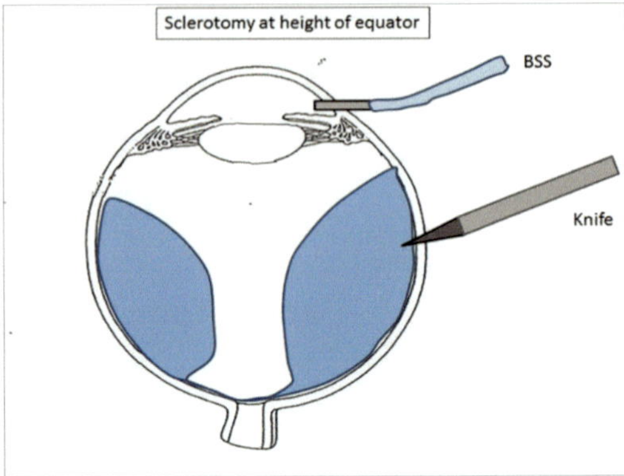

Fig. 29.2 Perform a 1–2 mm sclerotomy on height of the equator

Drainage of a serous choroidal detachment

Before performing a sclerotomy you should ascertain the location of the choroidal bullae in the eye (Fig. 29.2). They are usually located temporally and nasally.

A small sclerotomy of 2–3 mm in length is sufficient (Fig. 29.3). Place the sclerotomies between the insertion of the muscle and the equator. For example, if a temporal and nasal choroidal detachment is present, you should perform a temporal and nasal sclerotomy. The sclerotomy is located in the middle between the muscle insertion and equator. The sclerotomies should be 2–3 mm in length and extend in a radial direction. Once the sclerotomy is performed, clear fluid will flow out the sclerotomy. Repeat the maneuver on the nasal side if necessary.

The sclerotomies do not need to be sutured at the end of the surgery.

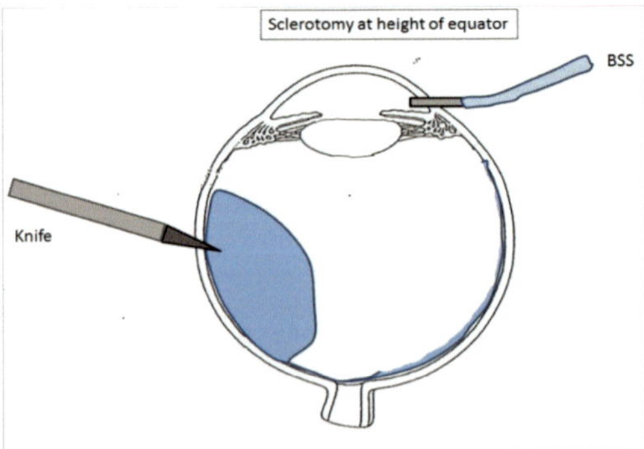

Fig. 29.3 The same maneuver on the other side

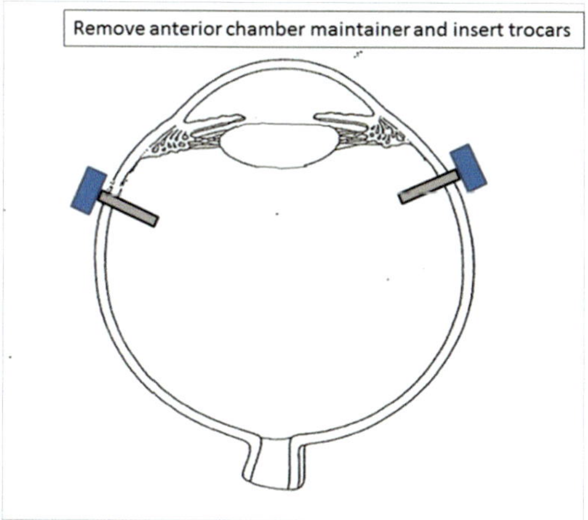

Fig. 29.4 Insert trocars and remove the anterior chamber maintainer

6. Insertion of trocars
When no more fluid flows out of the sclerotomy, you can try to insert the trocars at the pars plana if you have not done this before. Due to the detachment of the pars plana epithelium, this is a difficult procedure. Choose an area with little choroidal detachment. Use preferably 6 mm long trauma trocars from Alcon. Insert the trocar perpendicular and *not* lamellar. Check if the trocar is located in the vitreous cavity. If the trocar cannula is not in the vitreous cavity, it can be freed from the surrounding tissue with a membrane pic from the opposite trocar cannula. The same procedure can now be performed with the second trocar cannula. Remove the anterior chamber maintainer and insert a pars plana infusion line. Then insert a second trocar opposite to the infusion cannula. *Remark*: Double check several times during surgery the correct location of the trocar cannulas (Fig. 29.4).

7. Core vitrectomy
8. Injection of PFCL

If the choroidal detachment has regressed, a vitrectomy can be performed. You may need to insert a chandelier light. Then PFCL is injected,

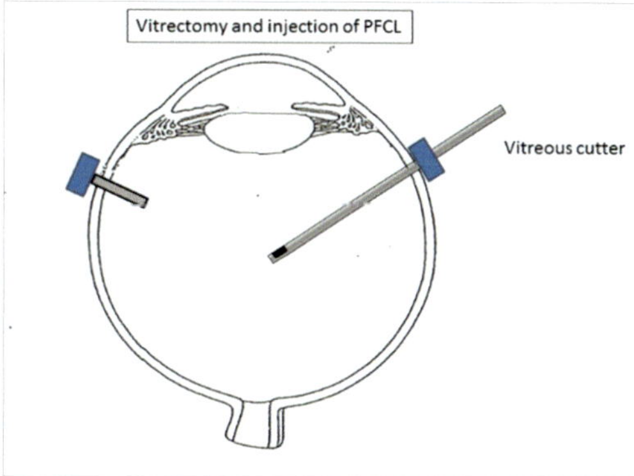

Fig. 29.5 Continue with a vitrectomy and instill PFCL (heavy water)

which pushes the residual suprachoroidal blood through the sclerotomies outside. You should now check the sclerotomies (flick the BIOM out and rotate the globe with the traction sutures) (Fig. 29.5).

9. Trimming of vitreous base
Perform a thorough trimming of the vitreous base because a long lasting or even permanent silicone oil tamponade is required.

10. Exchange of PFCL for silicone oil
If there is only a minor residual choroidal detachment, perform a PFCL/silicone oil exchange. The silicone oil is injected through the infusion cannula. Suture the sclerotomies with a Vicryl 8–0 stitch.

Postoperative course: The residual choroidal detachment will resorb within 3 months. We recommend a silicone removal after 3–6 months.

Surgical pearls no. 115
Hypotony: A hypotony is defined with an IOP < 6 mmHg. A choroidal detachment develops. A possible treatment is a drainage of the subchoroidal fluid and a permanent silicone oil tamponade.

Suprachoroidal Haemorrhage 30

Zoran Tomic and Ulrich Spandau

The expulsive haemorrhage is a haemorrhage in the suprachoroidal space (Diagram 30.1). Sometimes the term "suprachoroidal" is used synonymously to "subchoroidal". As a basic rule, these haemorrhages are removed from the scleral side and not transretinal.

As a general rule we wait 2 weeks with the vitrectomy so that the blood can liquefy. The surgery should be performed under general anaesthesia. Preoperative ultrasound is necessary to determine the shape and location of the choroidal haemorrhage. You have to perform a sclerotomy in the area of the highest choroidal detachment.

We describe the surgical procedure of a suprachoroidal haemorrhage without expulsion of intraocular tissue.

Instruments

1. 25-Gauge 4-port trocar system
2. BIOM
3. Anterior chamber maintainer
4. Vitreous cutter
5. Extra long 6 mm trocars, 25G from Alcon

You need instruments from the detachment set and the PPV set. The anterior chamber maintainer is an infusion cannula for the anterior chamber.

Tamponade

PFCL, 1000 or 5000csts silicone oil.

Main surgical steps

1. Limbal peritomy.

2. Place traction sutures beneath all four rectus muscles.

3. Insert an anterior chamber maintainer.

4. 3-4 mm sclerotomies between insertion of the muscle and the equator.

5. Expression of subchroidal blood.

6. Insertion of trocars.

7. Core vitrectomy.

8. Injection of PFCL.

9. Trimming of vitreous base.

10. Exchange of PFCL against silicone oil.

The surgery step-by-step

1. Limbal peritomy

2. Place traction sutures beneath all four rectus muscles

Perform a 360° peritomy and place traction sutures underneath all horizontal muscles.

Z. Tomic
Milos Klinika, Belgrade, Serbia

U. Spandau (✉)
St. Eriks Hospital, University of Stockholm, Stockholm, Sweden
e-mail: ulrich_spandau@yahoo.de

U. Spandau et al. (eds.), *Retinal Detachment Surgery and Proliferative Vitreoretinopathy*,
https://doi.org/10.1007/978-3-031-11946-0_30

Diagram 30.1 Diagram of the anatomy of suprachoroidal haemorrhage

Sclera
Haemorrhage in the suprachoroidal space
Choroid
Retina
Vitreous

3. Insert an anterior chamber maintainer

An inferotemporal paracentesis is performed, the anterior chamber maintainer is inserted, and the infusion line is opened (Figs. 30.1 and 30.2). Now the eyeball becomes normotensive. An infusion of the anterior chamber works particularly well when there is a pseudophakia. If the patient is phakic, try to insert the infusion cannula in an area of the pars plana where there is no choroidal detachment (ultrasound). When in doubt, place a 20-gauge sclerotomy using a long (6 mm) 20-gauge infusion port. It is of vital importance that the inner opening of the infusion port is in the vitreous cavity and not in the subretinal/suprachoroidal space.

4. 3–4 mm sclerotomies between insertion of the muscle and the equator

5. Expression of subchroidal blood

Before performing a sclerotomy you should ascertain the location of the SCH in the eye. You can confirm your ultrasound examination by inspecting the vitreous cavity with a light pipe. Search for the quadrant with the highest bullous choroidal detachment.

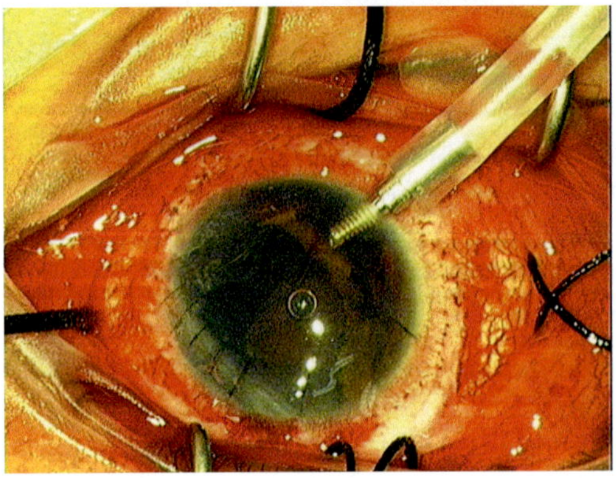

Fig. 30.1 Eye with a perforating trauma from a stick. In a first operation the temporal limbus was sutured with Ethilon 10–0 and the sclera with Vicryl 8–0. Prior to the second operation a 360-degree suprachoroidal haemorrhage was detected. Now four traction sutures were placed beneath the four horizontal muscles. An anterior chamber maintainer was inserted to stabilize the eye

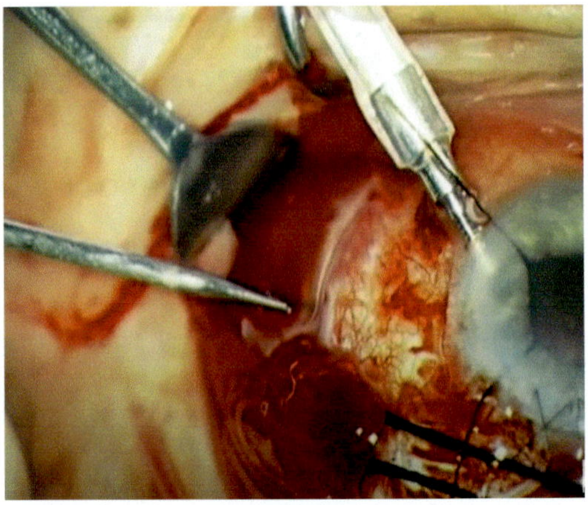

Fig. 30.2 A different case with SCH and endophthalmitis after complicated cataract surgery. With a 20G V lance a 3 mm sclerotomy is performed between equator and muscle insertion. Note the anterior chamber maintainer

The sclerotomy should be 3–4 mm mm in length and extend in a radial direction (Fig. 30.2). Concerning the location of these sclerotomies there are different preferences. Some surgeons perform the sclerotomies 4 mm posterior the limbus, other place the sclerotomies equatorial, since there is more suprachoroidal blood. We place the sclerotomies between the insertion of the muscle and the equator. For example, if a temporal and nasal choroidal detachment is present, you should perform a temporal and nasal sclerotomy. Once the sclerotomy is performed, liquefied blood and blood clots will flow out the sclerotomy (Fig. 30.3). Then examine the fundus with a light pipe from the limbus (Fig. 30.4). If residual blood is present then continue with expression of blood clots (Fig. 30.5).

If only liquefied blood flows out and no clots, you should enlarge the sclerotomy to 4 mm and compress the eyeball with two cotton swabs in the direction of the sclerotomies (Fig. 30.6). With this technique you can express big blood clots. Later on the 4 mm sclerotomies are closed with a Vicryl 8–0 X–sutures. You can leave

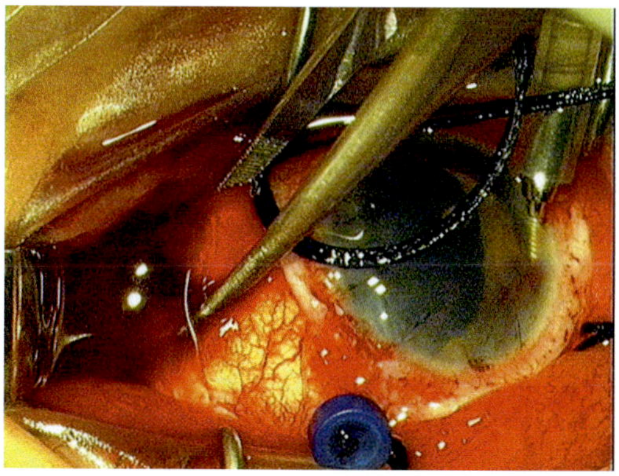

Fig. 30.3 Liquefied blood flows out of the second sclerotomy on the other side of the globe. Extract the blood by compressing the globe with a forceps or cotton swabs

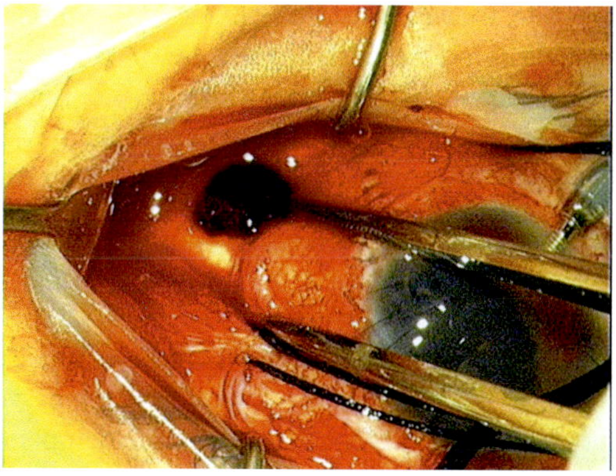

Fig. 30.6 If the sclerotomy is too small you cannot extract thick blood clots. Enlarge the sclerotomies to 4-mm incisions. This sclerotomy needs to be sutured with 1–2 Vicryl 8–0 cross sutures

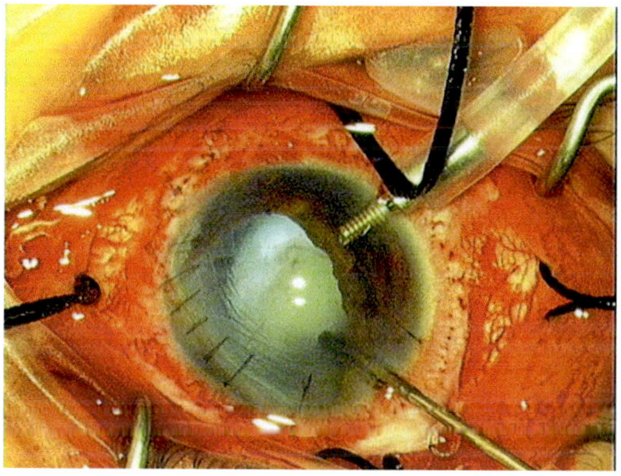

Fig. 30.4 Due to the choroidal detachment it is difficult to place trocar cannulas. With help of a light pipe, which is inserted through a paracentesis, the situation in the posterior segment is explored

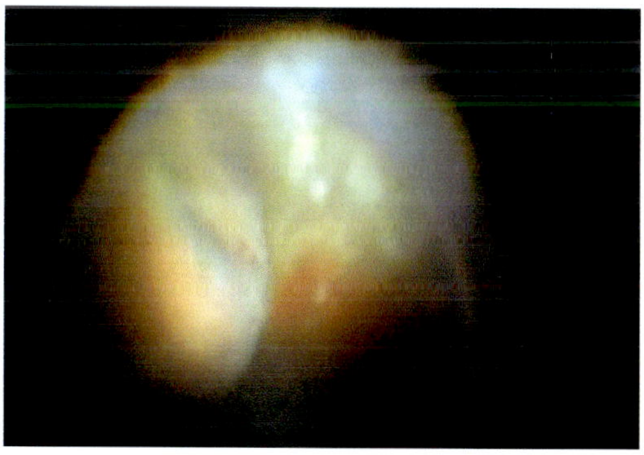

Fig. 30.5 The fundus can now be inspected. Much residual hemorrhage is present

2 mm sclerotomies open, so that residual blood can evacuate.

6. Insertion of trocars

When no more blood flows out of the sclerotomy, you should try to insert the trocars at the pars plana. Due to the detachment of the pars plana epithelium, this is a difficult procedure. Choose an area with little choroidal detachment and select a sutureable, longer infusion cannula (see above). We use 6 mm long trauma trocars from Alcon (Fig. 30.7). Check if the trocar is located in the vitreous cavity. Remove the anterior chamber maintainer and insert a pars plana infusion line. Then insert a second trocar

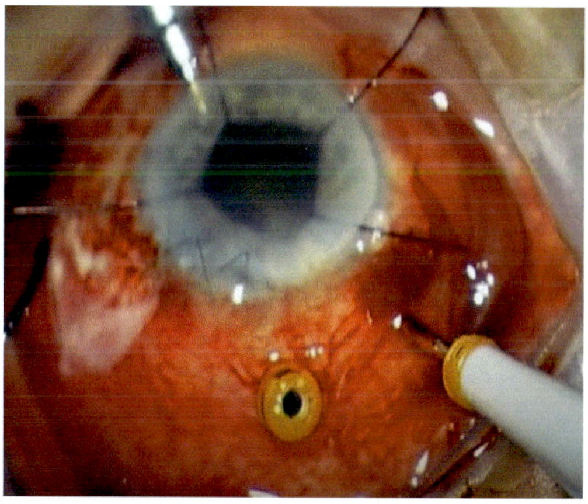

Fig. 30.7 Insert the trocar cannulas on the opposite side of the choroidal hemorrhage

opposite to the infusion cannula. If the trocar cannula is not in the vitreous cavity, it can be freed from the surrounding tissue with a membrane pic from the opposite trocar cannula. The same procedure can now be performed with the third trocar cannula.

Pits and Pearls

Subepithelial location of trocars: Especially in eyes with choroidal haemorrhage an initially correctly placed trocar cannula may move subepithelially during a later stage of the operation. Double-check the trocars several times during surgery.

7. Core vitrectomy

8. Injection of PFCL

If the choroidal detachment has regressed, a vitrectomy can be performed. You may need to insert a chandelier light. Then PFCL is injected, which pushes the residual suprachoroidal blood through the sclerotomies outside. You should now check the sclerotomies (flick the BIOM out and rotate the globe with the traction sutures). If little or no blood flows out in an area with a high choroidal detachment, try to expel blood clots with a forceps or cotton swabs.

9. Trimming of vitreous base

Perform a thorough trimming of the vitreous base in trauma patients, in particular the anterior part of the vitreous base which extends over the ciliary body. Otherwise the eye will develop cyclitic membranes which grow on the ciliary body and result in hypotony. Cyclitic membranes are very difficult to remove. The development of cyclitic membranes will increase if you use silicone oil as a tamponade.

10. Exchange of PFCL for silicone oil

If there is only a minor residual choroidal detachment, perform a PFCL/silicone oil exchange (Fig. 30.8). This surgical maneuver is shown in great detail in the next chapter. The silicone oil is injected through the infusion

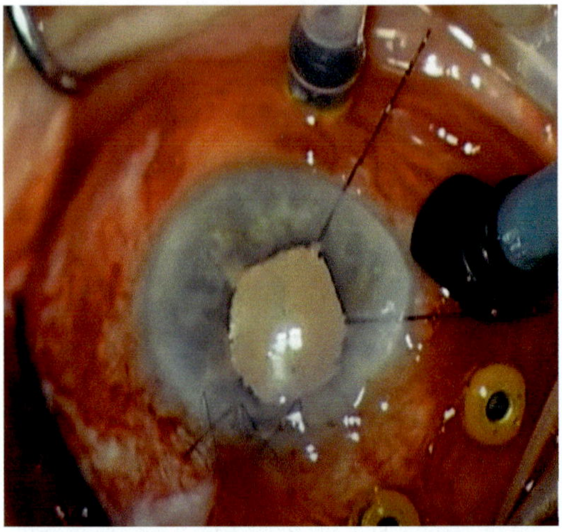

Fig. 30.8 Note the DORC infusion in the superior trocar cannula. PFCL is directly exchanged against silicone oil

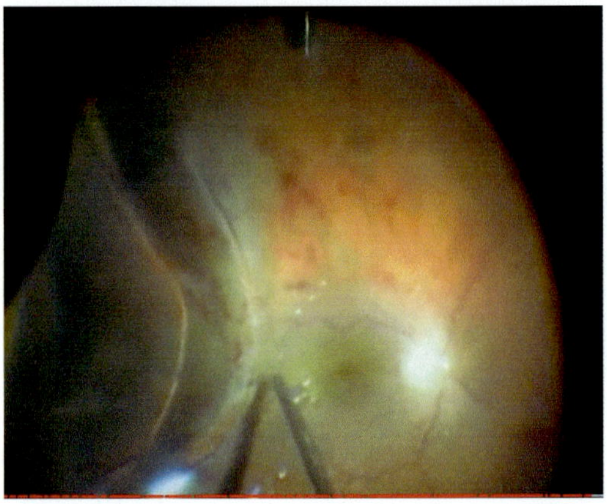

Fig. 30.9 The SCH is reduced, the posterior pole is free from blood and silicone oil is injected. The residual blood will be resorbed within 4–8 weeks

cannula (Fig. 30.9). Suture the sclerotomies with an 8–0 Vicryl suture.

After a few weeks an underfill of the silicone oil will occur. A silicone oil removal can be performed after approximately three months if no hypotony has developed. If you want to extend the tamponade, then inject additional silicone oil.

Surgical Techniques for Silicone Oil and PFCL

31

Zoran Tomic and Ulrich Spandau

Silicone oil is an excellent temporary tamponade but a poor permanent tamponade. It causes high IOP, emulsifies and may result in an optic atrophy. Silicone oil should be avoided in fresh and primary detachments. Silicone oil is indicated in recurrent detachments, complicated PVR detachments, diabetic tractive detachments and traumatic detachments. But even in these cases try to remove the silicone oil after three months.

Silicone oil tamponades can be performed with 25-gauge and 27-gauge technology. It is straightforward to use 1000 csts and 5000 csts silicone oil. In case of 27G we use a 25G trocar cannula for oil injection and extraction. You can inject the oil into a BSS-filled or an air-filled eye. But an injection into a BSS-filled eye is difficult because the two liquids are difficult to distinguish. We, therefore, recommend the exchange of air against silicone oil for routine cases.

1000 csts silicone oil: We use in almost all cases 1000 or 1300 csts silicone oil. The duration is 2–6 months. The emulsification is acceptable, and an IOP increase can be treated with antiglaucomatous drops.

Z. Tomic
Milos Klinika, Belgrade, Serbia

U. Spandau (✉)
St. Eriks Hospital, University of Stockholm, Stockholm, Sweden
e-mail: ulrich_spandau@yahoo.de

5000 csts silicone oil: 5000 csts silicone oil causes less ocular hypertension and less emulsification than 1000 csts silicone oil. It is therefore suitable for a permanent tamponade. We use 5000 csts silicone oil for eyes which require a permanent tamponade such as ocular hypotony, trauma cases and PVR detachments.

Heavy silicone oil: The heavy silicone oil Densiron Xtra (Fluoron) is a bit tricky to remove, because the silicone oil is heavier than BSS and the final oil bubble may fall onto the posterior pole. We remove Densiron Xtra 6–12 weeks after injection.

Duration of silicone oil tamponade

Duration of **light** silicone oil tamponade:

Retinal detachment: Six to twelve weeks.

Duration of **heavy** silicone oil tamponade:

Inferior detachment: Six weeks.

31.1 Silicone Oil Injection

The surgical method of choice regarding silicone oil exchange is the injection of silicone oil into an air-filled eye. This applies for light and heavy silicone oil. The injection of silicone oil into a PFCL filled eye is also possible but technically more difficult. This applies for light and heavy silicone oil. Also heavy silicone oil (Densiron Xtra) can be exchanged with PFCL. The risk that heavy silicone oil and PFCL will blend during

U. Spandau et al. (eds.), *Retinal Detachment Surgery and Proliferative Vitreoretinopathy*,
https://doi.org/10.1007/978-3-031-11946-0_31

Diagram 31.1 Diagram of the location of liquids during an air x silicone oil exchange

Intraoperatively	Postoperatively	
Air	Silicone oil	Vitreous cavity
Silicone oil	Water	

the short exchange time is low and both fluid phases can be well distinguished.

Diagram 31.1 shows the location of the fluids in the vitreous chamber during an air x silicone oil exchange. Air is lighter than silicone oil. During surgery, the silicone oil is injected into the air-filled vitreous cavity. Depending on the amount of injected oil more or less water will be localized at the inferior pole after surgery.

Regarding surgery: For injection of all types of silicone oil we use the 23G or 25G cannula (Alcon) (Fig. 31.1). Silicone oil injection is easy with chandelier light and a bit tricky without chandelier light. With chandelier light the intraocular air is released with an extrusion cannula. Without chandelier light the air pressure must be reduced to 10 mmHg to avoid intraocular high pressure.

31.1.1 Silicone Oil Injection with Chandelier Light (Under BIOM View)

Instruments:

23G or 25G metal cannula (Alcon).

Main surgical steps:

1. Prepare anterior chamber
2. Fluid against air exchange
3. Injection of silicone oil

The surgery step-by-step:

1. Prepare anterior chamber

Before you perform a fluid x air exchange, prepare the anterior chamber to prevent a silicone oil prolapse. The anterior chamber should have normal depth, and an iridectomy may be required (Fig. 31.2).

- *6 o'clock iridectomy for light silicone oils*: If aphakia or zonular lysis is present, create an Ando-iridectomy (6 o'clock) to prevent an increase in intraocular pressure. An Ando iridectomy prevents a secondary angle-closure because the aqueous can flow through the iridectomy at 6 o'clock into the anterior

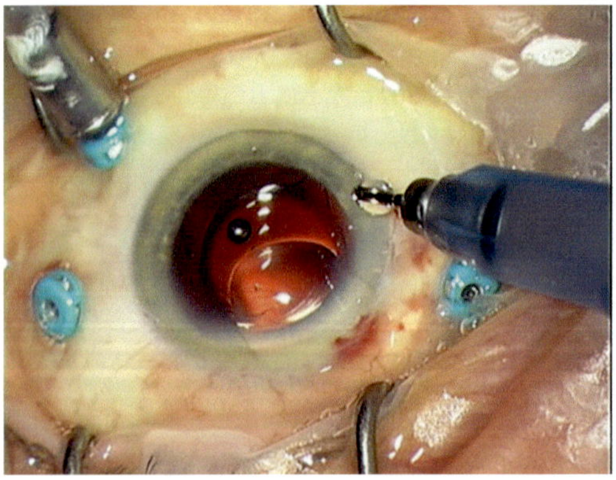

Fig. 31.1 We use a metal cannula (23G, 25G) for silicone oil and Densiron Xtra injection (Alcon)

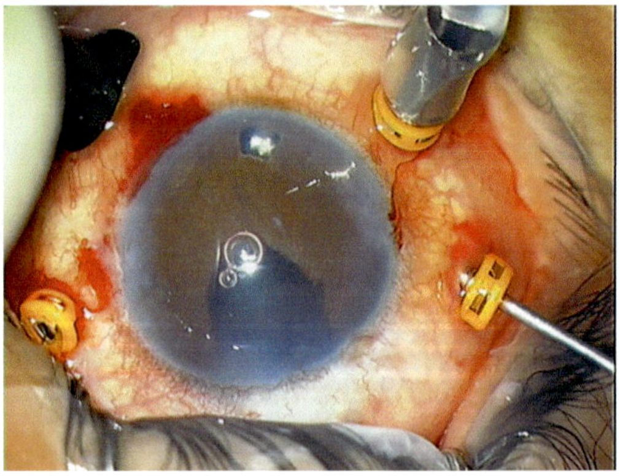

Fig. 31.2 A basal iridectomy. Place the vitreous cutter behind the iris and create an iridectomy with approximately 100 cuts/min. If the pupil is dilated then stretch the pupil at 6 o´clock with a forceps

chamber and press the oil bubble back into the vitreous cavity. Work bimanually: Draw the pupillary edge at 6 o'clock with an intravitreal forceps. Place the vitreous cutter (low cut rate: about 200 cuts/min) with the opening forward behind the iris at 6 o'clock, aspirate the iris and then cut a hole.

- *12 o'clock iridectomy for heavy silicone oils*: Densiron Xtra® (Geuder) is a heavy silicone oil and will tamponade the inferior retina. If an iridectomy is needed, it must be performed at 12 o'clock. Perform the iridectomy optimally in a perfluorocarbon liquid (PFCL) or water filled eye, i.e. before silicone oil injection.
- *Methylcellulose in anterior chamber*: If a large zonular lysis is present, inject now methyl cellulose into the anterior chamber; it can be left there postoperatively. It holds the anterior chamber silicone oil free. There will be only a slight postoperative rise of IOP.

2. Fluid against air exchange

3. Injection of silicone oil

The infusion line must remain in place during the complete surgery because the air streaming in keeps the eye normotensive (Figs. 31.3, 31.4 and 31.5). Attach a 23G or 25G metal cannula (Alcon) to a silicone oil syringe. The oil falls from the anterior onto the posterior pole, i.e. the eye is filled from the back to the front. At the same time the surgeon must release the air with a backflush instrument from a trocar. When the last air bubble disappears behind the lens, stop the air infusion and remove the residual air bubble. Then inject silicone oil until the globe is hypo- to normotensive. During this procedure, check for a positive venous pulse. If the globe is hypertensive then release oil by removing a valve or by simply cutting the infusion line.

31.1.2 Silicone Oil Tamponade Without Chandelier Light

Reduce the air pressure to 10 mmHg (Figs. 31.6 and 31.7). Inject the silicone oil. The second hand holds the light pipe. When the posterior segment is 90% filled with silicone oil, stop the injection. Flick out the BIOM, place an extrusion cannula behind the lens and inject the final 10% silicone oil. Wait until the last air bubble disappears behind the lens.

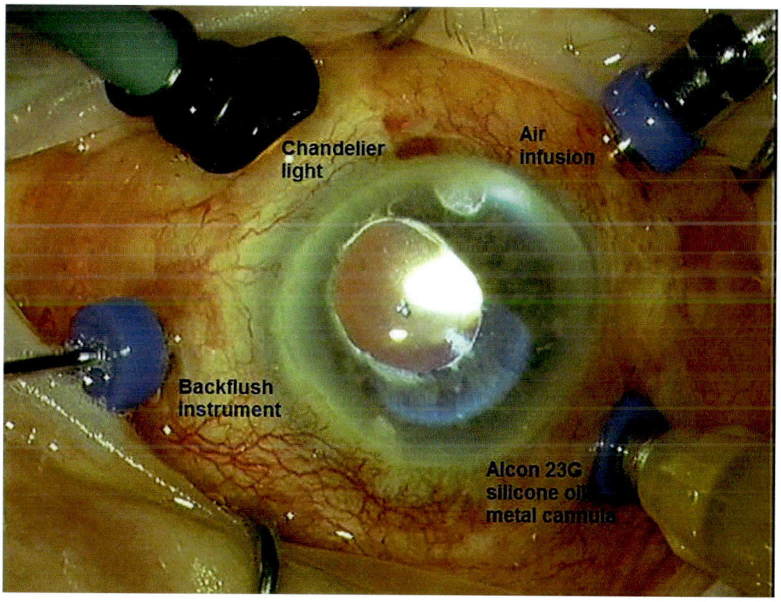

Fig. 31.3 Silicone oil injection **under** view to retina. Note that a chandelier light is required

Fig. 31.4 Setup for oil injection with view to retina

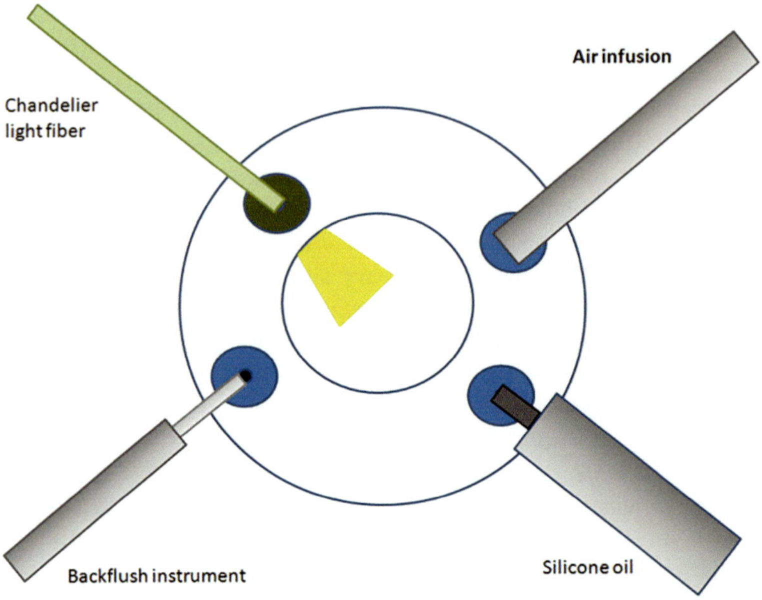

Fig. 31.5 You work bimanual in order to inject the silicone oil under view to retina

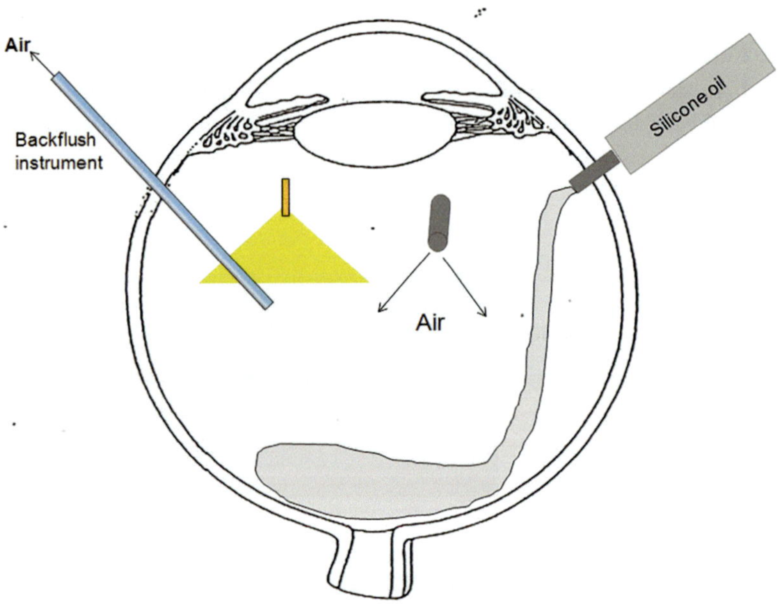

31.2 PFCL Against Silicone Oil Exchange (with DORC Infusion Line)

This situation is very different than the situation explained above. Why? The silicone oil is injected through the infusion line into the eye.

Surgery:

Instrument: (Figs. 31.8 and 31.9).

(1) 23G or 25G DORC infusion line with plastic cannula,

Remark: An infusion line with metal cannula (Alcon) does not work.

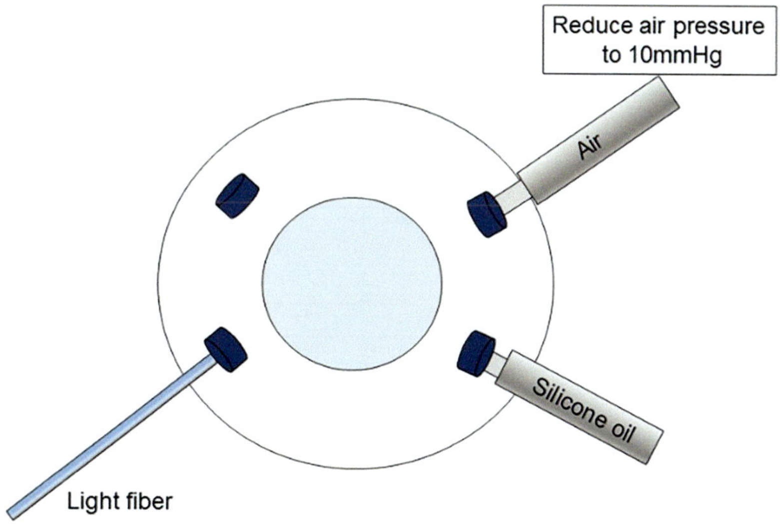

Fig. 31.6 Setup for silicone oil injection **without** chandelier light. **Remark**: Reduce the air pressure to 10 mmHg when injecting silicone oil

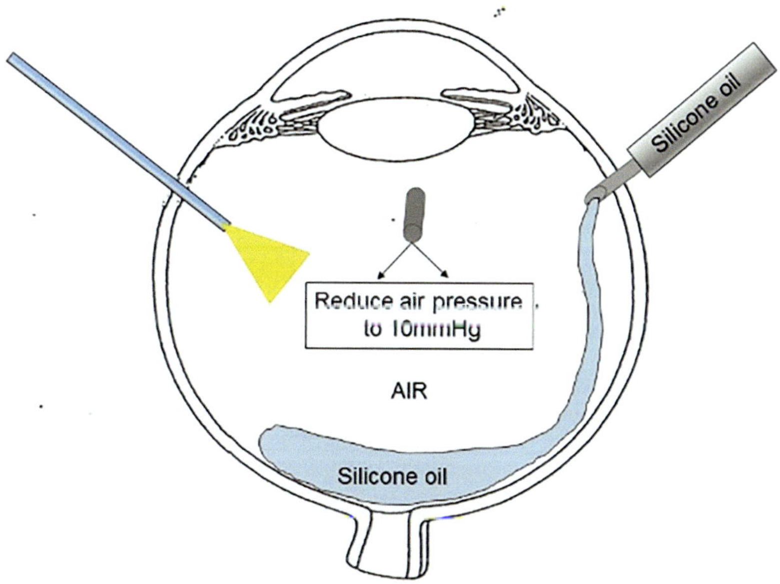

Fig. 31.7 If you use no chandelier light then reduce the air pressure to 10 mmHg when injecting silicone oil

The surgeon must work with the BIOM in order to remove the PFCL when injecting the silicone oil. There is only one method to inject the silicone oil:

Disconnect the infusion line from the BSS infusion and connect the infusion line to the silicone oil syringe. It is important to use a DORC infusion line (Fig. 31.9). An Alcon infusion line may fall off when injecting silicone oil (Fig. 31.8). Use instead a DORC infusion line which has a plastic cannula (Fig. 31.9). This infusion will remain stable in the infusion trocar when injecting silicone oil due to its special shape and different material of the DORC trocar cannula.

A chandelier light is not required. Hold the light probe in one hand and the backflush instrument in the other hand. Inject the silicone oil with active injection modus into the vitreous cavity. Hold the flute needle in the beginning above the PFCL bubble in order to aspirate the

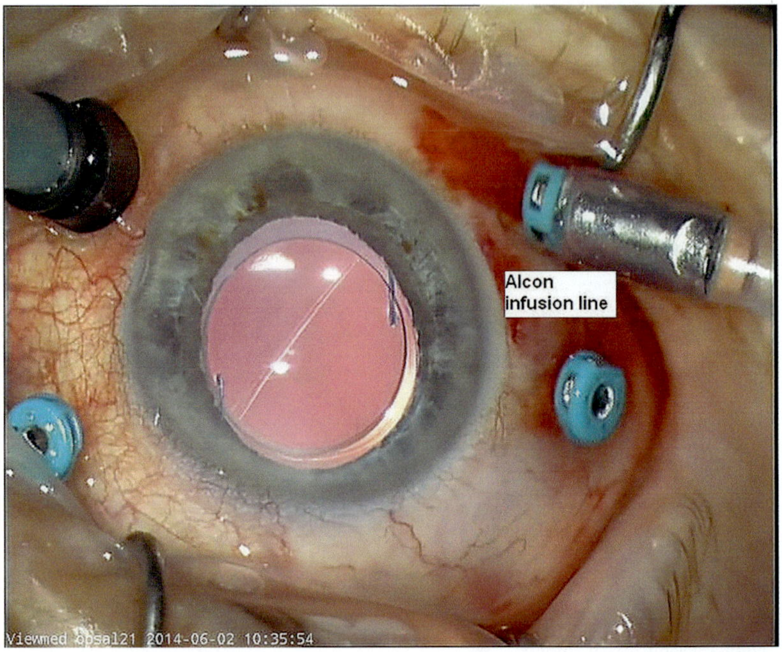

Fig. 31.8 PFCL x silicone oil exchange. An Alcon infusion line cannot be used for injection of silicone oil because the infusion cannula detaches

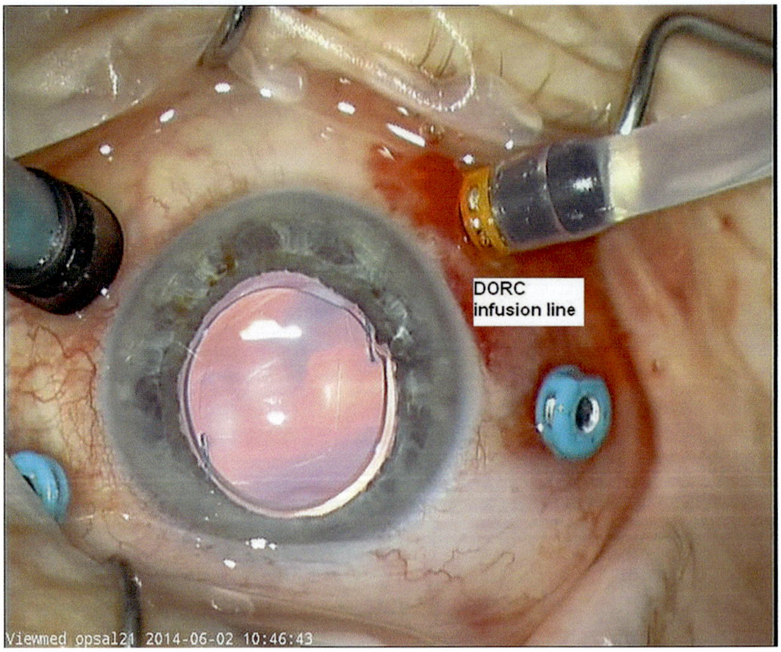

Fig. 31.9 PFCL x silicone oil exchange. Use instead a DORC infusion line with plastic cannula (not high-infusion line). The silicone oil is injected through the infusion line. The infusion line remains stable under injection of silicone oil

residual water (BSS) (Fig. 31.10). Then hold the flute needle into the PFCL phase (Fig. 31.11). Check the pressure of the eye a few times with an index finger. If the pressure is too high, stop the injection of oil and aspirate more PFCL. If the globe is hard (no venous pulse), remove at once a valve and let excess silicone oil flow out.

If subretinal fluid is present remove it by holding the tip of the flute needle in the break. Aspirate the subretinal fluid under the pressure of

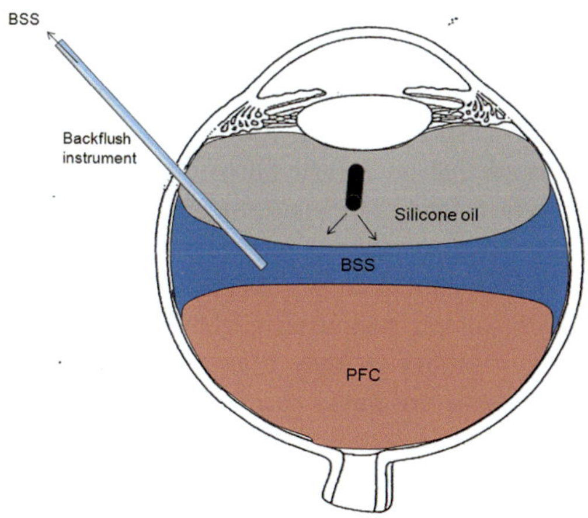

Fig. 31.10 PFCL x silicone oil exchange: Three fluid phases are present: PFCL on the posterior pole, silicone oil in the anterior pole and BSS in between. Remove first BSS

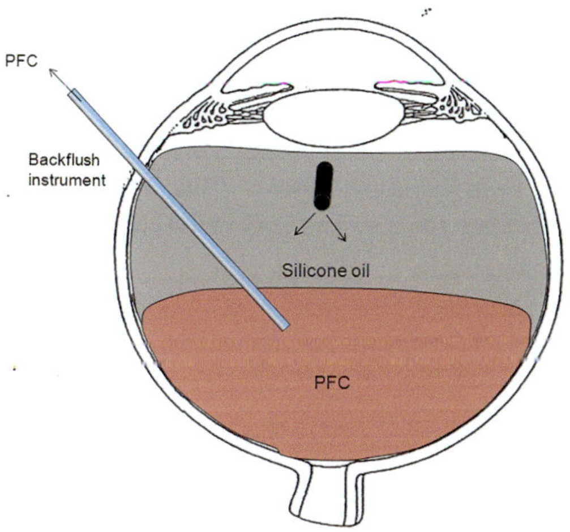

Fig. 31.11 Then remove the PFCL. The silicone oil is injected through the infusion line

the incoming oil and increase the pressure in the eye by injecting more oil. If the break is fully attached, you can complete the laser photocoagulation.

At the end of the aspiration you recognize clearly the PFCL meniscus and also the final PFCL-puddle at the posterior pole. The final PFCL bubble may be tricky to remove. It requires sufficient intraocular pressure. This can be achieved by injecting more silicone oil. Or alternatively, compress the globe with one finger in order to increase the intraocular pressure.

FAQ

What is the difference between PFCL x silicone oil and air x silicone oil exchange?

Do not confuse this method with air against silicone oil exchange. If you disconnect the infusion line with air and connect it to the silicone oil syringe then the eye will collapse. An air filled eye needs constant air infusion in order not to collapse. This is not the case in a PFCL filled eye. The eye is stable even if you disconnect the infusion line. In a PFCL x silicone oil exchange the silicone oil is injected through the infusion line.

I have problems to remove the final PFCL puddle. What to do?

(1) If unsure whether there still is some heavy liquid left behind, pause and wait. The heavy liquid will collect and the interface will be clearly visible after approximately 20 s.
(2) Removing the final puddle of heavy liquid is not an easy step. The danger is to aspirate retina into the flute needle at the posterior pole or to damage the optic disc. Either try to remove the final bubble "in one go" or let it collect over the optic disc. Then increase the pressure with the silicone oil injection and touch the bubble with the opening of the backflush instrument. For small remnant bubbles, indent the eye with your ring finger. This will give you a much better pressure control than the injection of silicone oil with the foot pedal. Aspirate the heavy liquid bubble and immediately cover the opening of your backflush instrument before withdrawing it from the eye, otherwise the heavy liquid bubble will drop back onto the posterior pole.

31.3 Silicone Oil, Densiron Xtra® Removal

The removal of silicone oil preserves the late complications such as emulsification and secondary glaucoma and restores the binocular vision in operated patient. The silicone oil can be removed when the retina is completely attached, chorioretinal scars are formed and the eye is not hypotensive. We remove the silicone oil 1.5–3 months after injection. We remove silicone oils as fast as possible in young patients (4–6 weeks). We are more tolerant with silicone oil in patients over 80 years and trauma eyes.

The most dreaded peroperative complication is a SCH (subchoroidal hemorrhage). The risk for this complication is especially high in myopic patients and patients eating anticoagulant medication.

The most common postoperative complication after silicone oil is a hypotony. For this reason, we prefer small sclerotomies and end surgery always with an air tamponade.

Remember that about 10–20% of patients undergoing silicone oil removal will need additional surgery at a later stage, e.g., for retinal redetachment or recurrent vitreous hemorrhage. The *silicone oil removal* procedure is an ideal opportunity to deal with any lesser or larger problems during the surgery. Therefore, perform a careful examination preoperatively for appropriate planning of the surgical steps. Exclude first a retinal detachment. Try to identify PVR membranes, which are a lot more difficult to see when silicone oil is still in situ. Be always prepared that additional vitreoretinal manipulations or even a "silicone oil exchange" may be necessary.

Before starting surgery identify which *type of silicone* oil has been used. Light silicone oils are easy to remove as they float on water. Heavy silicone oils are rather more difficult to remove because they are heavier than water.

Which gauge? 25G and even more 27G is an excellent choice for silicone oil removal because the risk of postoperative hypotony is significantly reduced. We use therefore a hybrid system with two 27G trocars and one 25G trocar. The 25G trocar is used for the removal of all types silicone oil (1000 csts, 5000 csts and Densiron Xtra).

What is the fastest silicone oil removal cannula?

The fastest extraction cannulas are the Alcon and the DORC plastic cannula (Fig. 31.12). Much slower are the 23G and 25G metal cannulas from Alcon (Fig. 31.13).

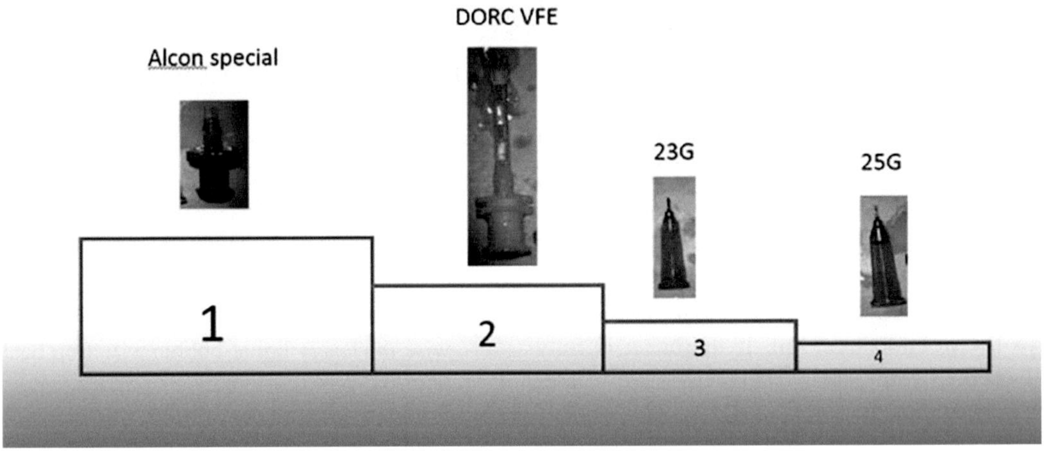

Fig. 31.12 The fastest extraction cannula is from Alcon, followed from DORC´s cannula. The slowest cannula is the 25G metal cannula from Alcon

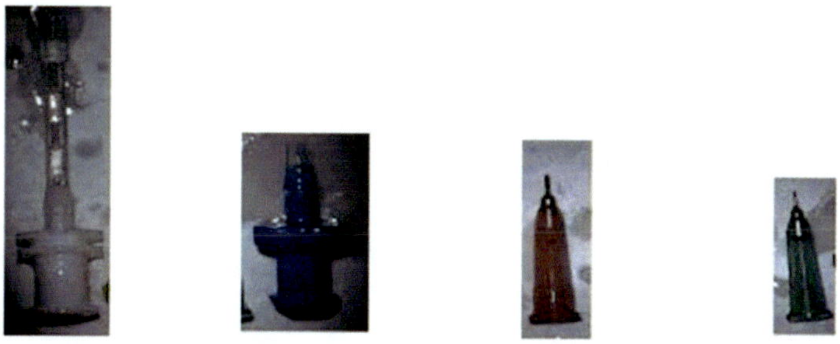

	DORC VFE	Alcon special	Alcon 23G	Alcon 25G
1000 csts	43 sec	18 sec	1,38 min	2,48 min
5000 csts	2,47 min	1,10 min	6,46 min	12,20 min

Fig. 31.13 The extraction time for 5000 csts silicone oil is 5 × longer than for 1000 csts silicone oil

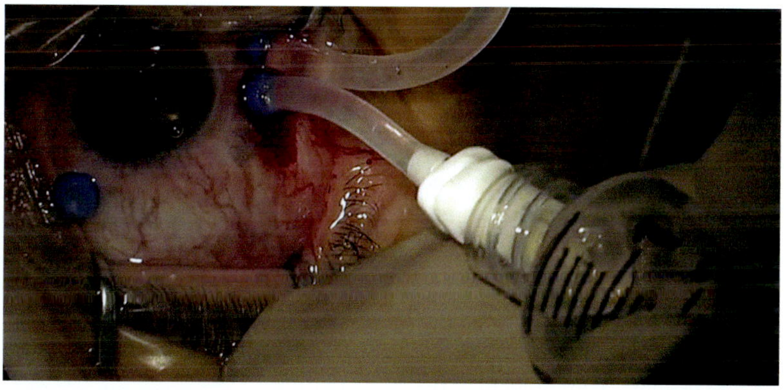

Fig. 31.14 Silicone oil removal with a silicone tube (VFE, DORC). We use it for 5000 csts silicone oil

Extraction time 1000 csts versus 5000 csts silicone oil.

The extraction time for 5000 csts silicone oil is 5 × longer than for 1000 csts silicone oil (Fig. 31.12).

Conclusion

- For 1000, 1300 csts silicone oil and Densiron Xtra we use the 25G metal cannula (Alcon).
- For 5000 csts silicone oil we prefer the plastic adapter from Alcon or DORC or alternatively the 23G metal cannula from Alcon.

31.3.1 Light Silicone Oil (1000, 1300 and 5000 Csts) Removal

For silicone oil extraction we use a hybrid system of 27G and 25G to minimize postoperative hypotony and avoid suturing. The silicone oil extraction is done via the 25G trocar. In case of 5000 csts we use the plastic adapter (VFE from Dorc or Alcon) (Figs. 31.14 and 31.16) and for 1000/1300 csts we use the 25G metal cannula (Fig. 31.15).

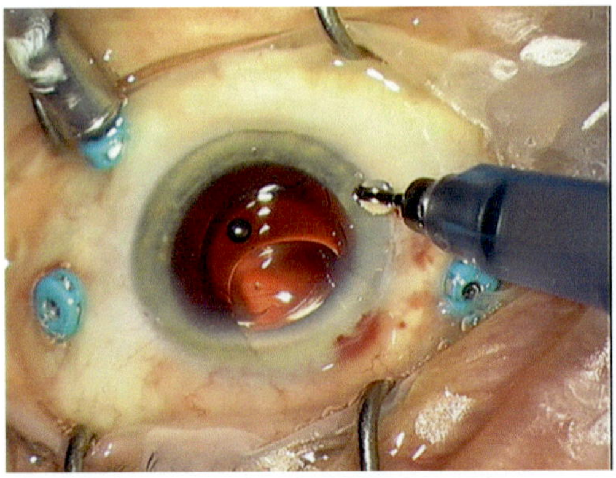

Fig. 31.15 1300 csts silicone oil or Densiron Xtra removal with a 25G metal cannula (Alcon)

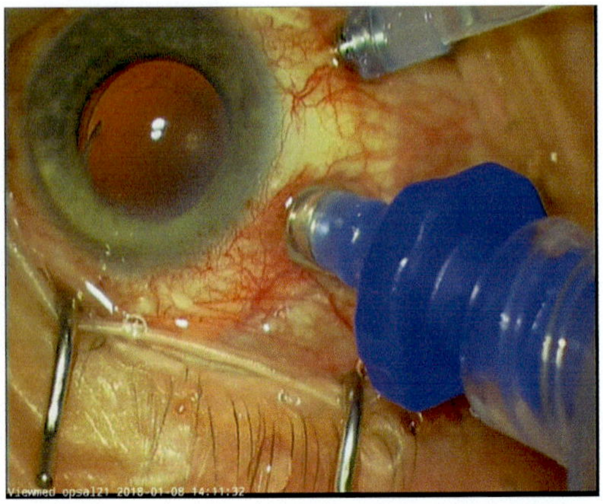

Fig. 31.16 This is the fastest silicone oil extraction cannula available. It fits to all gauges and the valve is removed prior use (Alcon). We use this adapter for 5000 csts silicone oil

31.3.2 Heavy Silicone Oil (Densiron Xtra®) Removal

For Densiron Xtra removal we use also a hybrid system of 27G and 25G. For removal of Densiron Xtra there are 2 extraction cannulas available:

(1) *Short 25G metal cannula* (Fig. 31.15, *Alcon*): This cannula can be used with all modern vitrectomy machines (EVA, Constellation or Stellaris) (Fig. 31.16).

(2) *23G metal 10 mm cannula* (Figs. 31.17 and 31.18, *DORC*): A good alternative is a longer 23G metal cannula from DORC. Especially recommended for long myopic eyes where you easily loose contact with the oil bubble this cannula is recommended.

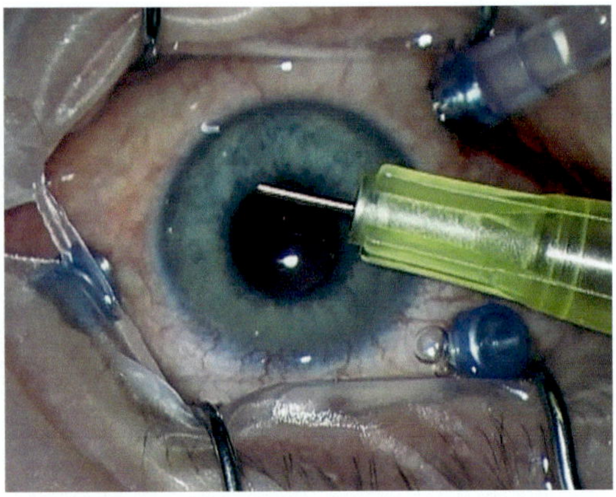

Fig. 31.17 Densiron Xtra removal with a long 23G metal cannula (DORC), good for myopic eyes

The main surgical steps:

Instruments

1. 3-port trocar system (two 27G trocars and one 25G trocar), 120D lens
2. Silicone oil 1000 csts: Active aspiration with 25-Gauge metal cannula (Alcon)
3. Silicone oil 5000csts: Active aspiration with Alcon special cannula
4. Densiron Xtra®: Active aspiration with 25-Gauge metal cannula (Alcon) OR 23G extrusion cannula (DORC)
5. 25G Charles flute instrument

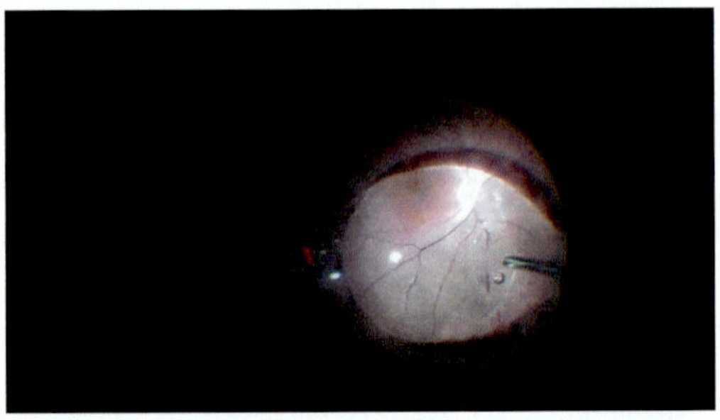

Fig. 31.18 Removal of Densiron Xtra with a 10 mm long 23G metal cannula from DORC

Possible tamponade
Air or gas.

Individual steps

1. **3-port system**
2. **Active silicone oil removal**
3. **Fluid against air exchange**
4. **Air against fluid exchange**
5. **Flush anterior chamber with BSS**
6. **Air tamponade**
7. **Removal of trocars**

The surgery step-by-step

1. 3-port system
2. Active silicone oil removal
Insert the 25G metal cannula into the 25G trocar and aspirate the silicone oil. In the beginning of the procedure the *infusion line is often clogged*: The reason of the clogged infusion line is silicone oil within the infusion because you compress the globe with the silicone oil cannula. Countermeasures are: (1) Do not compress the globe during silicone oil removal. You will otherwise press the silicone oil into the infusion line. (2) Increase the IOP to 40–50 mmHg until the BSS comes. Then reduce back to 25 mmHg.

Remark for heavy silicone oil (Densiron Xtra) removal.
Remove the silicone oil bubble as one would with conventional silicone oil, always staying in touch with the bubble with active suction (Fig. 31.18). The residual bubble will stay connected to the short cannula through the "siphoning" effect, will move upwards towards the cannula and can easily be removed this way. Be aware that the cannula has constant contact to the Densiron Xtra bubble. If you lose contact, then the residual bubble will fall on the posterior pole. In this case, fasten a 25G Charles flute cannula onto the silicone oil syringe and aspirate the residual bubble. Small remnant bubbles at the posterior pole can then be collected with the backflush instrument. The removal time is approximately 5 min.

3. Fluid against air exchange
Then perform a fluid x air exchange under view of the BIOM. Take the backflush instrument and try to "fish" residual oil from the water surface at the water/air interface (meniscus). In case of 23G a passive suction is sufficient but in case of 25G and 27G an active suction is required. If there is a bigger residual oil bubble, it will be time consuming to remove it with the flute needle. In this case, attach the backflush instrument to the silicone oil syring or use a vitreous cutter to aspirate the residual bubble.
4. Air against fluid exchange
This maneuver may cause big complications, so be cautious. Hold the backflush cannula behind the lens. DO NOT use active aspiration. Use ONLY passive aspiration. After you switched to BSS infusion the globe will fill slowly with fluid. If scleral folds occur, close the opening of the backflush cannula until the scleral folds disappear; then release the opening again. The water x air exchange should be performed approximately three times.
5. Flush anterior chamber with BSS
6. Internal search for retinal breaks
If you see silicone oil bubbles in the anterior chamber, then flush the anterior chamber with BSS and remove the silicone oil bubbles. Subsequently, check for peripheral tears or membranes, treat these pathologies and perform a tamponade if necessary.
7. Air tamponade
In order to prevent a postoperative hypotony an air tamponade is strongly recommended.
8. Removal of the trocars
Remove the trocars as usual. In all cases, we instill a simple air tamponade in order to seal the sclerotomy sites. The air tamponade prevents or reduces the postoperative hypotony.

Surgical pearls no. 45
A dreaded complication is a retinal and even sometimes *choroidal injury from the infusion fluid*. This happens during an air x BSS exchange: The vitreous cavity is filled with air and you switch back to BSS. If you now aspirate *actively* with a Charles flute needle within the air phase, you will create an under-pressure and the infusion fluid will stream will great force into the eye damaging the retina and choroid. In addition, the under-pressure may cause a rupture of

choroidal vessels. In order to avoid this, aspirate only *passively*. You can control the intraocular pressure on your own by closing the side opening of the Charles flute needle with your index finger.

Surgical pearls no. 46
Suprachoroidal hemorrhage (SCH). If a SCH develops you should react quickly. First perform a fluid/air exchange and in case of valveless trocars close all ports with plugs to increase the intraocular pressure. This should stabilize the situation. Then inject silicone oil and terminate surgery.

Surgical pearls no. 47
The disadvantage of 25G and especially 23G is the postoperative hypotony. In case of 23G and 25G you need an air tamponade and in myopic eyes you even need to suture the sclerotomies. The air tamponade and sutures are not necessary for 27G. It is therefore recommended to use a hybrid system: 27G trocars for infusion and light fiber and a 23G or 25G trocar for oil removal.

Surgical pearls no. 48
When *removing Densiron Xtra®* with a short cannula, it is important not to lose contact with the bubble before it starts "floating up" towards the cannula. If you lose contact with the bubble and it is too small to be reached with the short cannula, you need to proceed with a backflush cannula (which takes a long time) (Fig. 31.19).

Surgical pearls no. 49
Passive removal of light silicone oil: This method is time-consuming but avoids strong aspiration, which might lead to a suprachoroidal hemorrhage. Insert three 23-Gauge trocars. Remove the valves of both instrument trocar cannulas, open the infusion and let the oil evacuate passively. The eye must be positioned so that the silicone oil flows in the direction of the open trocar cannulas.

Surgical pearls no. 50
Always check the anterior chamber for *residual oil bubbles*. In particular, in cases with secondary glaucoma, it is advisable to flush the chamber angle to remove residual bubbles.

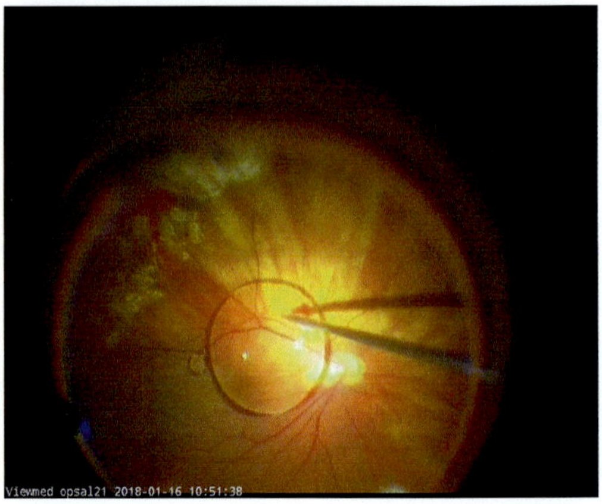

Fig. 31.19 If you lose contact with the Densiron bubble then attach a 25G extrusion cannula to the silicone oil syringe and remove the residual bubble

Surgical pearls no. 51
In pseudophakic patients with an intact posterior capsule, perform a *posterior capsulotomy with the vitreous cutter* via the pars plana at the end of the procedure. These patients will otherwise almost always develop a thick posterior capsular fibrosis and a YAG-capsulotomy is more difficult in eyes in which the retrolental vitreous has been removed.

Surgical pearls no. 52
"*Sticky silicone oil*" has sometimes been described after removing conventional or heavy silicone oils. This describes patches of silicone oil that are firmly attached to the retina and cannot be removed with suction alone. In our experience, this is most commonly caused by residual vitreous cortex in the area of adhesion and the best prevention of sticky silicone oil is a complete removal of this layer during the primary surgery. If you are faced with "sticky" silicone oil, try to fill the eye with PFCL. This usually dissolves the sticky patches of oil that can then be removed with conventional suction.

Part VII
International Video Cases

All videos of this part are found in a playlist on my youTube channel:
https://youtube.com/playlist?list=PL0dKYclPD7yNSVWL4zlBcgvrDlWUCyCv9
Chapter 32: **Video Case Reports**
Armada (Spain)
Cabrera (Spain)
Calzada (USA)
Cubero
Elgohary (Kingston Hospital)
Espejo
Faus
Fernandez-Sanz
García-Martinez
Ghasemi (Iran)
Gonzalez
John Kitchens (USA)
Kazaikin (Russia)
Kusaka (Japan)
Koch (France)
Lara (Spain)
Marticorena
Nadal (Spain)
Relimpio
Ruiz-Casas (Spain)
Tomic (Serbia)
Veckeneer (Belgium)
Zarranz.

Video Cases Reports

32

Diego Ruiz-Casas

The video case reports include a written case description, a fundus drawing, and the video. All videos of this chapter can be found in a playlist (International VR surgeons) of my YouTube channel: https://www.youtube.com/playlist?list=PL0dKYclPD7yNSVWL4zlBcgvrDlWUCyCv9

All Video-Cases According to Topics

PREVENTION OF PVR.

32.21: TOMIC3.

MACULAR PVR.

32.8: FERNANDEZ-SANZ.

32.5: ELGOHARY.

POSTERIOR PVR.

32.14: MARTICORENA.

32.7: FAUS.

32.25: VECKENEER.

32.17: RUIZ-CASAS1.

ANTERIOR PVR.

32.13: LARA.

32.12: KOCH2.

32.4: CUBERO.

PVR UNDER OIL.

32.3: CALZADA.

SUBRETINAL PVR.

32.11: KOCH1.

32.26: ZARRANZ.

32.2: CABRERA.

32.9: GARCÍA-MARTINEZ.

32.22: TOMIC4.

32.1: ARMADA.

TRAUMA.

32.10: GONZALEZ.

RETINECTOMY.

32.20: TOMIC2.

32.18: RUIZ CASAS2.

32.16: RELIMPIO

32.24: TOMIC6.

32.6: ESPEJO.

32.19: TOMIC1.

32.15: NADAL.

32.23: TOMIC5.

D. Ruiz-Casas (✉)
Retina Department Hospital Ramón Y Cajal, Madrid, Spain
e-mail: drdiegoruizcasas@gmail.com

U. Spandau et al. (eds.), *Retinal Detachment Surgery and Proliferative Vitreoretinopathy*,
https://doi.org/10.1007/978-3-031-11946-0_32

32.1 Chronic Retinal Detachment with Anterior and Posterior PVR and Peripapillar Subretinal Strands in a Napkin Ring Configuration

Felix Armadá-Maresca

32.1.1 Case Description (Fig. 32.1)

A 72-year-old patient with total retinal detachment (RD), stiff retina, anterior PVR, posterior epiretinal membranes (ERM), and extensive peripapillar subretinal strands in a napkin ring configuration. He had been operated elsewhere 9 months before but due to RD recurrence, it was decided not to operate again. Best-corrected visual acuity (BCVA) was light perception (LP). He had a transparent cornea and was pseudophakic with 180° posterior synechia.

32.1.2 Surgery (Fig. 32.2)

A 4-port 23G pars plana vitrectomy (PPV) was performed (EVA vitrectomy system with valvulated microcannulae and TDC cutter).

Intense retinal rigidity was observed due to massive subretinal proliferation. An access retinotomy was performed on the inferior-nasal retina to remove peripapillar subretinal membranes but complete removal was unsuccessful. A second superior-nasal retinotomy was then performed to achieve complete subretinal band removal.

Afterward, several ERM were observed and removed from the macular area.

Then a 270° relaxing retinectomy (from 5 to 12 h) was performed to deal with retinal stiffness due to intraretinal PVR. The retina was reattached with heavy liquid (PFCL), and 360° endophotocoagulation was completed under heavy liquid.

Finally a direct PFCL/5000cs Silicone oil (SO) exchange (PSX) was performed. First, PFCL was injected until it flowed back through the disconnected infusion line and then SO was injected through the infusion line at a 3-bar pressure while PFCL was aspirated by active extrusion (stopping aspiration when IOP dropped).

32.1.3 Follow-Up

The patient was instructed to remain face down for 10 days after surgery. Two months after surgery BCVA was of counting fingers, and the retina remained attached.

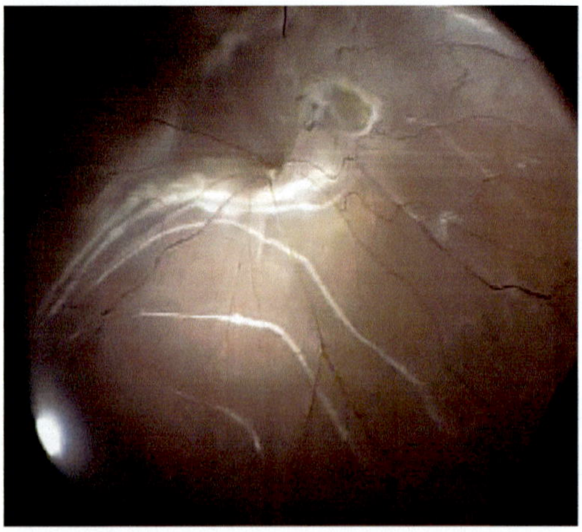

Fig. 32.1 RD with subretinal strands

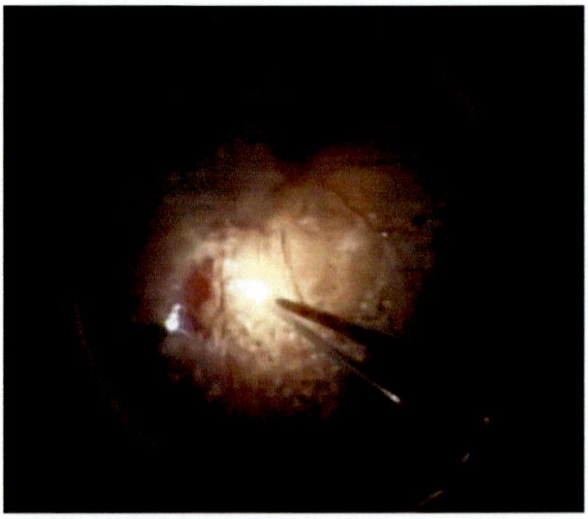

Fig. 32.2 Retina attached under silicone oil

32.2 Retinal Detachment with PVR, Subretinal Strands, and Luxated IOL

Francisco Cabrera Lopez

32.2.1 Case Description (Fig. 32.3)

55 y/o pseudophakic patient (cataract surgery 1 year ago) and previous uveitis history was referred due to visual acuity (VA) loss for 6 months. He presented a RD PVR CP9 with intraocular lens (IOL) and capsular bag luxation.

32.2.2 Surgical Procedure

4-port 23G pars plana vitrectomy (PPV) was performed. First the luxated IOL was released from the lower fibrotic vitreous base (VB) with vitreous cutter and forceps. Then the IOL was displaced into the anterior chamber (AC) with 2 end-grasping forceps and removed through a limbal incision.

Afterward posterior epiretinal membranes (ERMs) were removed bimanually using forceps + vitreous cutter or two forceps. A subretinal band was also removed through a pre-existing retinal tear at XI with forceps using endoilluminator as a fulcrum.

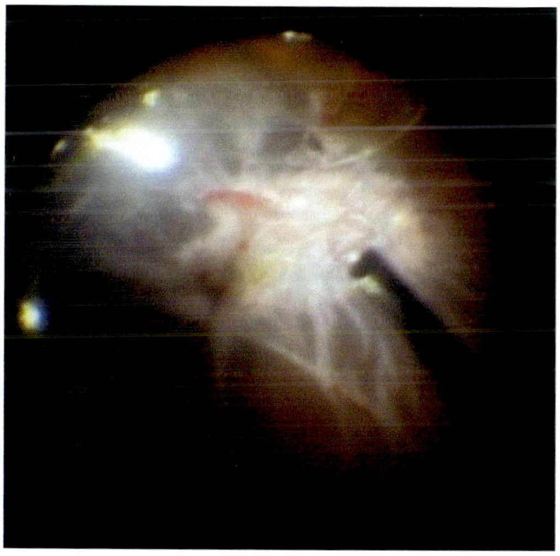

Fig. 32.3 Preoperative RD with PVR and luxated IOL

Then, heavy liquid (PFCL) was used to reattach the retina draining chronic thick subretinal fluid (SRF) through peripheral tears at VII and XI h.

The lower fibrotic posterior hyaloid (PH) at VB insertion was also removed bimanually with forceps and scissors.

Finally a 360° laser cerclage, and PFCL/Air exchange (FAX) followed by Air/5000cs Silicone Oil exchange (ASX) were performed.

Silicone Oil (SO) was left for 6 months and cornea got cloudy. Thus SO removal was done using an Eckardt temporary keratoprosthesis (TKP) after removing the cloudy cornea and releasing anterior synechiae. The retina remained attached without SO but.

PFCL bubbles in the vitreous cavity were found, which were removed with a dual bore cannula. A macular ERM was peeled with end-gripping forceps. There were also a few subretinal PFCL bubbles that were removed through micro retinotomies (made with a 23G Pick) using active suction with a silicone tip cannula. Finally the donor corneal graft was sutured.

32.2.3 Follow-Up (Fig. 32.4)

The retina was completely attached without tamponade, and BCVA was 0.2 after the two surgical procedures.

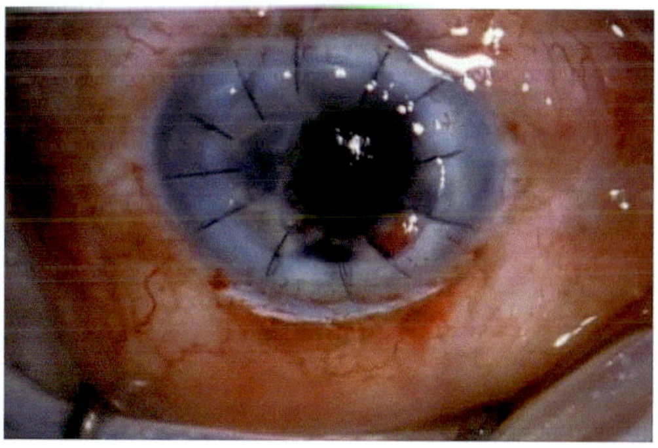

Fig. 32.4 Postoperative retinal reattachment and corneal graft

32.3 PVR Reoperation Under Silicone Oil

Jorge I. Calzada

32.3.1 Case Description

The technique presented in the video is my preferred approach for pars plana vitrectomy (PPV) reoperation for recurrent retinal detachment (RD) when silicone oil (SO) is already inside the vitreous cavity. Instead of standard 3-port PPV, in these cases I do not use an infusion cannula, so we call it "2-port PPV under oil". The endoilluminator is introduced through one port, and the active instrument is introduced through the second port. Intraocular pressure (IOP) is managed by intermittently injecting silicone oil (SO) into one of the superior cannulas. Care is taken to avoid unnecessary loss of SO passively through the ports by having an instrument or a plug inside the port at all times. Even with an open port the high viscosity of SO leads to very slow flow of oil out of the eye, helping maintain the IOP within target range.

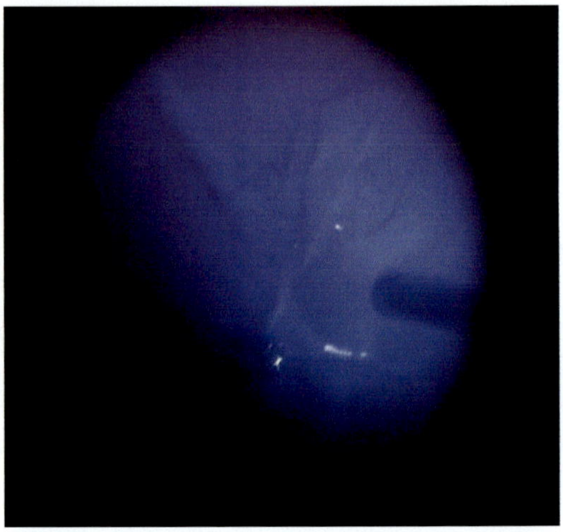

Fig. 32.5 Retinal membrane peeling under silicone oil

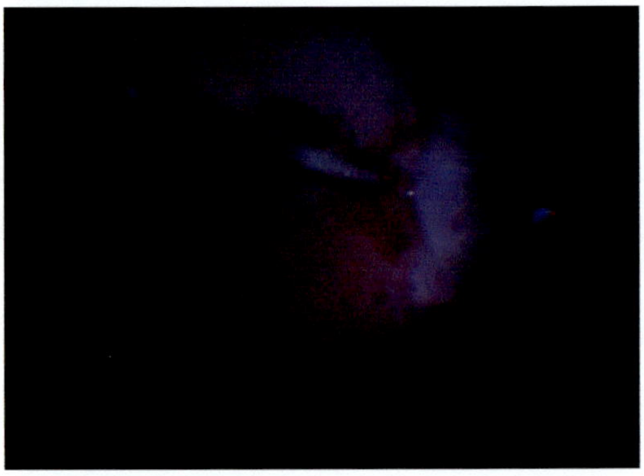

Fig. 32.6 Interface vitrectomy with subretinal fluid drainage under silicone oil

32.3.2 Surgery Description (Figs. 32.5 and 32.6)

The most critical steps of two-port PPV are epiretinal membrane (ERM) peeling, peripheral interface vitretomy, retinectomy, and subretinal fluid (SRF) aspiration. Most cases, like the one in our video, begin with forceps membrane peeling. I usually prefer to identify and peel ERMs initially in the posterior pole and continue the peeling dissection to the periphery. Peeling under SO has advantages and disadvantages. If a meniscus of aqueous fluid is present under the SO and over the retina, identification of the plane of the peeling may be difficult. Continued experience with this technique improves the ability of the surgeon to properly grasp the ERM as intended. Once a membrane is grasped and peeling is initiated, the reflection of the SO over the ERM actually facilitates the visualization of the sheet of proliferative vitreoretinopathy (PVR) membranes. In the video presented, one can clearly visualize the leading edge of the ERM as it is been lifted off of the retina and extended toward the retinal periphery.

During PVR reoperation under SO, complete removal of retinal traction and drainage of SRF leads to immediate reattachment of the retina. If all identifiable ERMs are peeled and the retina still remains detached, the usual next step is peripheral retinectomy. Intraocular cautery should be used to delineate the area of retinectomy and to decrease bleeding from the site of the retinectomy. Intraocular hemorrhage in two-port PPV under SO can be a problem sometimes, since the blood does not diffuse through the SO in the vitreous, leading to a localized clot. This local hemorrhage can either impede visualization of the retina that requires dissection or retinectomy or can extend into the subretinal space and track posteriorly to a submacular hemorrhage. Meticulous hemostasis during dissection is particularly important with this technique.

Subretinal fluid (SRF) drainage can be performed directly through a retinal break under the silicone oil (SO). As SRF is drained, SO may need to be injected into the eye to maintain adequate IOP. The steps of peeling, retinectomy, SRF aspiration, and SO injection may be repeated as needed until the retina is attached. At this point, laser retinopexy can be performed through the SO with an intraocular laser probe.

A significant advantage of this general technique is total duration of surgery when compared to other more involved procedures. The patient's tolerance for the procedure and the low levels of inflammation postoperatively are also benefits. This technique can be combined with phacoemulsification in a phaco/vitrectomy approach for simultaneous management of a cataract. Pars plana lensectomy in an oil-filled eye with the two-port PPV approach may be very difficult, though, and in my opinion is best avoided.

32.4 Retinal Detachment with PVR CP6 and Hypotony

Juan Manuel Cubero Parra

32.4.1 Case Description (Fig. 32.7)

72 y/o woman with recurrent retinal detachment (RD) under silicone oil (SO) in her right eye. She had been operated of pars plana vitrectomy (PPV) because of RD and macular hole three times.

The right eye was pseudophakic, and it was diagnosed of atrophic age-related macular degeneration (AMD) 6 months ago.

Snellen's best-corrected visual acuity (VA) was light perception (LP) without projection.

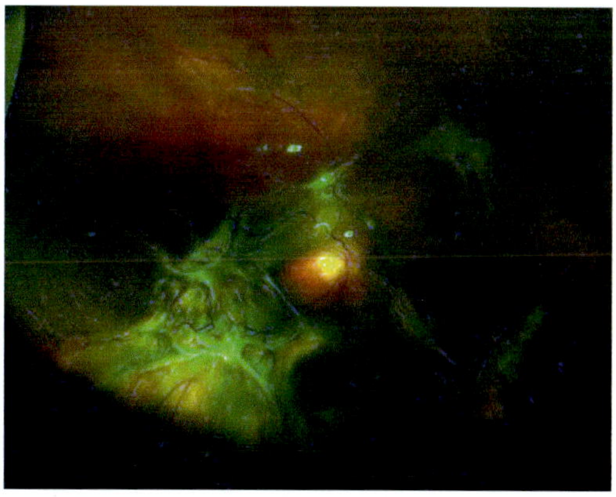

Fig. 32.7 Preoperative RD

Slit-lamp examination revealed anterior chamber cells ++, and posterior-superior synechia with pigment on intraocular lens (IOL) and inferior iridectomy.

IOP was 4 mmHg.

Fundus examination showed RD with epiretinal membranes (ERMs) on the macula and temporal quadrant with severe inferior retinal stiffness.

The left eye was amaurotic because of a RD 40 years ago.

32.4.2 Surgery Description

23G PPV with an accessory light infusion was conducted under general anesthesia.

First, SO was removed and macular ERMs were peeled bimanually with two forceps. One forceps was used to grasp the ERM and the other one to dissect it bluntly from the underlying retina. ERMs with extreme retinal adherence were segmented using forceps and scissors.

Posterior hyaloid (PH) remnants were found on the upper retina, and they were detached up to the posterior vitreous base (VB) by pulling with two forceps to avoid retinal tearing. The scarred PH remnants at VB were dissected bluntly with two forceps in order to relieve circumferential traction.

Then, heavy liquid (PFCL) was used to reattach the retina but inferior retinal stiffness prevented it. Thus, an inferior retinectomy was performed to relax anterior–posterior traction. Diathermy was applied to the cutting area, and the vitreous cutter was used to remove the stiff anterior retina and anterior vitreous remnants to avoid any traction at ciliary body and hypotony.

A subretinal clot was moved to the retinectomy edge sweeping it smoothly with a silicone tip cannula and extracted with the vitreous cutter. Subretinal membranes at the retinectomy edge were removed directly with forceps.

Finally, the vitreous cavity was filled with PFCL to reattach the retina and laser photocoagulation was applied to the retinectomy border. 5000cs SO was left as tamponade using a PFCL/Air exchange (FAX) followed by an Air/Silicone Oil Exchange (ASX).

32.4.3 Follow-Up (Fig. 32.8)

The patient was instructed to stay on prone position during the day, and on left lateral decubitus at night, for a week.

After a 4-month follow-up, the retina was attached under SO.

Best-corrected VA was counting fingers (CF) due to macular atrophy, but the patient was able to recognize colors and orient herself in an unknown room without help.

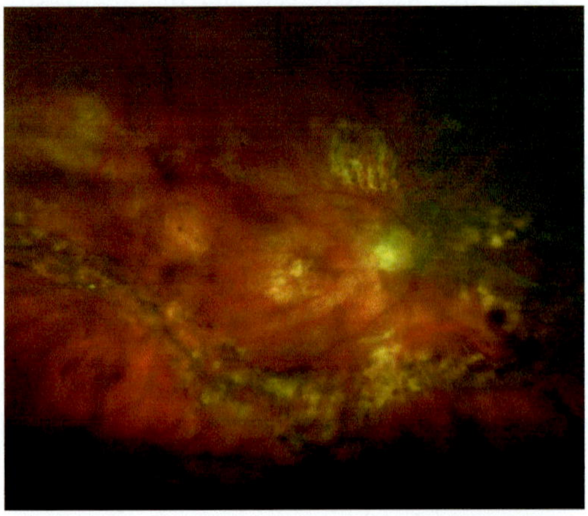

Fig. 32.8 Postoperative retinal attachment under silicone oil

32.5 Macular PVR Membranes Developing Acutely After Macula-On Retinal Detachment Surgery

Mostafa Elgohary

32.5.1 Case Description (Fig. 32.9)

A Caucasian female patient in her late 60 s presented with a macula on retinal detachment (RD) in her left eye. During the surgery she was found to have multiple U-shaped tears along the attachment of the posterior hyaloid (PH) to the posterior vitreous base (VB). She was highly myopic (nearly –9) and also had RD in the right eye treated with vitrectomy, cryotherapy, and SF6 gas tamponade.

Pars plana vitrectomy (PPV) proceeded as normal. I checked complete posterior vitreous detachment (PVD), and I treated the tears with cryotherapy and performed Fluid/Air exchange (FAX) followed by Air/Gas SF6 tamponade (AGX).

She attended her first and second postoperative follow up visits and was awaiting her final follow up at about 4 months. The retina was attached, and her visual acuity was 6/9. She presented to Eye Casualty at about 8 weeks postoperatively complaining of blurred and distorted vision in the left eye. The visual acuity (VA) was 6/12 and OCT showed that she had early signs of an epiretinal membrane (ERM). She was listed to have PPV and peeling of ERM in 6 to 8 weeks.

Almost 2 weeks later she returned to Eye Casualty with macula-off recurrent RD and her VA had gone down to hand movements. She was taken straight for surgery on the same day.

32.5.2 Surgery Description (Fig. 32.10)

During surgery, it was found that she had developed a significant macular PVR membrane, which had centrifugally contracted and opened up the treated breaks and caused recurrence of the RD.

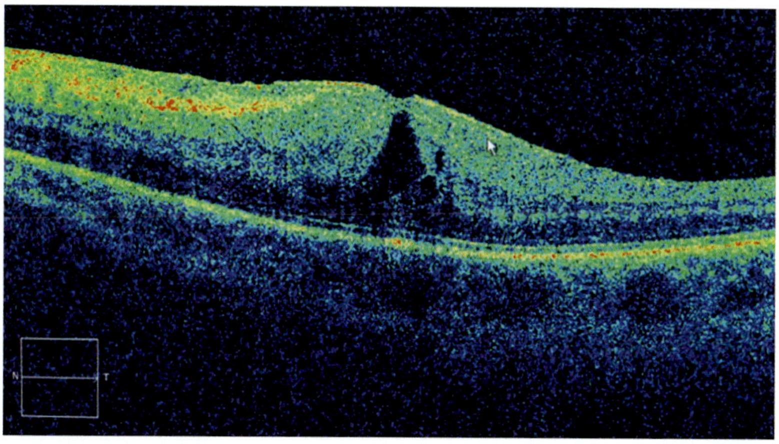

Fig. 32.9 Epiretinal membrane

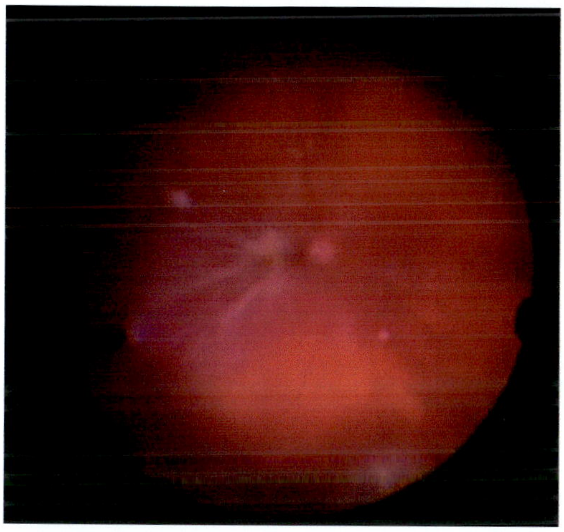

Fig. 32.10 RD with PVR

I used Trypan Blue to improve visualization of the ERM and internal limiting membrane (ILM) and a contact lens to improve my stereopsis. I started the peeling posteriorly, between the disc and fovea, proceeding first toward the fovea until the thick band of the membrane was off the fovea and then proceeded away from the fovea. I felt that there was some remnants of the PH that probably had not detached fully during the first surgery and that this was the predisposing factor for the development of the PVR membrane and led to opening of the breaks and therefore recurrence of the RD.

Further peeling was performed along the axes that were not directly transferring the force to the fovea. Once the membrane was clear of the macula and close to the arcade, I then used the wide-field (128D) lens to complete the peeling. I then performed FAX until the retina was attached removing the subretinal fluid (SRF) remnants with heavy liquid (PFCL), and applied laser to the edges of the opened breaks. I carried out AGX and used C3F8 tamponade.

32.5.3 Follow-Up (Fig. 32.11)

Postoperatively, VA improved to 6/12 as the cataract developed. After cataract surgery VA was 6/9.

32.6 Long-Standing Retinal Detachment with PVR and Hypotony

Francisco Espejo Arjona

32.6.1 Case Description (Fig. 32.12)

This pseudophakic patient suffered a previous ocular trauma and uveitis. He presented a complete closed funnel retinal detachment (RD), stiff and thickened retina, and choroidal thickening. The eye was hypotonic (IOP = 1 mmHg), and visual acuity (VA) was light perception (LP). Surgery was delayed twice due to skin rash and conjunctivitis.

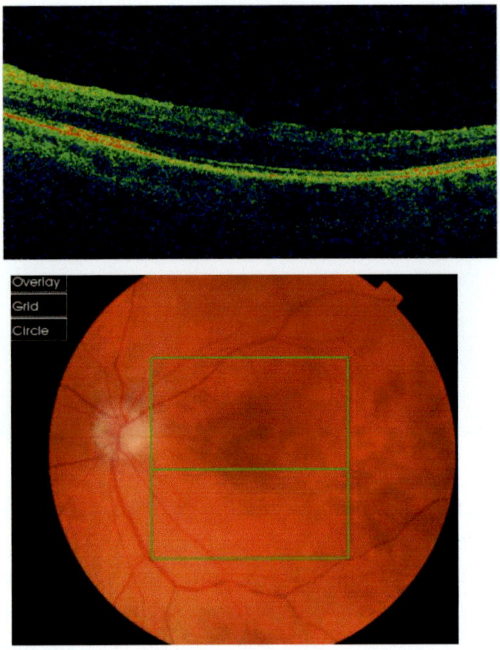

Fig. 32.11 Postoperative OCT and fundus picture

32.6.2 Surgery Description (Fig. 32.13)

A 23G Pars plana vitrectomy (PPV) and 360º retinectomy without buckling was indicated.

A scarred posterior hyaloid (PH) attached at posterior vitreous base (VB) edge was found during surgery. This PH plaque induced massive circumferential traction and hindered posterior epiretinal membrane (ERM) removal; it was segmented and removed with the vitreous cutter. The last scarred PH remnants at VB insertion were gently removed bimanually with forceps and scissors. PH dissection and PFCL injection opened the retinal funnel, but a thickened posterior retina was now observed.

Posterior ERMs and ILM were stained with Brilliant Blue and removed with forceps. However, after ERM and ILM peeling, the posterior retina still looked wrinkled because of intraretinal PVR precluding retinal reattachment.

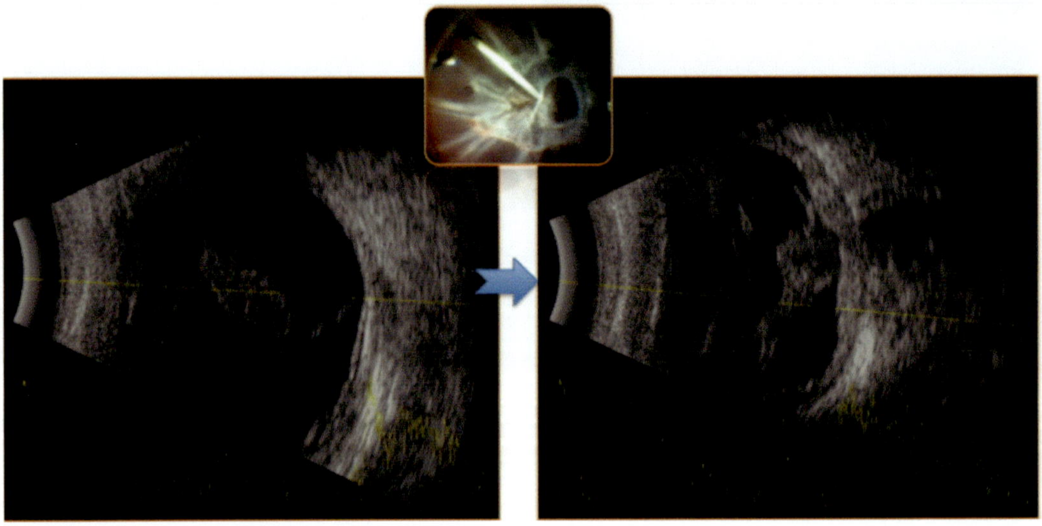

Fig. 32.12 Preoperative ultrasound. Closed funnel RD

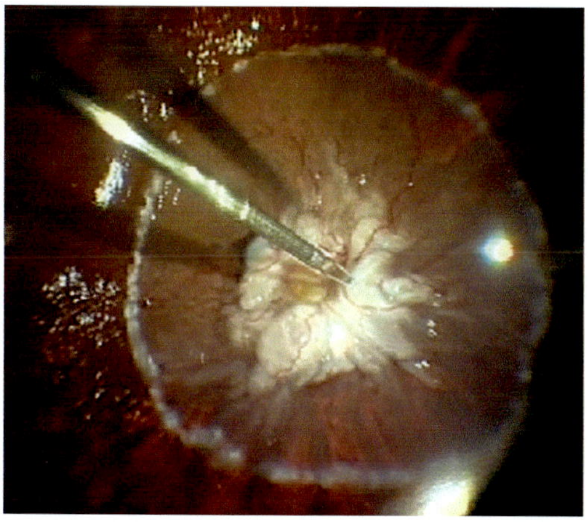

Fig. 32.13 360 retinectomy

A 360° retinectomy was performed to relieve anterior–posterior traction due to retinal shortening and allow retinal reattachment. First, heavy liquid (PFCL) was used to stabilize the macular area and avoid retinal rotation. Afterward, diathermy all around the cutting area was performed to avoid subretinal bleeding. Then retinectomy was performed at posterior VB edge where many retinal tears were found. The retina was cut with the vitreous cutter, but four retinal bridges were left uncut to avoid retinal displacement or rotation. Finally PFCL was injected again up to the retinectomy edge, and the retinal bridges were eventually cut. The posterior retinal folded back due to intrinsic contraction, it looked thickened and cystic, but no subretinal membranes were found. Choroidal was also observed.

The retina was attached with PFCL. However, the posterior retina still looked wrinkled and it did not stretch despite retinal massage with a soft tip cannula and ERM remnants removal.

Photocoagulation of the retinectomy edge was performed with 3 laser rows, and a PFCL-BSS/Air exchange (FAX) was used to reattach the retina, drying carefully the retinectomy edge to avoid retinal slippage. Once the retinal edge was flat and dry, the rest of PFCL was removed at optic nerve and an Air/5000cs silicone oil (SO) exchange (ASX) was performed.

32.6.3 Follow-Up

The retina remained attached under oil, but IOP was low and best-corrected VA was hand motion (HM).

32.7 Peripheral RD with Initial Immature Membranes Over 360° Peripheral Retina

Fernando Faus Guijarro

32.7.1 Case Description (Fig. 32.14)

52 y/o man previously operated (three times) of RD who presented with a new complete peripheral macula ON retinal detachment (RD) because of posterior PVR. Best-corrected visual acuity (VA) was 0,4.

Despite macula attachment peripheral RD was due to immature epiretinal membranes (ERMs) covering the whole retinal surface.

32.7.2 Surgery Description (Fig. 32.15)

A 23G pars plana vitrectomy (PPV) was conducted under local anaesthesia plus sedation.

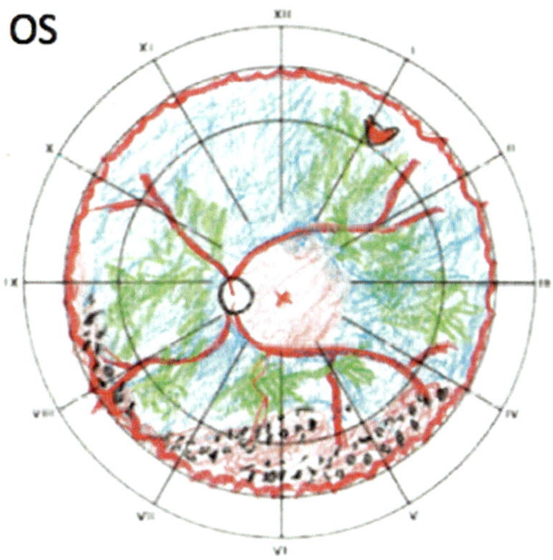

Fig. 32.14 Peripheral RD

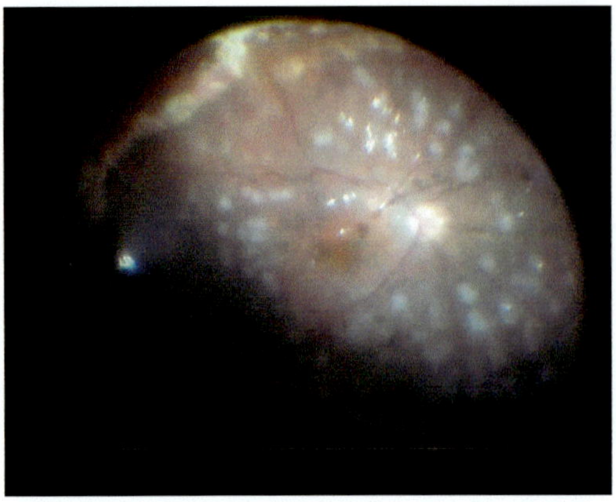

Fig. 32.15 Retinal attachment under silicone oil

Initially a little vitrectomy was performed because the patient had been previously vitrectomized and there were almost no peripheral vitreous remnants. Then heavy liquid (PFCL) (perfluoroctane) was used to preserve macular attachment during surgery.

ERMs were stained with two-dye mixture (Brilliant Blue G plus trypan blue used for cataract surgery) after fluid/air exchange (FAX). Dye was left in the eye for two minutes to get complete peripheral retina proliferations staining. During the staining time smooth eye movements were done so that dye reached the whole peripheral retina, obtaining a nice visualization of all immature membranes.

Air/fluid exchange (AFX) was performed, and the dye was washed up.

Then, ERM peeling was carefully performed under fluid. During the peeling the light probe was moved to illuminate tangentially on the retinal surface and facilitate the visualization of immature membranes. PFCL was injected twice to stabilize the retina and peel from posterior to anterior trying to eliminate the PVR membranes as much as possible.

Finally FAX was performed to reattach the retina and remove subretinal fluid (SRF) completely. Panretinal photocoagulation was applied, and air/silicone oil exchange (ASX) was performed leaving heavy silicone oil (Densiron) as tamponade.

32.7.3 Follow-Up

Densiron was removed 4 weeks later without complications. BCVA was 0,4, and the retina remained attached.

32.8 Localized Inferior Retinal Redetachment Due to PVR CA4 with Macular ERM

Guillermo Fernandez Sanz

[ ] **Video: 32.8 Fernando-Sanz.**

32.8.1 Case Description (Fig. 32.16)

A 52-year-old man who came to the clinic as a follow up of a macula on rhegmatogenous retinal detachment (RD) surgery (23 G vitrectomy + cryotherapy + endolaser + SF6 26%) performed 2.5 months ago in right eye (RE). He had a couple of episodes of inflammatory flare up during this time as he was tapering his steroid drops and these were treated by increasing the frequency of instillation of the drops. He complained of recent appearance of distortion and decreased visual acuity (VA) of his RE over the previous 2 weeks.

Snellen best-corrected visual acuity (BCVA) of the RE was 0.1 (1 month prior it had been of 0.7) and 1.00 in the left eye (LE). Slit-lamp examination revealed a clear cornea, deep anterior chamber, no anterior chamber cells, and a mild-moderate nuclear opacity of lens. Intraocular pressure (IOP) was 10 mmHg in RE and 12 mmHg in LE. RE fundus examination showed a thick epiretinal membrane (ERM) on the superior half of the macula with significant traction and epiretinal pigment (macular PVR). Optical coherence tomography (OCT) confirmed the ERM. The retina looked mostly attached with cryo and laser scars, but there was a fibrotic vitreous skirt and vitreous base (VB) on the nasal periphery (from 1–7 h) that was lifting the retina infero-nasally (localized RD) with no break seen.

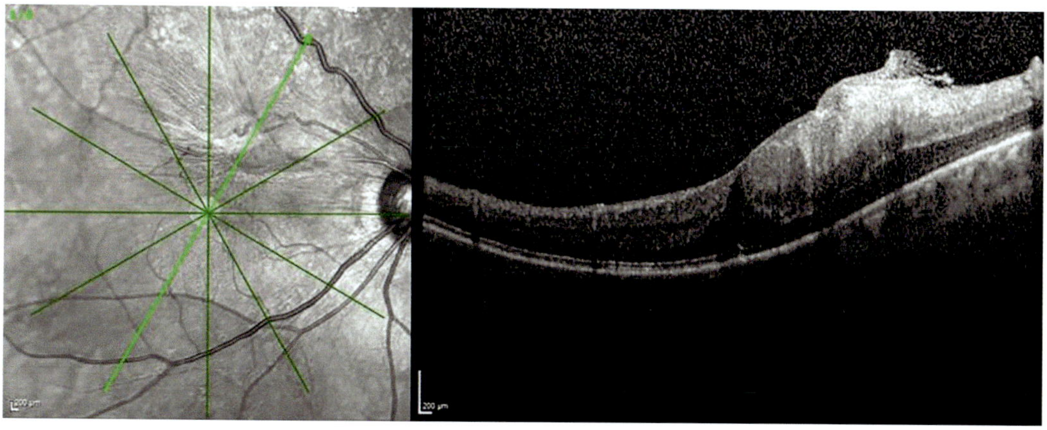

Fig. 32.16 Preoperative OCT of RE. BCVA was 0.1, and it showed a thick ERM affecting the superior half of the macula

Surgical treatment was indicated, with combined 360° buckle + vitrectomy + ERM/ILM peel + C_3F_8 in RE. Leaving cataract surgery for a future surgery once the final axial length was determined.

32.8.2 Surgery

Surgery was conducted under general anesthesia. 360° conjunctival peritomy was performed, creating radial relaxing incisions at 3 and 9 o'clock to prevent tearing of the conjunctiva. The rectus muscles were slung with 2/0 black silk sutures. An encircling band (model 240) was passed under the rectus muscles, and it was fixed with a sleeve in the supero-temporal quadrant. 5/0 nylon sutures were passed in each quadrant to fix the band approximately around the equator of the eye (12 mm posterior to the limbus).

Three ports for 23-Gauge pars plana vitrectomy (PPV) were used. Staining of the ERM and ILM (ILM Blue, DORC) was done directly since it was a vitrectomized eye. A flat disposable macula lens was placed (1284 DD, DORC), and 23 GA asymmetric peeling forceps (Storz) were used to start the peel of the ERM. At a certain point the traction exerted while peeling seemed excessive so 23 GA endgripping forceps (Storz) were used to start an in block peel of ILM and ERM. The ILM was re-stained, and the peel was completed.

Vitrectomy was enhanced with the help of the indent created by the buckle. The indentation seemed a bit low, so the band was tightened. Triamcinolone was injected intravitreally to highlight any vitreous remnants. A peripheral retinotomy was performed with the cutter, on the apex of the indent in the supero-nasal quadrant, to drain the subretinal fluid (SRF) since no break had been identified.

A 360° scleral depressed search was done, and cryotherapy was given to any suspicious areas.

Fluid/Air exchange (FAX) was performed with internal drainage of SRF through the peripheral retinotomy. Complete attachment of the retina was observed under air. 360° laser was applied, and cryotherapy of the retinotomy was performed. The supero-temporal sclerotomy was sutured with 8/0 vycril, and an Air/Gas C_3F_8 14% exchange (AGX) was done. The other sclerotomies and conjunctiva were closed with 8/0 vycril. Finally, subconjunctival antibiotics and steroids were given.

32.8.3 Follow-Up (Fig. 32.17)

The patient was instructed to posture face down during the day and to sleep on his right side for the initial 7 days after surgery. After this, posture was free during the day and limited to the

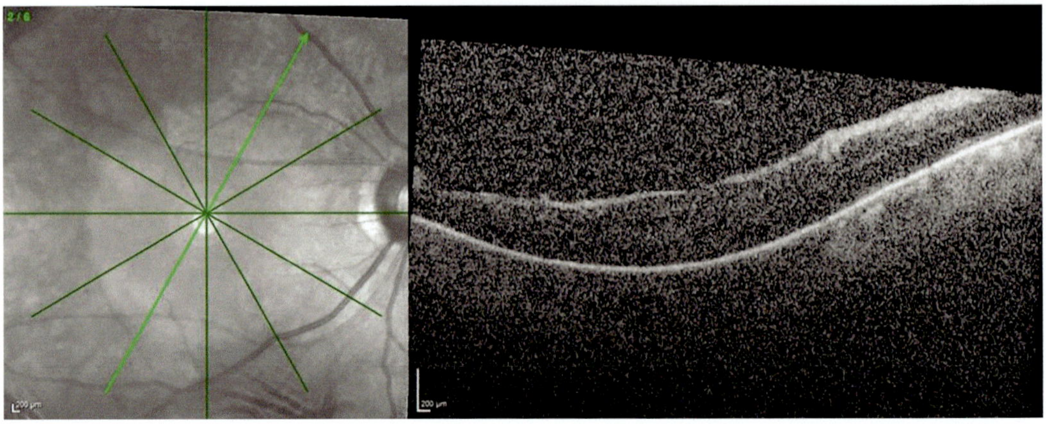

Fig. 32.17 OCT RE. Ten weeks post-operation. BCVA was 0.3. No signs of ERM and partial recovery of the normal foveal contour was noted

nighttime when he had to keep on sleeping on his right side for another 2 weeks.

After 10 weeks, complete reattachment of the retina was achieved in the absence of intraocular gas. Snellen BCVA of the RE was 0.3. Slit-lamp examination revealed a clear cornea, deep anterior chamber, anterior chamber cells ±, posterior synechiae at 3 and 12 h, and a moderate nuclear opacity with moderate subcapsular sclerosis of lens. IOP was 10 mmHg in RE. RE fundus examination showed no gas, good indentation of buckle 360º, laser scars on the buckle 360º, complete reattachment of the retina, and macula with good appearance.

Optical coherence tomography revealed no ERM and no macular edema.

32.9 PVR RD with Napkin Ring, Subretinal Membranes and Subretinal Clot

Jesus Ramon Garcia Martinez

32.9.1 Case Description (Fig. 32.18)

A 65 y/o woman was referred from another hospital with a history of three failed retinal detachment (RD) surgeries in her left eye. She was previously treated with scleral buckle and vitrectomy + gas tamponade, but she developed RD with proliferative vitreoretinopathy (PVR). Vitreous base (VB) contraction and anterior retinal pulling due to anterior PVR in nasal quadrants with several retinal holes were observed, there were also peripapillary subretinal membranes in a napkin ring configuration and a subretinal clot in the superior quadrant. Her visual acuity (VA) was counting fingers at 50 cm in LE and 0,7 in RE. Slit lamp examination revealed corneal clouding, a posterior chamber intraocular lens (IOL) and posterior capsule fibrosis and opacification with atrophic iris.

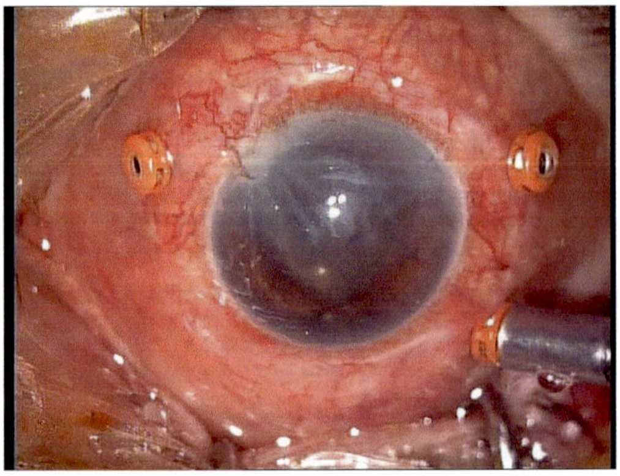

Fig. 32.18 Anterior segment with cloudy cornea and posterior chamber IOL with capsular fibrosis and opacification

32.9.2 Surgery Description (Figs. 32.18, 32.19, 32.20)

Surgery was conducted under retrobulbar anesthesia and sedation. 23G transconjunctival pars plana vitrectomy (PPV) with and an accessory chandelier light was performed using a contact wide field viewing system (Landers wide field vitrectomy contact lens).

At the beginning, corneal epithelium, IOL, and fibrotic capsular bag were removed because they precluded a correct retinal visualization.

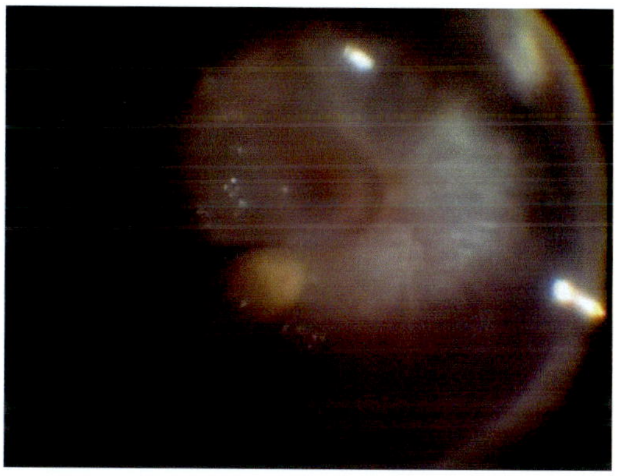

Fig. 32.19 Image of the fundus with subretinal clot in the superior arcade, subretinal membranes, moth-eaten aspect of peripheral retina, and anterior PVR at the nasal quadrant

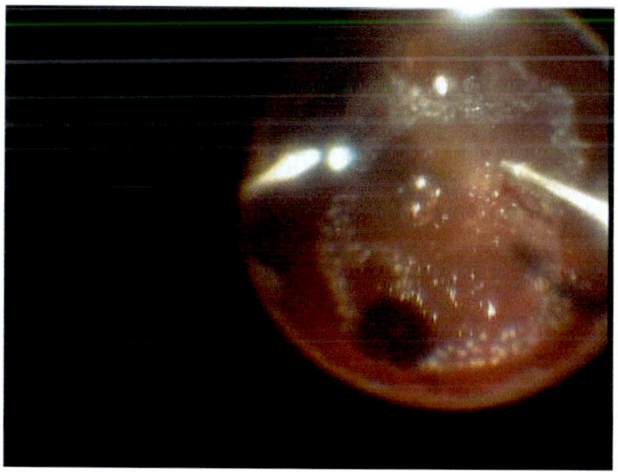

Fig. 32.20 Final result with complete retinal attachment

Initially, heavy liquid (PFCL) was carefully injected to stabilize and fixate posterior retina and assess equatorial retina behavior. The retina at VB had a moth-eaten aspect and the anterior retinal tissue looked fibrotic at nasal and superior retinal quadrants, thus a circumferential relaxing/access retinotomy, posterior to the scarred retinal tissue was performed. Prior to performing the retinotomy, PFCL was aspirated to avoid PFCL bubbles migration into the subretinal space and diathermy was done, then the retina was cut with the vitreous cutter. The retinotomy was large enough to allow adequate access to subretinal membranes.

The best way to remove subretinal membranes is bimanually. Forceps are used to grasp the membrane and gently pull it to determine whether it will strip free. A cannula, vitreous cutter, endolight, or other forceps can be used to support the membrane tangentially and avoid traction on the retina.

Once the subretinal membranes were extracted, the subretinal clot was lifted grasping it with forceps. Subretinal clot was attached strongly to the anterior retina, and two forceps were needed to pull it out gently from the retina, then it was removed with the vitreous cutter.

After all membranes were removed, the retina was reattached with PFCL, injecting it over the retinal edge, and 360° three-row laser photocoagulation was performed at the retinal edge under PFCL.

After the retina was reattached silicone oil was chosen as a tamponade in this case with an almost 360° retinotomy. A direct PFCL-Silicone oil exchange was performed to prevent retinal slippage. Direct PFCL-silicone oil exchange (PSX) was set in the vitrectomy console. First, infusion line was disconnected and PFCL was injected until it passed through the disconnected infusion line. At this moment, silicone oil was injected through the temporal superior microcannula and PFCL aspirated with a soft tipped cannula through the other superior microcannula. At the end, the soft tip cannula was placed over the optic nerve or far away from the macula to remove all the PFCL.

32.9.3 Follow-Up

Patient was instructed to avoid face-up position for the initial ten days after surgery. Complete attachment of the retina was achieved, but visual acuity improvement was very poor due to corneal clouding and chronic macular edema. The patient refused further surgical interventions.

32.10 Retinal Detachment in Perforating Ocular Trauma

Fernando Gonzalez Gonzalez

32.10.1 Case Description

Perforating ocular trauma caused by a fire weapon (slug shotgun) in a 62-year-old male patient without any personal or ocular history of interest. The entrance wound was in the superior pars plana, and the exit wound was suspected to be temporal and retroequatorial.

Best-corrected visual acuity (BCVA) was light perception and projection. No intraocular structures were observed due to dense vitreous hemorrhage. Intraocular pressure (IOP) was 4 mmHg.

CT scanner showed a foreign body allocated in the retroequatorial extraocular inferior-temporal orbit.

32.10.2 Surgical Procedure (Fig. 32.21)

Exploration surgery was conducted under general anesthesia. After conjunctival peritomy, a 3 mm superior pars plana wound was observed and sutured, but no exit wound was found. Then, according to CT scan images, lateral rectus muscle was deinserted to access retroequatorial sclera where the exit wound was found and sutured.

Once the ocular globe was closed, a 23G pars plana vitrectomy (PPV) was performed. The lens was removed preserving lens capsule due to the complexity of the case to improve visualization. A retinal detachment (RD) with subretinal bleeding and a temporal exit wound were observed. Vitreous shaving, lifting posterior hyaloid (PH) as much as possible up to vitreous base (VB), was performed. Then, the retina was attached with heavy liquid (PFCL) and the exit wound treated with laser. Finally silicone oil (SO) was left as tamponade performing fluid-PFCL/Air exchange (FAX) followed by Air/Silicone oil exchange (ASX). No retinectomy/chorioretinectomy was performed due to bad visualization to reduce iatrogeny leaving it for a second procedure if necessary despite a likely redetachment due to PVR.

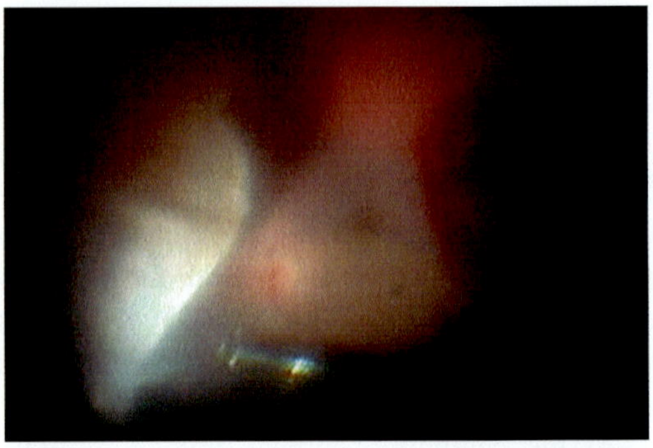

Fig. 32.21 Perforating ocular trauma with RD and exit wound

The postoperative evolution was satisfactory achieving a retinal reattachment; however, two weeks later an expected redetachment was observed in the temporal area. A second surgery under local anesthesia was performed.

First, a 2.5 mm encircling band was sutured at equator to relax a likely scarred VB. Then 23G PPV was performed lifting PH thoroughly up to VB in order to avoid redetachment and aggressive PVR, initial scarred PH membranes at VB were removed with vitreous cutter and forceps. *The exit wound was already separated from the retina and supported by the buckle, thus no retinectomy or chorioretinectomy were performed because there was no retinal traction from the wound.*

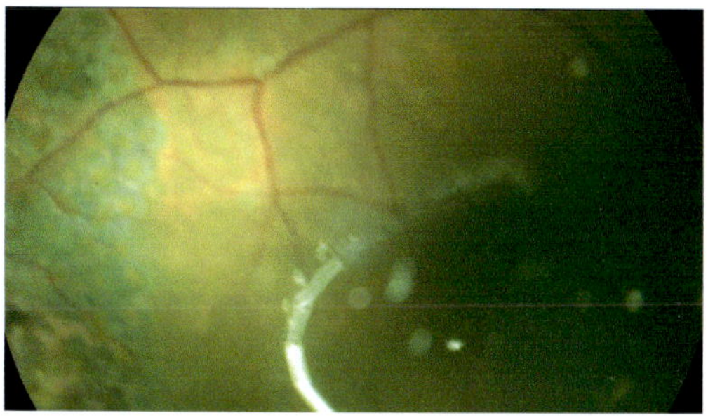

Fig. 32.22 Retina attached under SO

32.10.3 Follow-Up (Fig. 32.22)

The evolution was favorable getting a complete retinal reapplication. A secondary intraocular lens (IOL) implantation surgery in sulcus was performed, achieving 20/60 BCVA.

We would like to highlight in this cases that early intervention, with vitrectomy lifting PH to VB, improves considerably the prognosis of these cases.

32.11 Inferior Retinal Detachment with Subretinal Strands

Philippe Koch

32.11.1 Case Description (Fig. 32.23)

This 22 years old military man came back from war with a head blunt trauma associated to a full right eye retinal detachment (RD) since more than two weeks. Multiple strands of subretinal PVR were observed in the fundus (including under the macular area) and associated to series of inferior retinal breaks extending from 3 to 7 o'clock in the periphery.

32.11.2 Surgical Procedure (Fig. 32.24)

Viewing modes: Slit-Lamp from Zeiss.

Noticeable instruments: 23G vertical scissors from Eyetech, 23G ILM pick from synergetics, and 23G ILM forceps from Dorc.

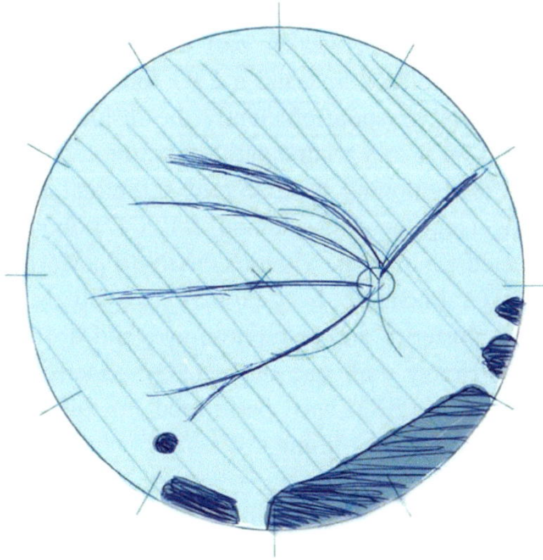

Fig. 32.23 RD with subretinal strands

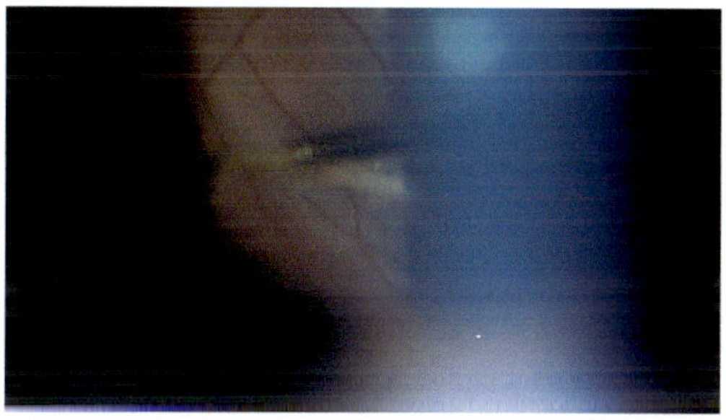

Fig. 32.24 Subretinal strand removal

A 2-port 23G pars plana vitrectomy (PPV) was thus performed and posterior vitreous detachment (PVD) was obtained using the vitreous probe. A heavy liquid (PFCL) bubble was then injected to secure the retina during peripheral vitrectomy. As observed in the video, a cautious vitrectomy was performed using the Dorc peristaltic pump to avoid grasping the retina while shaving the vitreous, even using a cut-by-cut method. Peripheral retinal breaks were then enlarged inferiorly to help removing subretinal fluid (SRF) and tobacco dust. PFCL was then removed to work on the subretinal PVR. As shown in one example of subretinal band removal, the retina is dissected using a vertical scissor parallel to the subretinal strand and a 23G ILM pick is then inserted subretinally to allow a lateral mobilization of the strand prior to pull on it. Normally, the weaker part of the subretinal cord will release first and a 23G forceps would then allow grasping efficiently the residual cord to pull on it in a contralateral direction.

After removing the different subretinal PVR cords using the same method, a PFCL bubble is injected again in the vitreous cavity to perform a laser treatment of the periphery as well as on every posterior access retinotomy. And a direct PFCL/Heavy silicone oil (SO) (Densiron) exchange (PSX) was performed to allow a complete vitreous filling.

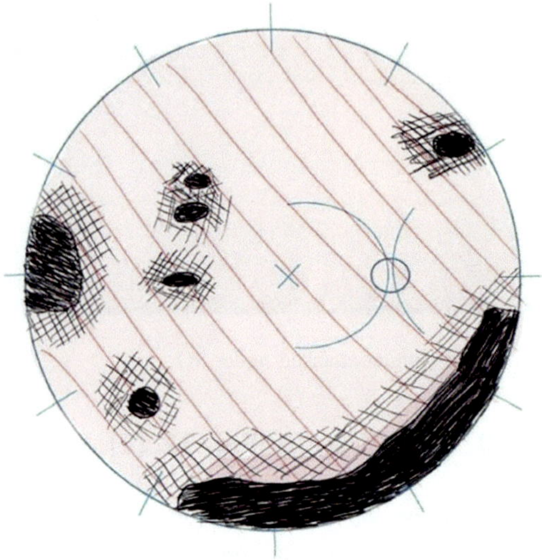

Fig. 32.25 Postoperative retinal reattachment

32.11.3 Follow-Up (Fig. 32.25)

In this young patient, heavy SO removal was performed 6 weeks after surgery and retina is still attached 18 months after surgery with a best corrected visual acuity (BCVA) of 20/100, even following this sub-macular cord removal.

In conclusion, the use of a 23G ILM pick subretinally frequently allows weakening the subretinal strands prior to removing them from the subretinal space with conventional forceps. This action is more respectable of the subretinal anatomy by pulling in a counter direction, opposite to the site of attachment of the residual PVR cord. Sometime, multiple subretinal openings are required to weaken the cord at different places prior to its removal.

32.12 Retinal Detachment Under Silicone Oil with PVR

Philippe Koch

32.12.1 Case Description (Fig. 32.26)

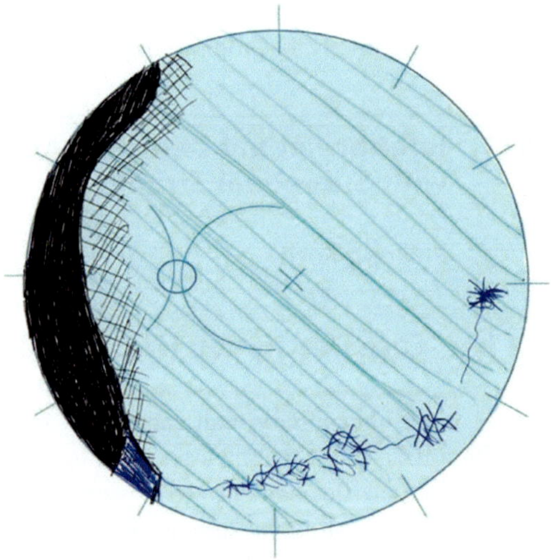

Fig. 32.26 RD with inferior PVR

This is the case of 49 years old man who presented 5 months ago with a history of ocular trauma and a decreased visual acuity (VA) since 10 days. Examination showed a full retinal detachment (RD) of the left eye due to a giant retinal tear (GRT) extending from 7 to 11 o'clock associated to multiple risk factors of PVR (massive vitreous bleeding, hypotony, choroidal detachment, and tobacco dust). The patient was operated with a 23G pars plana vitrectomy (PPV), a laser treatment around the GRT, and silicone oil (SO) injection at the end of surgery to reposition the retina.

Even with an appropriate tamponade using SO, the patient developed one month after his first surgery a massive inferior PVR CA3, contracting the retina from 4 to 7 o'clock and opening again the initial tear at 7 o'clock. He was thus immediately re-operated to stabilize the situation.

32.12.2 Surgical Procedure (Fig. 32.27)

Viewing modes: Slit-Lamp & Resight from Zeiss.

Noticeable instruments: 23G Diamond duster, 23G ILM pick from synergetics, and 23G ILM forceps from Dorc.

The procedure started with a SO removal through a 2-port 23G PPV and an active extrusion. A wide-angle viewing system allowed to visualize the PVR areas contracting the retina inferiorly, as confirmed by a trypan bluc staining.

Complete vitreous shaving was checked using a vitrectome probe, and a diamond-duster and 23G forceps were then used to try to detach anterior epiretinal membranes (ERMs). However, ERM attachment was too strong and these attempts were inefficient using these conventional methods. As a contrary, the use of an ILM-pick allowed a smooth dissection and detachment of this ERM until being peeled using forceps.

A second set of ERM dissections was then performed to show how this pick can be helpful to weaken and dissect the anterior PVR prior to remove it from the retina using forceps.

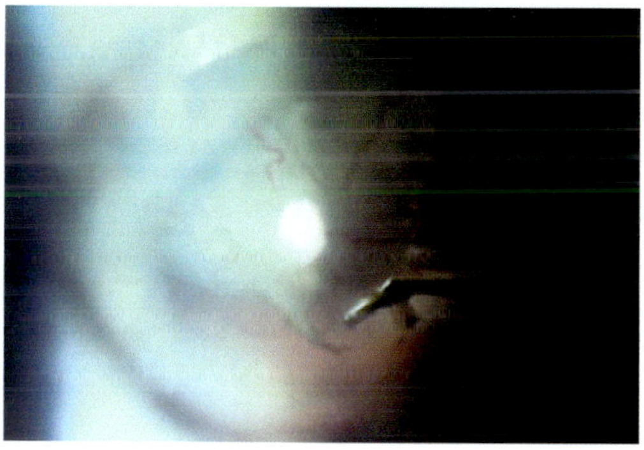

Fig. 32.27 Anterior PVR dissection

As observed at the end of surgery, the inferior retina was mobile again and laser was applied inferiorly from 3 to 8 o'clock under heavy liquid (PFCL) to secure the retina prior to perform a direct PFCL/Heavy SO (Densiron) exchange (PSX).

32.12.3 Follow-Up (Fig. 32.28)

8 weeks later, a new surgery was performed to remove Densiron and the retina remained attached. Another two months after surgery, the patient is recovering with a flat retina and a best-corrected VA (BCVA) of 20/200.

In conclusion, in some tricky situations, ILM pick is becoming a powerful instrument to weaken and dissect the PVR from the retina and then detach it with forceps. By slightly moving it laterally, this instrument achieves to weaken the PVR. However, in some situations, PVR cannot be dissected even using this method and a peripheral retinectomy is preferred, particularly in cases were retinal breaks occur while peeling the PVR.

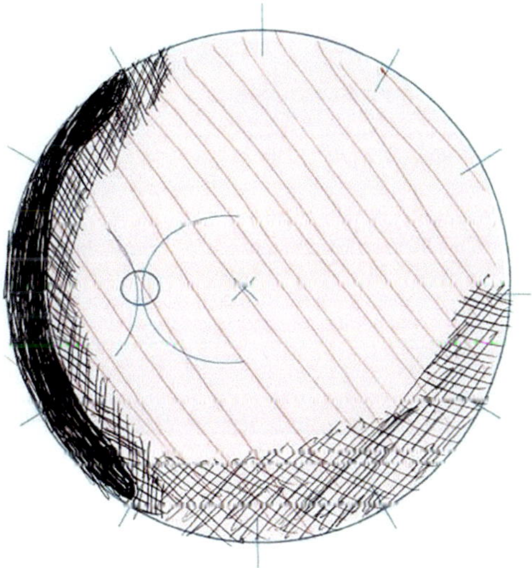

Fig. 32.28 Postoperative retinal reattachment

32.13 Chronic Retinal Detachment with PVR

Francisco J. Lara Medina

32.13.1 Case Description (Fig. 32.29)

68y/o male affected by a chronic pseudophakic retinal detachment (RD) of 6 months of evolution, vitreous haze, and localized upper anterior PVR CA1.

32.13.2 Surgical Procedure

Surgery started by placing a 2.5 mm scleral band 12 mm from the limbus. The band was fixed with scleral tunnels, avoiding the need for sutures and achieving a better integration with ocular surface.

Afterwards, 23G pars plana vitrectomy (PPV) was performed although vitreous turbidity hindered detached retina visualization. Once central vitreous was removed, superior vitreous base (VB) scarring and a retinal tear at V hours were observed. Posterior hyaloid (PH) remained adherent to the upper peripheral retina. Vitreous cutter without cutting was used to detach PH using anterior–posterior movements parallel to the retina. This maneuver should always be performed stabilizing detached retina with external scleral indentation. Indentation can be performed by an experienced assistant or preferably by the surgeon (using an auxiliary chandelier light).

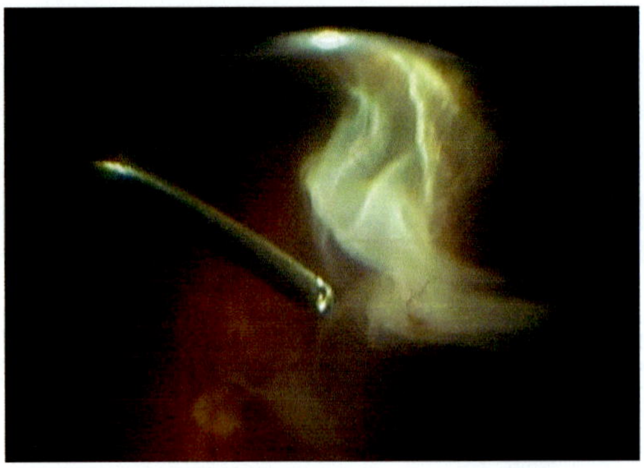

Fig. 32.29 RD with PVR CA1

Once PH was lifted, the vitreous cutter was used to segment scarred PH at VB. When the vitreous cutter could not dissect PH anymore, 23G ILM forceps were used instead. Anterior membranes and scarred PH at VB were completely dissected and removed bimanually with forceps and vitreous cutter. Forceps were used to lift the membranes and vitreous cutter to dissect them bluntly by backpressure movements. When a cleavage plane was obtained, PH traction was cut with the vitrectomy probe.

After dealing with localized anterior PVR, heavy liquid (PFCL) was injected to perform the reattachment test and remove thick subretinal fluid (SRF) through a pre-existing retinal tear. A pocket of persistent SRF in the nasal retina was removed with gentle massage toward the retinal tear by scleral indentation. Then, complete peripheral vitrectomy with indentation was performed.

Finally, the eye was filled with PFCL and laser photocoagulation was done on rhegmatogenous retinal lesions, especially on the retinal area where proliferations were removed. Fluid-PFCL/Air exchange (FAX) was performed followed by 360º laser-cerclage. C3F8 12% was left as tamponade.

32.13.3 Follow-Up (Fig. 32.30)

Retinal was completely attached without tamponade.

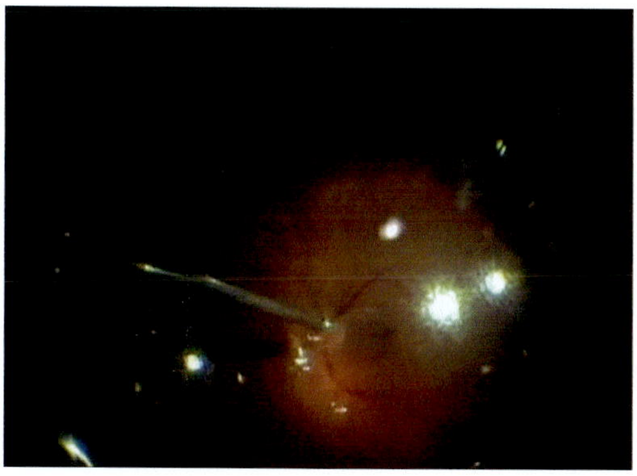

Fig. 32.30 Retina attached under air

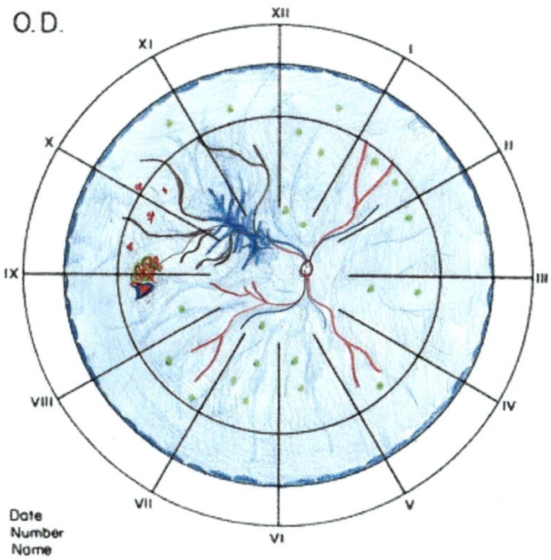

Fig. 32.31 Right eye. Retinal detachment case

32.14 Complete Retinal Detachment with PVR and Retinal New Vessels Secondary to Branch Retinal Vein Occlusion

Joaquín Marticorena Salinero

32.14.1 Case Description (Fig. 32.31)

A 79-year-old man who reported to the clinic because of decreased visual acuity of his right eye over the previous two weeks. Snellen best-corrected visual acuity (BCVA) of the right eye was counting fingers at 30 cm and 1.00 in the left eye. Slit-lamp examination revealed anterior chamber (AC) cells ++, and posterior synechia in 360º that were partially released after topical atropine administration. Nuclear opacity of lens and anterior capsule pseudoexfoliation were present. Right eye fundus examination showed asteroid hyalosis, complete rhegmatogenous retinal detachment (RD) with proliferative vitreoretinopathy (PVR), and presence of different foci of retinal new vessels (NV) at the temporal-superior quadrant secondary to ischemic branch retinal vein occlusion (BRVO). Surgical treatment was indicated, with combined phacoemulsification, intraocular lens (IOL) implantation and pars plana vitrectomy (PPV). Measurement of IOL was based on the keratometry of the right eye and axial length of the left eye after discarding previous anisometropia.

32.14.2 Surgery Description

Surgery was conducted under retrobulbar anesthesia and sedation. Release of posterior synechia, clear cornea phacoemulsification, and in-the-bag implantation of IOL was initially performed. Three ports for transconjunctival 23 Gauge PPV, and an accessory chandelier light were used. At the beginning, exploration of complete RD confirmed the presence of a single retinal tear adjacent to retinal NV in between temporal vascular arcades. During initial central vitrectomy, the absence of complete posterior vitreous detachment (PVD) was observed. Posterior hyaloid (PH) was still attached at the superior temporal quadrant where an epiretinal membrane (ERM) and fixed retinal star folds were present in the context of PVR. PH was also attached at different foci of retinal NV. PVD and partial ERM peeling at site of PVR was done after staining with brilliant peel and trypan blue (Membrane Blue Dual, DORC). Special care was taken during peeling in order to avoid iatrogenic retinal tears in an ischemic and very friable retina. Perfluorocarbon liquid (PFCL) was also used to exert counter-pressure during peeling. Bimanual maneuvers to detach PH were done with the help of an ILM-forceps and a diamond-dusted scraper. These permitted the creation of a dissection plane that allowed to perform segmentation of the PVR membranes and attached PH using the vitreous cutter. Dissection and endodiathermy to retinal NV adjacent to the retinal tear was done. Peripheral vitrectomy was performed under indentation with the light-pipe. Because of the posterior location of the retinal tear and presence of subretinal fluid (SRF) anterior to this lesion, the following maneuvers were performed before doing endolaser. First, vitreous cavity was filled with PFCL up to the level of retinal break. Then, a fluid-air exchange (FAX) was performed with internal drainage of SRF through the tear. Finally, additional PFCL was injected reaching an anterior plane of the tear while residual air was replaced by fluid. Thus, endolaser to the tear and sectorial laser to the ischemic retinal was done in complete absence of SRF. After laser, fluid-PFCL/air (FAX) and air/gas (C_3F_8 14%) exchange (AGX) were performed. Complete attachment of the retina was observed under PFCL and under air.

32.14.3 Follow-Up (Fig. 32.32)

Patient was instructed to posture sitting up, avoiding face-up position for the initial 10 days after surgery. After 9 weeks, complete reattachment of the retina was achieved in the absence of intraocular gas. Optical coherence tomography revealed no macular edema. Right eye BCVA was 0.4 with impaired central fixation.

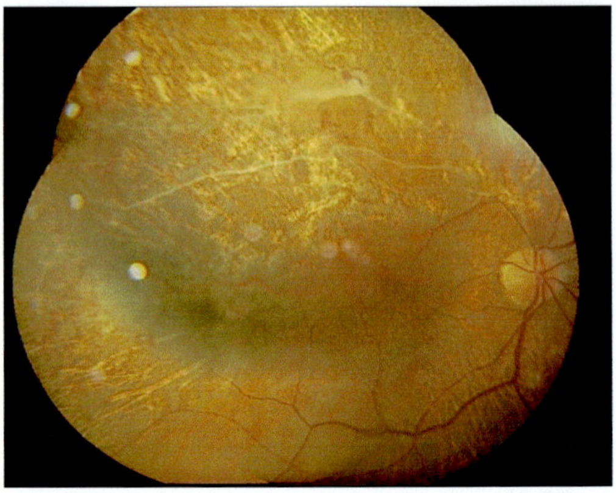

Fig. 32.32 Right eye. Nine weeks after surgery with complete retinal reattachment, sectorial endolaser scars at the temporal superior quadrant, and presence of hyalinized retinal vessels secondary to BRVO. Arrow showing remnants of dissected PVR membrane

32.15 Pediatric Retinal Detachment with PVR and Closed Funnel Retinal Configuration

Jeroni Nadal Reus

32.15.1 Case Description (Fig. 32.33)

3-year-old highly myopic patient (–12D) with a total retinal detachment (RD) due to giant retinal tear (GRT). RD showed initial PVR with

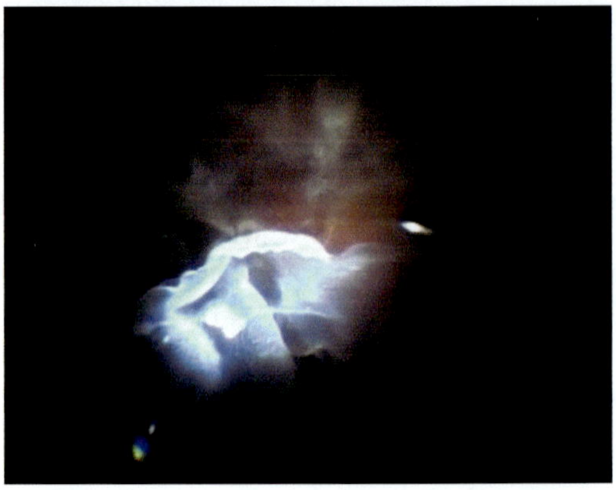

Fig. 32.33 Initial RD due to GRT with PVR CP1

epiretinal membranes (ERM) at macular area and rolled retinal edges. Best-corrected visual acuity (BCVA) was hand movements.

A 4-port 23G phaco/vitrectomy was carried out, macular ERM and ILM were peeled, and careful bimanual posterior hyaloid (PH) detachment up to vitreous base (VB) was completed with two forceps. The retina was reattached with heavy liquid (PFCL) and endolaser was applied to the GRT edge. PFCL/Air exchange (FAX) followed by Air/Silicone Oil exchange (ASX) were performed leaving 5000cs Silicone Oil (SO) as tamponade. Despite meticulous initial surgery with preventive ILM peeling and PH detachment up to VB insertion, PVR evolved inducing a complete RD under silicone oil.

32.15.2 Surgery Description (Fig. 32.34)

A 4-port 23G pars plana vitrectomy (PPV) was performed to deal with RD with PVR CP12 + CA12 in a closed funnel retinal configuration.

First SO was removed, and the closed retinal funnel was opened with viscodissection in order to be able to reach the posterior pole. Then, posterior ERMs were removed bimanually with 2 forceps and the macular area was stabilized with PFCL. The peripheral retina was extremely stiff due to intraretinal PVR, and a relaxing 360° retinectomy was done to relax anterior–posterior traction. The posterior retinal remnant was attached with PFCL, but it was still contracted, so retinal massage with a silicone tip cannula and retinal stretching with two forceps were fulfilled to relax circumferential retinal traction.

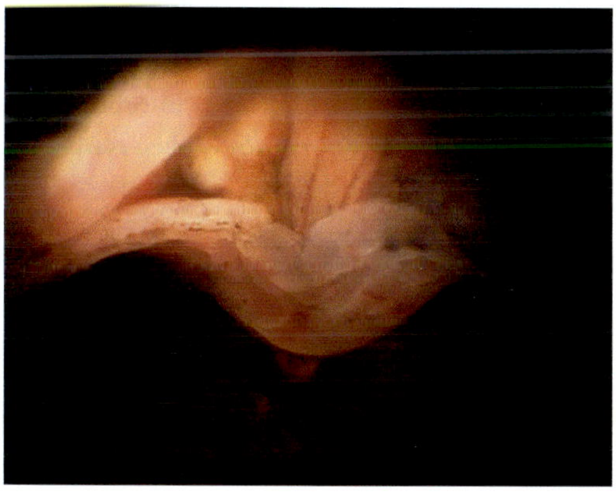

Fig. 32.34 RD PVR CP12 + CA12 in closed funnel retinal configuration

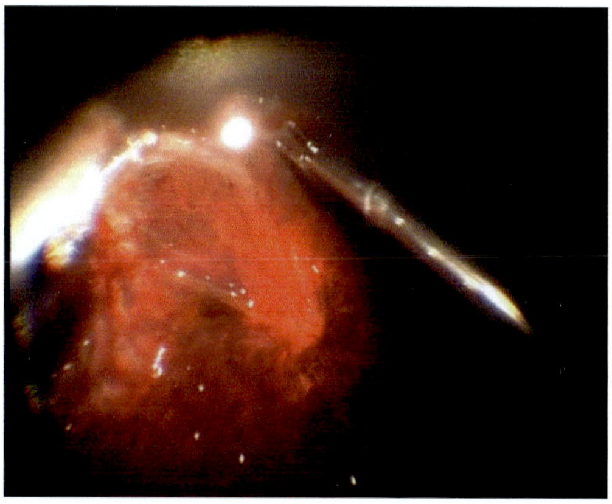

Fig. 32.35 Retina attached under PFCL

Finally a complete retinal attachment under PFCL was achieved and 360° endolaser at the retinectomy edge applied. FAX followed by ASX were performed leaving 5000cs SO as tamponade.

32.15.3 Follow-Up

The patient was operated to remove SO 8 months after surgery, the retina remained attached without tamponade, BCVA was 20/200, and IOP was 8 mmHg.

32.16 Retinal Redetachment PVR CA6 and Intraretinal PVR with Posterior Pole Breaks

Maria Isabel Relimpio Lopez

32.16.1 Case Description (Fig. 32.36)

A mentally challenged 7 years old boy who underwent a pars plana vitrectomy (PPV) on his left eye 1 month ago. Snellen best-corrected visual acuity (BCVA) of the right eye was 20/20 and left eye: Hand Moving.

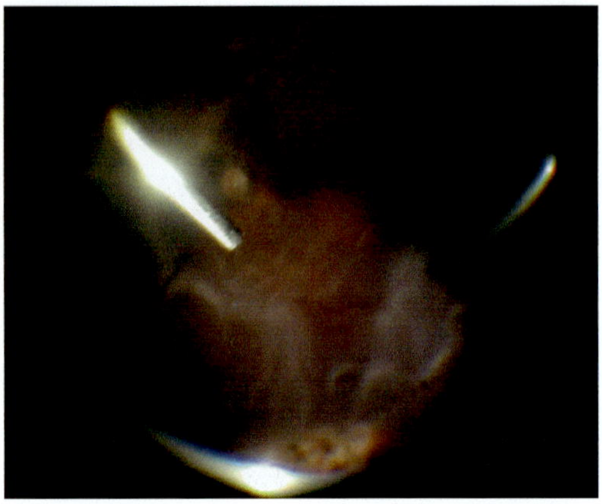

Fig. 32.36 RD with PVR CA6 and Intraretinal PVR

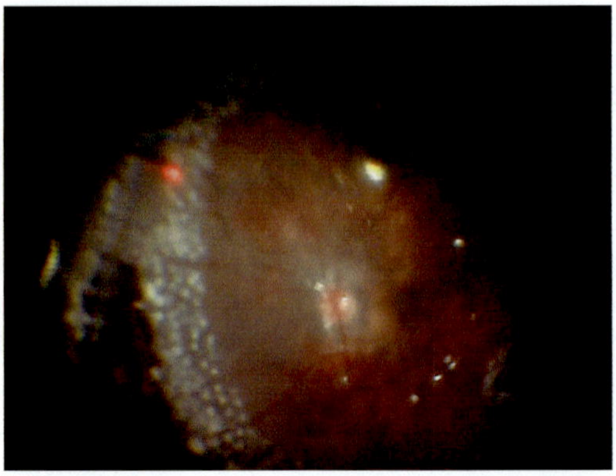

Fig. 32.37 Retina reattached under air

Left eye slit-lamp examination revealed aphakia, + cells in anterior chamber with no other complications. Eye fundus examination showed a complete rhegmatogenous retinal detachment (RD) with anterior PVR with the edge of the retina attached but a microbreak at posterior pole, which enlarged during the bimanual surgery and multiple breaks in the second surgery. A dexamethasone implant was still inside the eye (In aphakia cases I currently suture it at one sclerotomy).

32.16.2 Surgery Description (Fig. 32.37)

First surgery: PPV + peeling and delamination of epiretinal membranes + Retinectomy < 180º + tangential retinotomy due the intrinsic rigidity + Endolaser 360º + silicone oil 5000cs. An encircling band was already placed.

A three port 23G transconjunctival PPV was conducted under general anesthesia, using contact wide angle viewing system Anterior PVR at the edge of the previous treated breaks of the anterior failed PPV was observed.

First internal limiting membrane (ILM) and epiretinal membrane (ERM) peeling (stained with Dual Blue) were carried out under heavy liquid (PFCL) to avoid posterior PVR. It would have been better to peel ILM widely (I currently peel the ILM of the nasal area to decrease the risk of funnel shaped retinal redetachment).

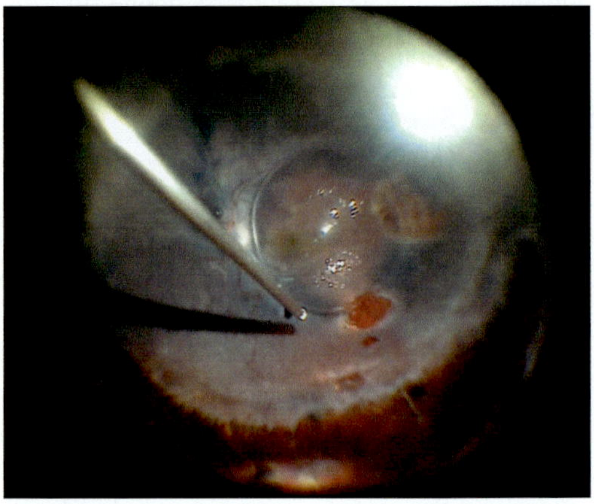

Fig. 32.38 Retinal redetachment due to intraretinal PVR

In the previous surgery, posterior hyaloid (PH) was detached up to equator (due to posterior vitreous base insertion (VB)) in order not to induce iatrogenic breaks. So, the remaining membranes and scarred PH at VB insertion were peeled off bimanually with forceps and a diamond-dusted silicone tip or scissors.

Then, the remaining contracted and devitalized retina anterior to the retinotomy was excised with the vitreous cutter. The edge of the retinotomy was treated with several rows of laser and BSS-PFCL/Air exchange (FAX) followed by Air/Silicone Oil (SO) exchange (ASX) were performed leaving 5000cs SO as a tamponade. In order to avoid retinal slippage during FAX, a soft silicone-tip needle should be place underneath the anterior edge of the retinotomy until it is completely dried.

After one month and a half the retina detached again due to some breaks at the posterior pole due to the rigidity of the retina.

Second Surgery: PPV + peeling and delamination of ERMs + 360° Retinectomy + Endolaser 360° + SO 5000cs.

A 360° retinotomy had to be performed to reattach the retina. Retinal suspenders were maintained during retinectomy to avoid retinal folding. Endodiathermy was applied on the vessels but it was a quite posterior retinectomy and bleeding from vessels trunks was harder to stop.

32.16.3 Follow-Up

Prognosis is grim in children for this kind of surgery. Vitreous is so attached and posterior in children that incomplete detachment of PH can induce complications. Bimanual surgery is necessary to remove all ERMs. ILM peeling prevents further tractions at the posterior pole with secondary breaks that can detach the retina again. Wide ILM peeling, extending it even in the nasal area, is a good maneuver to avoid postoperative retinal funnels avoiding a new redetachment.

32.17 Long-Standing Retinal Detachment with PVR CP6

Diego Ruiz-Casas

32.17.1 Case Description (Fig. 32.39)

A 70 year-old phakic woman complained of floaters and poor visual acuity (VA) (hand motion) for 3 months in her left eye. A long-standing retinal detachment (RD) with PVR CP6 was found. RD showed full thickness retinal contraction at the posterior pole, retinal starfolds close to the inferior vitreous base (VB), and mild VB contraction. The lens was clear with no significant cataract.

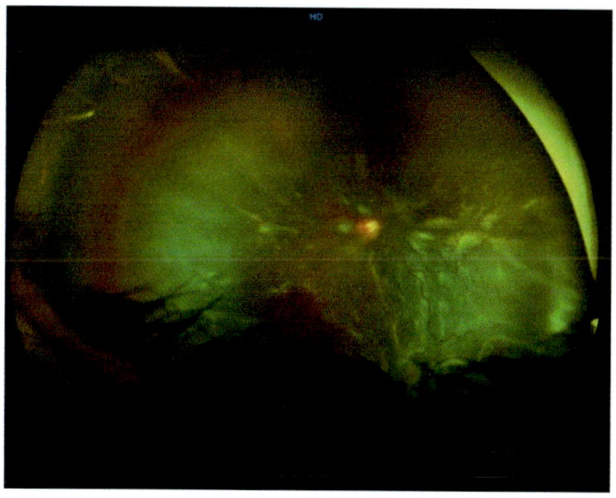

Fig 32.39 RD with PVR CP6

32.17.2 Surgery Description (Fig. 32.40)

23G Phaco/vitrectomy was indicated to get a complete vitrectomy and silicone oil (SO) tamponade. First, phacoemulsification and intraocular lens (IOL) implantation were carried out through a 2.75 mm corneal incision, with 5.5 mm CCC and anterior capsule polishing to avoid anterior capsular phimosis and opacification. Then, 23G 4-port pars plana vitrectomy (PPV) with chandelier light at 12 h (to allow direct illumination by the assistant) was performed.

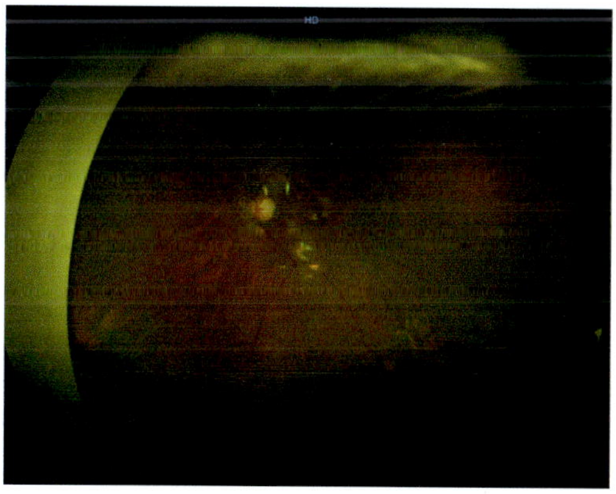

Fig. 32.40 Retina attached under silicone oil

Posterior hyaloid (PH) was detached and contracted forming an anterior fibrous plaque at the posterior border of the VB. PH was lifted up to VB in every quadrant and removed together with the attached anterior retinal flaps. The retinal tears were marked with diathermy trying to cauterize the everted retinal edges.

Internal limiting membrane (ILM) and epiretinal membranes (ERMs) were stained with Dual Blue and peeled under heavy liquid (PFCL) to hold the macular area and avoid shearing forces at optic nerve. First centripetal peeling movements were applied until the fovea was clean of ERM (not to induce a macular hole), and then taut ILM/ERM were peeled centrifugally, as far as possible, using direct visualization with contact macular lens or BIOM.

Next, mature starfolds were addressed removing ERMs from posterior to anterior. First a cleavage plane was found sliding an illuminated pick through the retinal valleys, and then ERMs were delaminated up to VB grasping ERMs with ILM forceps and dissecting them from the underlying retina with the blunt Illuminated Pik (Alcon Grieshaber).

An inferior starfold due to immature ERM was impossible to grasp directly or lift from a cleavage plane. To deal with it, a homemade sharp membrane pick was made by bending the tip of a 25G retrobulbar Atkinson needle. The sharp pick was moved anteriorly on the retinal surface until a cleavage plane was created. Afterwards, ERM delamination was performed the same way as mature membranes but complete ERM removal was impossible. Thus, ERM edges were grasped with two forceps (ILM + Serrated) and pulled apart to strip the ERM without tearing the retina, relaxing tangential traction completely. Then, ERM remnants were dissected up to VB using the blunt Illuminated Pick again.

Afterwards, vitreous shaving with self-indentation was performed, cutting PH at VB insertion as short as possible and debulking vitreous at VB (23G vitreous cutter was set to perform shaving = 300 mmHg max vacuum/7500 cpm/50/50 duty cycle).

A Complete vitrectomy was achieved dissecting anterior hyaloid (AH) at Salzman´s hiatus (SH) 360º and then shaving AH anteriorly to ciliary body and posteriorly to VB. The AH dissection (AHD) maneuver is of paramount importance to avoid anterior PVR and hypotony because it removes any traction from ciliary body to VB. AHD is done cutting AH at SH just over the VB anterior border (23G vitreous cutter was set to perform trenching = 400 mmHg max vacuum/500–1000 cpm/core duty cycle).

The retina looked completely relaxed after complete vitrectomy and ERM peeling. The retinal tear everted edges were removed with a microretinectomy and the anterior chamber (AC) depth was adjusted with BSS injection prior to performing PFCL-BSS/Air exchange (FAX) with a sandwich technique to remove all subretinal fluid (SRF). After FAX, BSS was dripped over the macular area to get rid of any PFCL remnant, and a superior sclerotomy (the one whose microcannula was to be removed last) was presutured. Then Air/Silicone Oil Exchange (ASX) was performed keeping air pressure at 30 mmHg until SO reached the infusion cannula. At that time, air infusion was stopped to avoid air bubbles and SO was injected until there were no air remnants behind the lens. Finally, all microcannulas and sclerotomies, but the last one, were removed and sutured, lid speculum was loosened to avoid unintentional eye pressure, IOP was adjusted to 15–21 mmHg by injecting SO and checking IOP with a Terry-Barraquer tonometer (Ocular Instruments), and the last microcannula was removed whilst the presutured sclerotomy was tied so that no SO leaked.

Complete SO filling is mandatory to get a good tamponade effect and avoid fluid compartments where PVR develops. To get a perfect SO filling the AC must keep its normal depth, vitreous has to be removed completely, no SRF must be left and IOP must be normal (15–21 mmHg) at the end of the case.

32.17.3 Follow-Up (Fig. 32.40)

The patient was instructed to keep a prone position for 24 h so that if a PFCL bubble migrated subretinally it did not collect in the macular area.

Retina was completely attached and SO removed in 3 months achieving 20/60 BCVA.

32.18 Retinal Detachment with PVR CP6 + CA9 and Traumatic Cataract

Diego Ruiz-Casas

32.18.1 Case Description

A 35 year-old phakic patient was operated elsewhere of retinal detachment (RD) due to superior giant retinal tear (GRT) with 23G pars plana vitrectomy (PPV) and 2.5 mm encircling band. He was referred due to redetachment observed with ultrasound. His visual acuity (VA) was light perception (LP). Intraocular pressure (IOP) was 3 mmHg.

Slit-lamp examination showed an intumescent cataract with an iatrogenic posterior circular tear at posterior lens capsule. A retinal detachment (RD) with stiff retina could be observed by ultrasound examination.

32.18.2 Surgery Description (Fig. 32.41)

4-port 23G Phaco-PPV was indicated to get a complete vitrectomy and anterior PVR dissection.

Phacoemulsification was carried out through a 2.75 mm corneal incision, with a 5.5 mm CCC to put an intraocular lens (IOL) at ciliary sulcus because posterior lens capsule was damaged. Hydrodissection broke posterior lens capsule and anterior lensectomy was performed with phacoemulsification handpiece and vitreous cutter, preserving anterior capsule to implant a 3-piece IOL at sulcus with the button-hole (BH) maneuver; luxating the IOL optic through the CCC and leaving haptics at ciliary sulcus.

Then, 23G 4-port PPV with chandelier light was performed. A RD with PVR CP6 + CA9 at inferior and nasal vitreous base (VB) was observed.

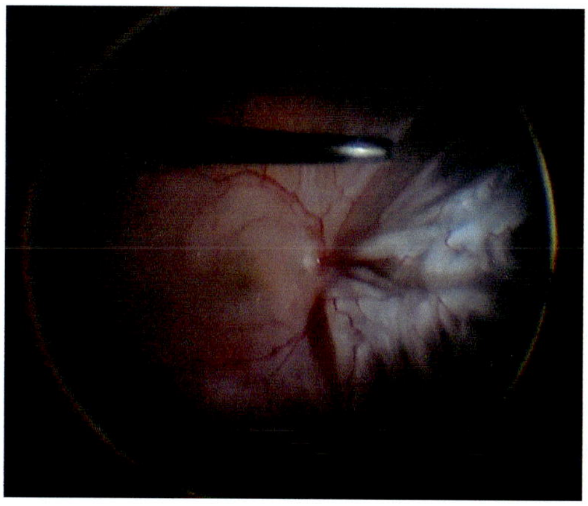

Fig. 32.41 RD with PVR CP6 + CA9

First, luxated lens remnants were removed with the vitreous cutter and posterior epiretinal membranes (ERMs) at posterior pole and macular ILM were stained with Dual Blue and peeled under heavy liquid (PFCL).

Then, anterior ERM were removed bimanually (2 forceps or pick + forceps) as peripheral as possible up to VB. However, a few nasal immature membranes were impossible to delaminate from retinal surface, and were left behind.

Next, anterior PVR due to VB scarring was dealt with. VB membranes were removed or segmented bimanually (2 forceps or pick + forceps) trying to relax VB circumferential centripetal traction. An encircling band was already in place and it was expected to support scarred VB and allow retinal reattachment.

Afterward, complete PPV was performed with self-indentation. First vitreous shaving was carried out, cutting scarred posterior hyaloid (PH) at VB insertion as short as possible and debulking vitreous at VB (23G vitreous cutter was set to perform shaving vitrectomy). Then, anterior hyaloid (AH) dissection at Salzman's hiatus (SH) 360° was completed (23G vitreous cutter was set to perform trenching vitrectomy).

The AH dissection (AHD) maneuver is important to avoid anterior PVR and hypotony. AHD relaxes any traction from ciliary body to VB and anterior retina. AHD avoids ciliary body scarring with subsequent hypotony if retinectomy is performed, by preventing detached pars plana epithelium and anterior retinal remnants folding anteriorly and being part of the ciliary scar tissue.

Silicone oil (SO) tamponade was planned and the iris-lens diaphragm was not sure to be competent, thus, and inferior iridotomy was performed and the anterior chamber (AC) was filled with dispersive viscoelastic to keep a normal AC depth.

Then, a reattachment test was performed with a Fluid (BSS)-PFCL/Air exchange (FAX) but the retina was too stiff, and retinal tears and scarred VB were posterior to buckle indentation precluding retinal reattachment. Therefore, an Air/Fluid exchange (AFX) was performed and a relaxing retinectomy was indicated. Retinectomy was performed under PFCL-BSS to improve visualization, control bleeding vessels and avoid subretinal blood collection and inadverted choroidal impacts. Diathermy was applied first and then the retina was cut with the vitreous cutter. Retinectomy extension was 200º, enlarging it well into healthy retina. The retina was cut with the vitreous cutter just posterior to VB insertion to avoid reproliferation. All bleeding points were cauterized, preretinal and subretinal clots removed, and the anterior retinal flap was completely shaved up to ora serrata to avoid inflammation, iris rubeosis or ciliary scar tissue from devitalized peripheral retina remnants.

Finally the retina was attached with PFCL, 360º endolaser was applied and FAX (with careful retinal edge drying to avoid slippage) followed by Air/Silicone Oil Exchange (ASX) were performed to fill the eye completely with 1000cs SO at 15–21 mmHg.

32.18.3 Follow-Up (Fig. 32.42)

The retina remained attached under SO, VA improved to 20/60 and IOP raised to 14 mmHg.

A new 23G PPV was performed 3 months later to remove SO and new ERMs.

SO was removed from vitreous cavity and AC emulsification, cleaning cells over the IOL as well. Anterior and posterior new or mature ERMs were removed bimanually with forceps and illuminated pick up to retinectomy edge. A few ERMs were so stuck to the retinal tissue they had to be segmented and left behind. 360º Endolaser was enlarged and FAX followed by Air/Gas exchange (AGX) performed to leave SF6 20% as tamponade.

The retina remained attached without tamponade, VA was 20/60 and IOP was 12 mmHg.

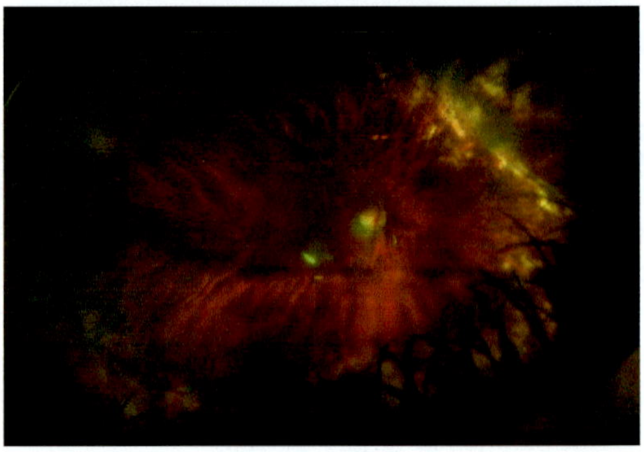

Fig. 32.42 Retina attached without tamponade

32.19 Retinal Detachment After Penetrating Ocular Trauma

Zoran Tomic

32.19.1 Case Description

46 y/o male, professional driver suffered a scleral laceration in his right eye by a piece of wood while chopping them. At admission the eye was hypotonic with deep anterior chamber (AC). Behind the transparent posteriorly dislocated lens there was a dense vitreous hemorrhage and ultrasound examination showed complete retinal detachment (RD). Wound exploration revealed scleral laceration in the upper temporal quadrant with uveal and retinal prolapse. The prolapsed tissue was excised and the wound sutured with Vicryl 7/0 interrupted X-sutures.

32.19.2 Surgery Description (Figs. 32.43, 32.44)

A week after the primary surgery, 23G pars plana vitrectomy (PPV) was performed. Peroperatively posterior lens dislocation, dense vitreous hemorrhage, complete retinal detachment with superotemporal and inferonasal giant retinal tear (GRT), epiretinal (ERM) and subretinal PVR and subretinal hemorrhage were observed.

They were treated with: 23G PPV, lensectomy, epiretinal membrane (ERM) peeling, retinectomy 360° to release posterior retina from peripheral vitreous base (VB) scar and sclerochoroidal wound, removal of subretinal membranes and hemorrhage, pupilloplasty, secondary retropupillary iris claw intraocular lens (IOL) implantation and silicone oil (SO) tamponade.

32.19.3 Follow-Up

Surgery was repeated two times in following two months due to reproliferation with ERM peeling and SO exchange. SO was successfully removed six months later. Initial best-corrected visual acuity (BCVA) was light perception only and final BCVA three months after silicone oil removal was 0,1–0,2 eccentrically. Unfortunately this result was not good enough for the patient to keep his professional driving license.

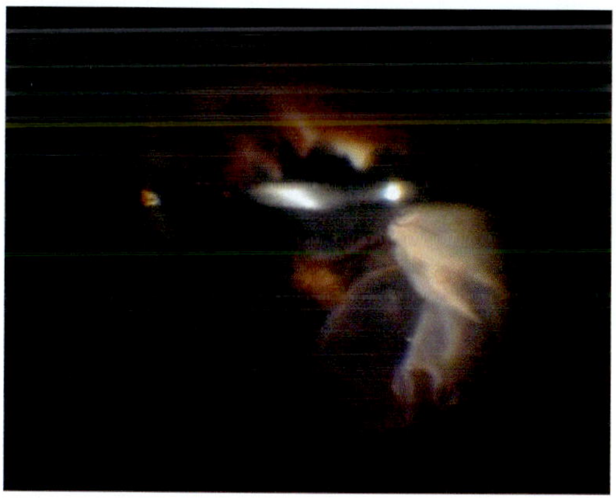

Fig. 32.43 Retinal detachment

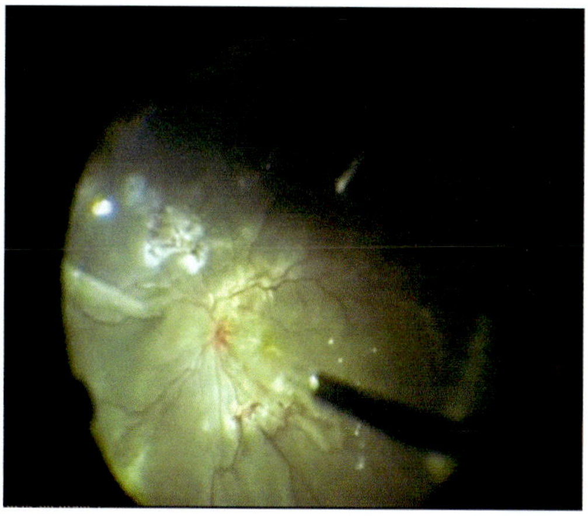

Fig. 32.44 Retinal reattachment

32.20 Retinal Detachment Under Silicone Oil with PVR CP2 + CA6

Zoran Tomic

32.20.1 Case Description (Fig. 32.45)

65 y/o male underwent a combined phacoemulsification with posterior chamber intraocular lens (IOL) implantation and pars plana vitrectomy (PPV) with silicone oil (SO) tamponade for retinal detachment (RD) in the right eye at another clinic. Was admitted for the treatment of inferior redetachment with PVR CP2 and anterior

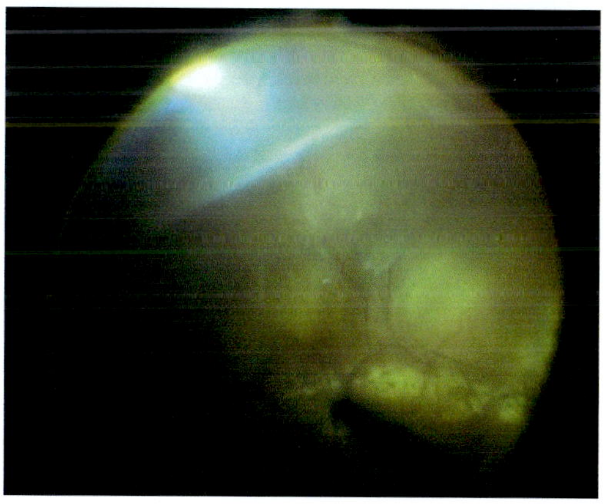

Fig. 32.45 Retinal detachment

PVR CA6, several retinal tears and SO under the retina. He lost the vision in his left eye due to secondary glaucoma after phacoemulsification with IOL implantation and PPV with SO tamponade for RD as well.

32.20.2 Surgery Description (Fig. 32.46)

23G PPV with SO removal, peeling of epiretinal membranes (ERM), scarred posterior hyaloid (PH) dissection at vitreous base (VB), peripheral circumferential 270° retinotomy and endolaser treatment were performed and retina was completely attached with heavy liquid (PFCL) and fluid-PFCL/Air exchange (FAX) followed by Air/Silicone Oil exchange (ASX) leaving 1000cs SO as tampoande.

32.20.3 Follow-Up

Three months after surgery SO was successfully removed. Initial best-corrected visual acuity (BCVA) at presentation was 0,04 and final BCVA two months after SO removal was 0,2.

32.21 Myopic Retinal Detachment Without Posterior Vitreous Detachment

Zoran Tomic

32.21.1 Case Description (Fig. 32.47)

12 y/o myopic male (–8, 25 D) was admitted for treatment of rhegmatogenous retinal detachment (RD) with macular involvement in his left eye after two weeks duration. Retinal tears were observed at 2 and 3 h.

32.21.2 Surgery Description (Fig. 32.48)

Lens sparing 23G pars plana vitrectomy (PPV) combined with encircling band was performed. Induction of posterior vitreous detachment (PVD) was made after triamcinolone staining, lifting posterior hyaloid (PH) up to vitreous base (VB), retina was attached with heavy liquid (PFCL) and fluid-PFCL/Air exchange (FAX), tears were treated with

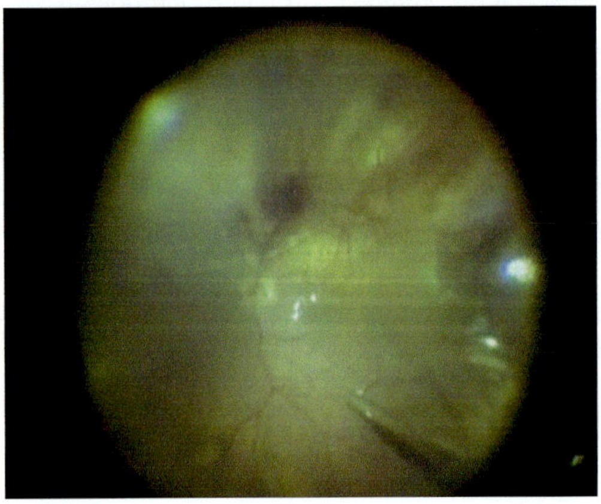

Fig. 32.46 Retinal reattachment

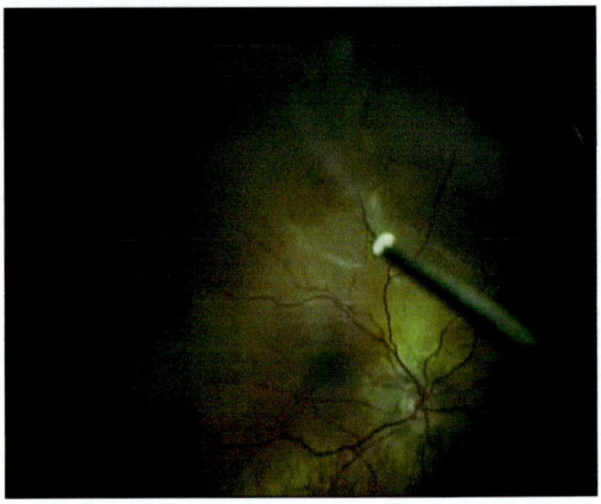

Fig. 32.47 Retinal detachment

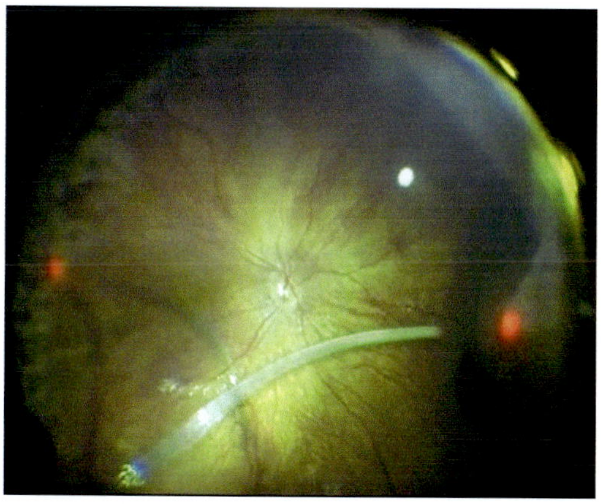

Fig. 32.48 Retinal reattachment

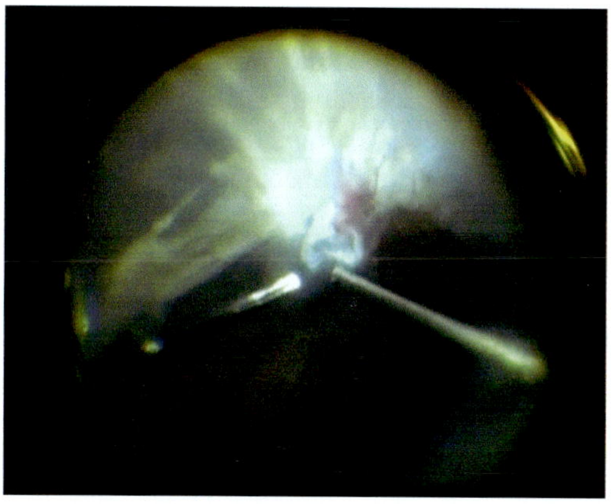

Fig. 32.49 Retinal detachment

endolaser and Air/Gas exchange was performed (AGX) leaving gas as tamponade.

32.21.3 Follow-Up

Initial best-corrected visual acuity (BCVA) was 0,3 and final BCVA three months after surgery was 0,5.

32.22 Retinal Detachment with PVR CA4 and Subretinal Strands

Zoran Tomic

32.22.1 Case Description (Fig. 32.49)

60 y/o male was admitted for the treatment of tractional-rhegmatogenous retinal detachment (RD) with PVR CA4 of three months duration. He underwent previously phacoemulsification with posterior chamber intraocular lens (IOL) implantation for complicated cataract after corneal ulceration.

32.22.2 Surgery Description (Fig. 32.50)

23G Pars plana vitrectomy (PPV) and peeling of epiretinal membranes (ERMs) and two subretinal strands were performed. Anterior epiretinal membranes, actually scarred posterior hyaloid (PH) at vitreous base insertion (VB) were removed bimanually with forceps and scissors. Subretinal membranes at VB were removed bimanually with two forceps through two access retinotomies. Peripheral tears were observed at 5,

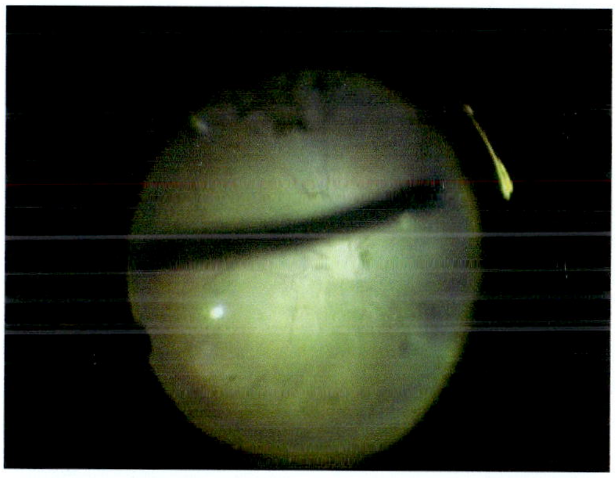

Fig. 32.50 Retinal reattachment

7 and 8 h and were treated with endolaser after retinal attachment with heavy liquid (PFCL) and fluid-PFCL/Air exchange (FAX) removing subretinal fluid (SRF) completely. Finally 1000cs silicone oil (SO) was injected with Air/Silicone oil exchange (ASX).

32.22.3 Follow-Up

Three months later SO was successfully removed. Initial best-corrected visual acuity (BCVA) was hand motions (HM) and final BCVA two months after SO removal was 0,1.

32.23 Traumatic Retinal Detachment with Retinal Incarceration and Ora Dialysis

Zoran Tomic

32.23.1 Case Description (Fig. 32.51)

30 y/o female was admitted for the treatment of traumatic retinal detachment (RD) in her right eye with vitreous hemorrhage and advanced PVR, twelve days after suturing of scleral laceration and removal of intraocular foreign body (IOFB) (glass) that was performed at another clinic.

32.23.2 Surgery Description (Fig. 32.52)

A combined phacoemulsification and intraocular lens implantation (IOL) with 23G pars plana vitrectomy (PPV) was performed. Peroperatively after removal of vitreous hemorrhage, a traction retinal detachment with retinal incarceration at laceration site and ora dialysis at opposite side (temporally) was observed.

A peripheral circumferential retinectomy 360° released the retina from the sclerochoroidal wound. Then the retina was unfolded, relocated and reattached with heavy liquid (PFCL). Endolaser 360° was done under PFCL. Finally a fluid-PFCL/Air exchange (FAX) was performed followed by Air/Silicone oil exchange (ASX) leaving 1000cs silicone oil (SO) as tamponade. At the end of the surgery retina was completely attached.

32.23.3 Follow-Up

Three months later, surgery was repeated due to development of subretinal PVR. After removal of subretinal strands, SO 5700cs was injected and no additional surgery was planned. Initial best-corrected visual acuity (BCVA) was light perception (LP) and final BCVA two months after injection of dense silicone oil was 0,1.

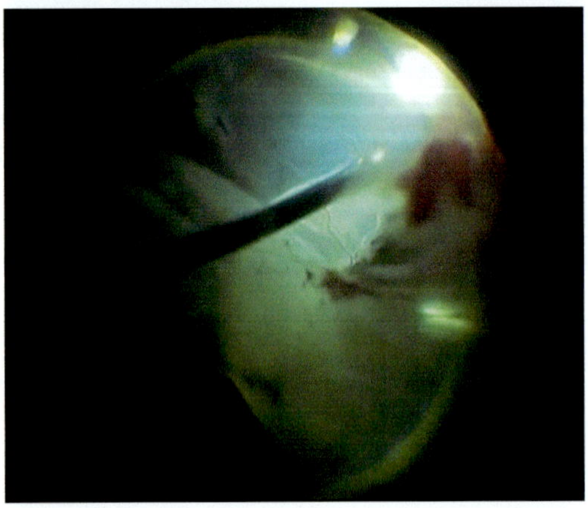

Fig. 32.51 Retinal detachment

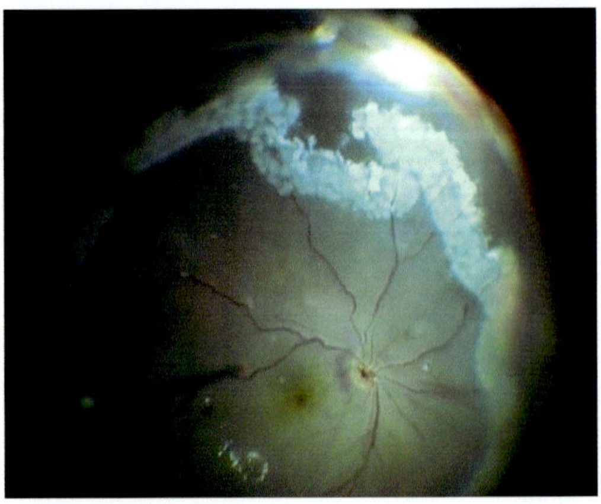

Fig. 32.52 Retinal reattachment

32.24 Traumatic Retinal Detachment CP12 + CA12 with Closed Funnel Shape

Zoran Tomic

32.24.1 Case Description (Fig. 32.53)

42 y/o male was hit by a piece of wood in his left eye. He didn't see more than light perception (LP) for the last six months and decided to ask for help by the beginning of the next year. Examination revealed mature traumatic cataract and funnel shape retinal detachment (RD) shown by ultrasound. Patient was informed about limited expectations and probable need for several surgeries.

32.24.2 Surgery Description (Fig. 32.54)

Combined phacoemulsification with intraocular lens (IOL) implantation and 23G pars plana vitrectomy (PPV) were performed in peribulbar anaesthesia. Peroperatively a closed funnel RD with PVR CP12 + CA12 and subretinal strands were observed. All visible epiretinal membranes (ERM) and scarred posterior hyaloid (PH) were removed up to vitreous base (VB). However, the retina remained contracted and shortened and a primary inferior circumferential retinectomy was performed. After it was done all visible subretinal strands were removed and the retina was attached completely with heavy liquid (PFCL) injection. Three rows of continuous endolaser were placed at the retinectomy edge and fluid-PFCL/Air (FAX) followed by Air/Silicone oil (ASX) exchange were performed to leave 1000cs silicone oil (SO) as tamponade.

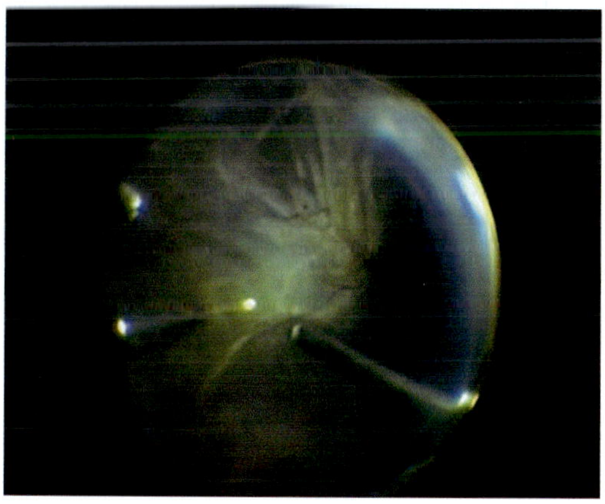

Fig. 32.53 Retinal Detachment

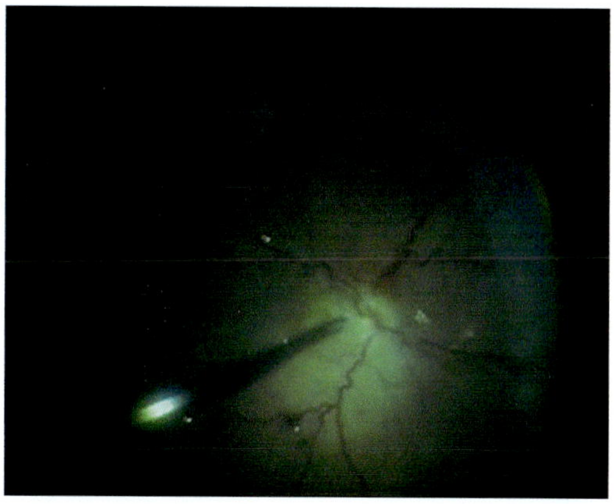

Fig. 32.54 Retinal reattachment

32.24.3 Follow Up

Retina was attached with a single surgery and four months later silicone oil (SO) was successfully removed. Initial VA improved from LP to 0,05 two months after SO removal.

32.25 Retinal Redetachment with PVR CP12

Zoran Tomic

32.25.1 Case Description (Fig. 32.55)

A 55 y/o male presented with an aggressive looking total retinal detachment (RD) with PVR in 4 quadrants 6 weeks post pseudophakic macula on RD treated with pars plana vitrectomy (PPV) and air. There were starfolds in 2 circumferential zones: first between posterior pole

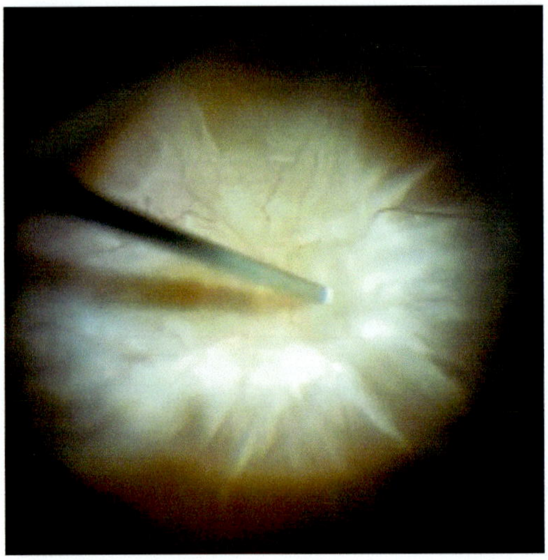

Fig. 32.55 Intraoperative picture

and equator, second anterior to equator near vitreous base (VB). There were no anterior PVR complications because ciliary body was free (complete vitrectomy was done during primary PPV).

32.25.2 Surgical Strategy

Start peeling centrally, posterior membranes are most often purely epiretinal (ERMs) so they can be peeled/freed completely from the underlying retina. As your peeling extends towards VB, be careful because the membranes tend to have deeper intraretinal extensions anteriorly. Complete removal without additional breaks may be impossible: the zone where epiretinal becomes intraretinal will be the retinotomy site. So the goal is to free as large an area of central retina as possible from ERMs. A retinotomy (as last resort) releases/rescues the "conquered" and "healthy" central area from the anterior retina that is beyond repair due to intraretinal PVR.

Understanding this fundamental difference between posterior ERMs (most likely originating from RPE seeding) and anterior (VB) membranes (rather Muller cell based) dictates surgical strategy (1,2).

Caveat: be patient, don't look at the clock, just think this is your only case for today and you have the day off tomorrow!!

Basic surgical setup: 23G 4-port (chandelier) PPV. Endgripping forceps, vertical scissors (very versatile: spatula, pick, scissors), soft tipped active backflush, membrane blue dual (trypan blue + brilliant blue). If this would have been a primary surgery with fresh PVR, an encircling buckle could have been an additional tool to try and avoid retinotomy in the acute phase.

32.25.3 Surgical Procedure

First, posterior ERMs were removed bimanually without retinal breaks. Fresh PVR membranes tend to stain poorly: repeat if necessary, preferably under air (despite high viscosity and density of the dye, in contracted retina with breaks, the dye tends to move subretinally: this can be toxic and it also reduces the contrast because everything tends to have a bluish hue afterwards).

Caution: Do not re-stain after extensive peeling: trypan blue will stain tissue damage that you have caused inadvertently, making further peeling of the stained tissue rather perilous.

As ERMs reach the VB they seem to be integrated intraretinally: you have reached the border between purely epiretinal and intraretinal PVR. Intraretinal PVR cannot be peeled without making breaks. Consequently the anterior traction can only be counteracted by broad indentation with an encircling buckle or with retinotomy (3).

Then, heavy liquid (PFCL) was injected (preferably perfluoroctane, as it is less heavy than decaline). It facilitated ERM engaging for additional peeling as the membrane is less "squashed". Thus, using directional endo-light and PFCL, posterior ERMs were removed easier (better visualization than chandelier). It also makes anterior ERMs peeling easier, because PFCL functions as 3rd hand stabilizing central retina whilst anterior ERMs are removed with one hand indenting and the other using forceps.

Afterwards, a relaxing retinectomy was performed to remove anterior ERMs and anterior–posterior traction due to retinal stiffness. Diathermy on large vessels was used at the border of the retinectomy (between peeled central retina and the redundant periphery). Retinectomy extension was calculated according to residual stiffness of the retina. Anterior retinal remnants were completely removed to prevent anterior retinal loop with hypotony or ischemia with rubeosis.

Finally the retina was attached. Rather than laser under heavy liquid and perform direct PFCL/silicone oil exchange (PSX): a fluid/air exchange (FAX) was performed first because the retina would settle in a more relaxed central position. This is a fundamental difference with large retinotomy (as in full macular translocation (FMT) or giant tear (GRT) cases) without PVR, in these cases retinal slippage has to be avoided with direct PSX. Very limited laser was done, just to the retinotomy border or even no laser at all is a correct option because extensive laser at this point is not going to prevent recurrent PVR and is sacrificing healthier retina (4).

32.25.4 Follow-Up

Retina remained attached without silicone oil

Appendix

Retinal Detachment with Epiretinal and Subretinal PVR Removal

Javier Zarranz-Ventura

Case Description (Fig. 32.56)

This is a case of redetachment following a failed primary repair with pars plana vitrectomy (PPV), laser retinopexy and heavy silicon oil for a subtotal retinal detachment (RD) with multiple temporal and inferior breaks. Now the retina is detached nasally and inferiorly under heavy oil due to an epiretinal proliferative vitreoretinopathy (PVR) and 2 subretinal PVR bands (a large nasal band and a small temporal band).

Surgical Procedure (Fig. 32.57)

As first step, the heavy oil was removed with the viscous fluid removal set using a 23G pack. Then, trypan blue was employed to stain the epiretinal membrane (ERM) that was peeled with an end-grasping forceps using a small heavy liquid (PFCL) bubble to counter-pressure the traction exerted with the forceps during the peel. Once this step has been completed, the superotemporal sclerotomy was enlarged to a 20G port, a retinotomy was performed with endodiathermy and a

Fig. 32.56 Preoperative RD

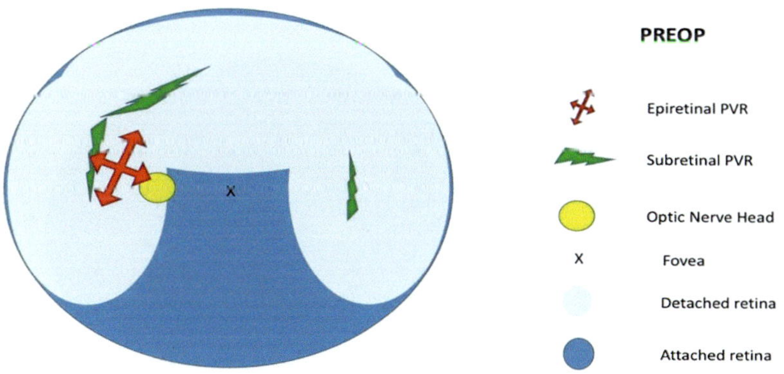

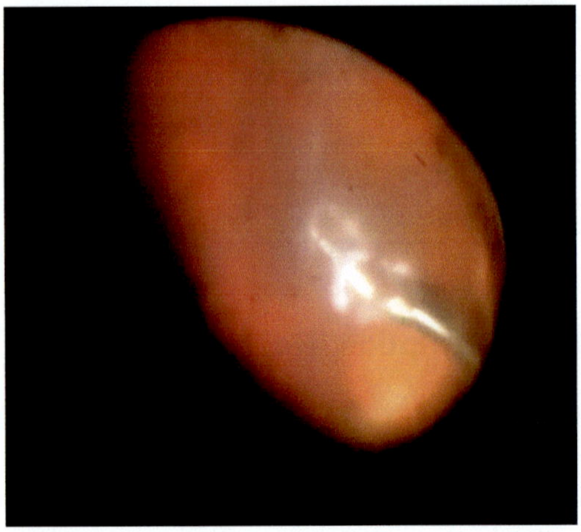

Fig. 32.57 Subretinal strand removal

passive-aspiration backflush cannula flute, and a 20G angled forceps was employed to remove the circumferential subretinal band of PVR nasally. A second retinotomy was performed with the same approach (endodiathermy + backflush cannula flute) to complete the band removal, and once the nasal band had been completely removed a temporal retinotomy was also performed and the small temporal subretinal band was removed too. A superior iridotomy was performed with the vitreous cutter through a temporal side port. The vitreous cavity was completely filled with PFCL and laser retinopexy was applied to all retinal breaks. Direct PFCL/Heavy Silicon Oil was performed and the surgery was completed.

Follow-Up (Fig. 32.58)

The retina was completely attached under heavy oil and after its removal.

List of Collaborators for Video Cases

Felix Armadá-Maresca, Ph.D. Head of the ophthalmology department at University Hospital La Paz, Madrid (Spain).

Francisco Cabrera Lopez, Ph.D. Head of Ophthalmology Department at Complejo Hospitalario Universitario Insular Materno-Infantil de Gran Canaria. Associate Professor of Ophthalmology at Universidad de Las Palmas de Gran Canaria, (Spain).

Jorge I. Calzada, M.D FACS. President, Charles Retina Institute, Memphis, Tennessee (USA).

Juan Manuel Cubero Parra, M.D. Vitreo-Retina Unit Hospital la Arruzafa, Córdoba (Spain).

Mostafa Elgohary, MB ChB M.Sc., M.D FRCSEd FRCSI FRCOphth. Consultant Vitreoretinal Surgeon at Kingston Hospital (UK).

Francisco Espejo Arjona, M.D. Ophthalmology department (Vitreo-Retina and Ocular Oncology). Virgen Macarena University Hospital, Seville (Spain).

Fernando Faus Guijarro, Ph.D. Universitary Hospital Miguel Servet, Zaragoza (Spain).

Guillermo Fernandez Sanz, M.D, DiSSO. Director of the Retina Service Fundacion Jimenez Diaz University Hospital & Ruber Juan Bravo Hospital, Madrid (Spain).

Fig. 32.58 Postoperative retinal attachment

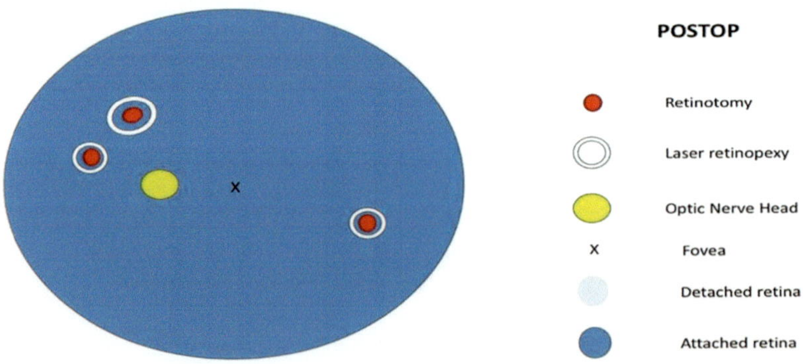

Jesus Ramon Garcia Martinez. Ph.D. Director of the retina service. Hospital La Paz Madrid and Oftalvist, Madrid (Spain).

Fernando Gonzalez Gonzalez, Ph.D. Retina unit, Hospital Perpetuo Socorro, Complejo Hospitalario Universitario Badajoz (CHUB). Ophthalmology department coordinator Hospital Quiron Salud CLIDEBA. Badajoz, (Spain).

John Kitchens, M.D Partner, Retina Associates of Kentucky (USA).

Dr. Philippe Koch, M.D, Ph.D, FEBO, EVRTS, EVRS Board Member & Congress Coordinator. Professor at Orsay-Paris South University. Brussels (Belgium).

Carlos Mateo, Ph.D. IMO Instituto de Microcirugía Ocular, Barcelona, Spain.

Khalil Ghasemi Falavarjani, M.D. Associate Professor of Ophthalmology, Diseases and Surgery of the Retina and Vitreous. Eye Department, Iran University of Medical Sciences, Tehran (Iran).

Victor N. Kazaykin, Ph.D. IRTC "Eye Microsurgery" Ekaterinburg Center, Ekaterinburg (Russia).

Prof. Shunji Kusaka. Department of Ophthalmology Kindai University Sakai Hospital (Japan).

Joaquín Marticorena Salinero, Ph.D. Department Ophthalmology Complejo Hospitalario Universitario de A Coruña (CHUAC), A Coruña (Spain).

Jeroni Nadal Reus, Ph.D. Head of the retina department at Centro de Oftalmología Barraquer, Barcelona (Spain).

Maria Isabel Relimpio Lopez, M.D. Vitreo-Retina surgeon specialist & Research director. Virgen Macarena Hospital/Santa Angela de la Cruz, VIAMED Hospital. aMIRAS Ophthalmology Clinic founding partner. Seville (Spain).

Marc Veckeneer, Ph.D. VR surgeon, ZNA Middelheim Hospital, Antwerp (Belgium).

Javier Zarranz-Ventura M.D, Ph.D, FEBO. Institut Clínic of Ophthalmology (ICOF). Hospital Clínic of Barcelona (Spain).

References

1. Lewis GP, Charteris DG, Sethi CS, Fisher SK. Animal models of retinal detachment and reattachment: identifying cellular events that may affect visual recovery. Eye. 2002;16:375–87.
2. Charteris DG, Downie J, Aylward GW, Sethi C, Luthert P. Intraretinal and periretinal pathology in anterior proliferative vitreoretinopathy. Graefes Arch Clin Exp Ophthalmol. 2007;245:93–100.
3. Veckeneer MAH. Improving the outcome of rhegmatogenous retinal detachment repair by adding pieces to the puzzle. Erasmus University Rotterdam. Chapter 3. 2015. ISBN 978-94-6228-695-5
4. Veckeneer M, Maaijwee K, Charteris DG, van Meurs JC. Deferred laser photocoagulation of relaxing retinotomies under silicone oil tamponade to reduce recurrent macular detachment in severe proliferative vitreoretinopathy. Graefes Arch Clin Exp Ophthalmol. 2014;252:1539–44.

Part VIII

Postoperative Follow-Up and Complications and Tipps and Tricks for RD Surgery

All videos of this part are found in a playlist on my youTube channel:
https://youtube.com/playlist?list=PL0dKYclPD7yMn861X0g-aHCS6KZ5NcH1N

Chapter 33: **After Surgery and Complications**
Iridectomy
Iris-IOL capture
Complication lasernecrosis
Managing Dry Macular Folds after Vitreoretinal Surgery Dr. Mateo
Chapter 34: No video
Chapter 35: No video.

After Surgery and Complications

33

Zoran Tomic and Ulrich Spandau

Positioning (Figs. 33.1 and 33.2): In case of gas and silicone oil tamponade we position the patients for 1 week. In case of 1000 csts and 5000 csts silicone oil we position in the same way as with a gas tamponade. In case of Densiron 68 the patient is advised to sleep on the back (supine) and free positioning under the day.

Eye-drops: For all retinal detachment cases we prescribe Atropine 1% × 1 and cortisone drops × 5 for 2 weeks. In case of postoperative uveitis we inject subtenonal triamcinolone (whole ampule). In case of an IOP between 21 and 30 mmHg we prescribe antiglaucomatous drops and if the IOP >30 mmHg we prescribe Acetazolamid × 2–4. Young patients with silicone oil tamponade have often increased IOP and require Acetazolamid for a longer duration.

Follow-up:

Retinal detachment with vitrectomy: 1 day post OP, 1 week postop for IOP measurement and 2 weeks post OP.

Retinal detachment with episcleral buckling: 1 day postop, if the retina is attached once more 2 weeks postop.

Electronic supplementary material The online version of this chapter (10.1007/978-3-031-11946-0_33) contains supplementary material, which is available to authorized users.

Z. Tomic
Milos Klinika, Belgrade, Serbia

U. Spandau (✉)
St. Eriks Hospital, University of Stockholm, Stockholm, Sweden
e-mail: ulrich_spandau@yahoo.de

U. Spandau et al. (eds.), *Retinal Detachment Surgery and Proliferative Vitreoretinopathy*, https://doi.org/10.1007/978-3-031-11946-0_33

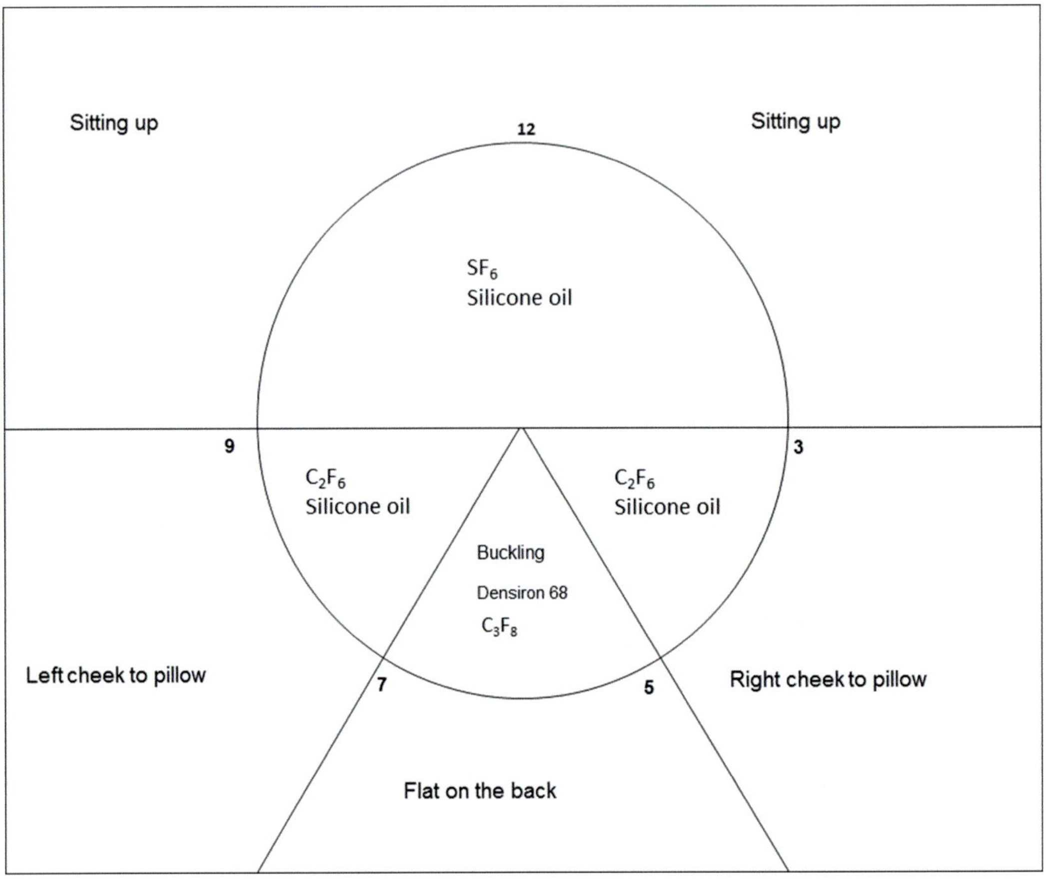

Fig. 33.1 Tamponade and posture for retinal detachment depending on the location of the break

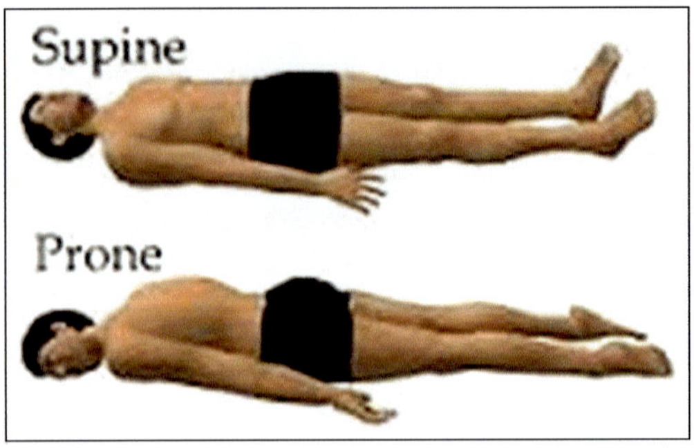

Fig. 33.2 Supine (on the back) and prone (face down) position. Photocourtesy wikipedia

Caution for silicone oil removals: They have a rather high detachment risk and a PVR detachment quickly develops. We see these patients 1 day postop and, 1 week postop.

Table 33.1 Peroperative complications

Choroidal detachment	Subepithelial location of infusion trocar
Prevention	• In case of ocular normotony check the location of the infusion trocar during surgery
Treatment	• Remove the infusion, replace it in an instrument trocar and wait until the choroidal detachment disappears • In case of ocular hypotony use 6 mm trauma trocars from Alcon
Iatrogenic tears	Dissection of adherent membranes
Prevention	Bimanual peeling
PFCL under retina	If the breaks that come in contact with PFCL are still under traction
Prevention	Remove traction before injecting PFCL
Treatment	1. Active suction with a 41-gauge cannula 2. Inject BSS in the macular area and displace PFCL inferiorly

Table 33.2 Early postoperative complications

Fibrin formation	(1) After synechiolysis; Use of iris retractors (2) After combined phaco/vitrectomy surgery
Treatment	(1) Steroid drops (2) tPA into the anterior chamber, 3 6 µg
Increased IOP	(1) Retained viscoelastica after combined surgery (2) Failure in preparing a proper gas concentration (3) Overfilling of silicone oil
Treatment	(1) Release of viscoelastica through existing side ports (2) Removal of some silicone oil (3) Antiglaucomatous drugs
Haemorrhages	• From the retinotomy edge • From ciliary processes behind the inf. Iridectomy
Prevention	Meticulous haemostasis of the retinotomy edge Inspection of the inferior iridectomy
Treatment	Removal of preretinal/intraocular blood
Air travel (**Fig. 33.3**)	Air and gas expand at a travel height of 10 km and a cabin pressure correlating to a height of 2 km
Prevention	Assess amount of gas before air travel. If 4 optic disc diameter fit between optic disc and air bubble then air travel is safe

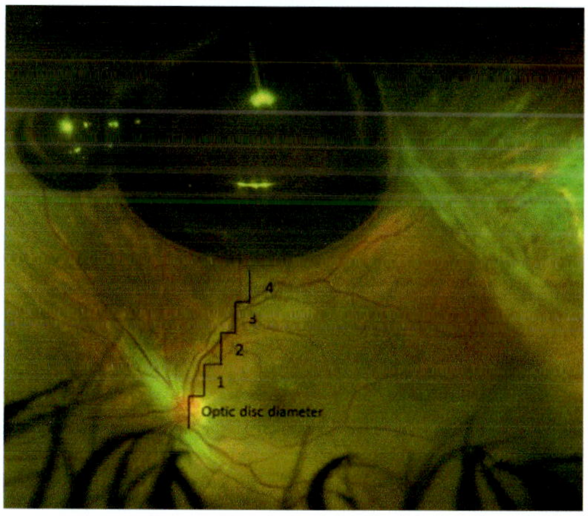

Fig. 33.3 Measure the distance from optic disc to the apex of the gas bubble. If the distance is >4 times opic disc diameter then air travel is safe

The complications are divided in **peroperative** (**Table 33.1**), **early postoperative** (**Table 33.2**) and **late postoperative complications** (**Table 33.3**).

Table 33.3 Late postoperative complications

Recurrent PVR	The most common cause for ultimate failure of the PVR surgery
Prevention	• Meticulous dissection of all membranes • Anti-inflammatory medication
Cataract	• Prolonged exposure to gas or silicone oil • Mechanical injury of the lens capsule • Lens capsule damage by infusion fluid
Prevention/treatment	Combined phaco/vitrectomy
Macular folds	Postoperative submacular fluid with gas tamponade and face down position
Prevention	(a) Avoid submacular fluid (b) Posterior drainage retinotomy (c) Avoid immediate face down position after surgery
Treatment	(a) Induction of retinal detachment through subretinal BSS injection (b) Reattachment with PFCL (c) Massage of macular folds
Video: Managing Dry Macular Folds after Vitreoretinal Surgery Dr. Mateo	
Subretinal Silicone Oil	If the breaks or retinotomy are still under traction
Prevention	Before injecting oil assess retinal traction by fluid x air exchange or attachment under PFCL
Treatment	1. Remove silicone oil and release traction by enlarging retinotomies or removal of membranes 2. Inject oil again after traction is relaxed
Inferior recurrent detachment	Cyclitic PVR membranes at the inferior pole cause an inferior recurrent detachment
Prevention	1. Remove PVR membranes 2. Avoid PVR through atraumatic surgery 3. Encircling band
Treatment	• Densiron 68 • Retinotomy • Inferior circumferential buckle
Iris rubeosis	Partially detached retina
Prevention	Prevent partially detached retina
Treatment	• Injection of anti-VEGF • Removal of detached retina
Hypotony under silicone oil	• Silicone oil presses vitreous against ciliary body resulting in fibrotic membranes and ciliary body insufficiency • Pars planitis • Large retinotomies
Prevention	• Meticulous vitreous base shaving
Treatment	• Removal of fibrotic membranes from ciliary body • Anti-inflammatory drugs
Iris bombé in silicone filled eye	Posterior synechiae
Prevention	…
Treatment	Basal iridectomy and removal of posterior synechiae
Video: Basal iridectomy	
Iris -IOL capture (Fig. 33.4)	• Gas tamponade presses the IOL forward, the IOL is located before the iris. Then anterior synechiae form between iris and anterior capsule. A pupillary block occurs
Prevention	• Not too large rhexis
Treatment	• Removal of anterior synechiae and reposition of IOL

(continued)

Table 33.3 (continued)

Recurrent PVR	The most common cause for ultimate failure of the PVR surgery
Video: Iris-IOL capture	
Ocular hypertension under silicone oil	• Secondary glaucoma even in underfill • Overfill of silicone oil
Prevention	Avoid overfill
Treatment	Silicone oil removal Aqueous shunt device (e.g. Ahmed valve)
Laser necrosis (Video) (Figs. 33.4, 33.5 and 33.6)	Occurs most commonly in the inferior pole and causes a retinal detachment
Prevention	Reduce laser power (until minimal white bleaching) and a laser duration = 200 ms
Treatment	PFCL + laser posterior to the necrosis + Densiron 68 (alternatively inferior buckle)
Video: Complication laser necrosis	

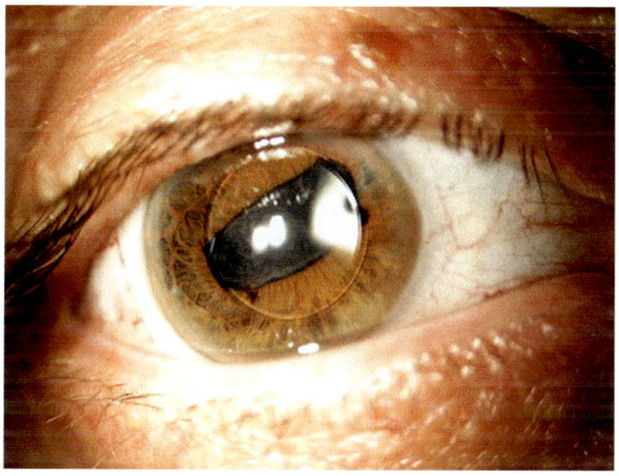

Fig. 33.4 Iris-IOL capture after vitrectomy with gas tamponade (see video)

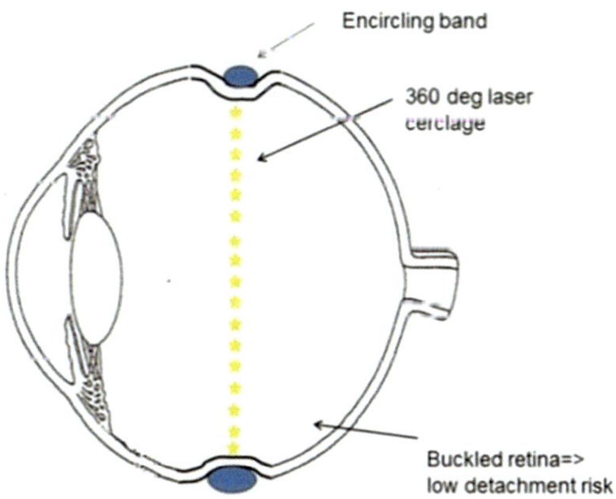

Fig. 33.5 360° laser cerclage is safe if an encircling band is present and the laser cerclage is performed on the impression of the encircling band. A retinal detachment due to lasernecrosis is unlikely (see video)

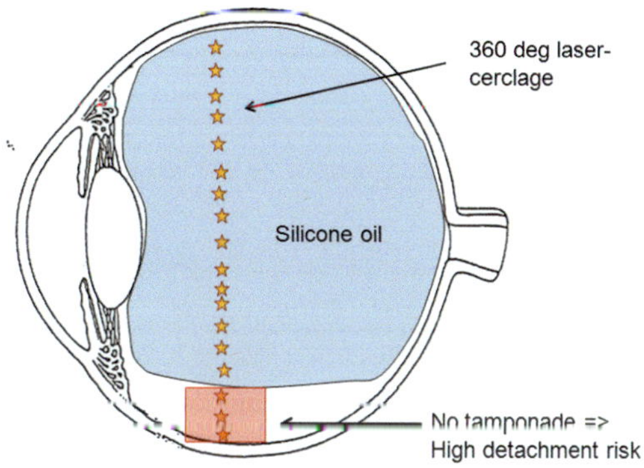

Fig. 33.6 360° laser cerclage is not safe if an encircling band is absent. A retinal detachment due to lasernecrosis is likely at the inferior pole

Postoperative Complications After Vitreoretinal Surgery

34

Zora Ignjatović

34.1 Changes of the Cornea

During vitrectomy itself, keratopathy can develop, especially if the operation is prolonged or the operated eye is already at an increased risk of corneal problems (dry eye, diabetes, etc.).

Epithelial edema can progress to such an extent that the haze requires corneal scraping to enable the surgeon to finish the intervention.

Smaller or larger corneal erosions (Figs. 34.1 and 34.2) might also occur during the postoperative period. These eyes must be carefully monitored because the effects of topical corticosteroids or other risk factors can impair the healing process, and also cause the ulceration (Fig. 34.3) with delayed scar formation (Figs. 34.4 and 34.5); finally, infection may also develop [4]. The patient can experience symptoms ranging from severe unpleasant itching to significant pain.

Therapeutically the best option is placing a therapeutic contact lens if there is no chemosis of the conjunctiva; which is not uncommon in the first days after the operation. Alternatively, the eye can be patched until epithelialization occurs.

It is recommended to reduce the administration of topical corticosteroid drops in the first few days and at the same time monitor and treat possible inflammations (caused by discontinuation of the usual therapy). If there is significant inflammation, sub-Tenon injection of Triamcinolone is recommended, avoiding dexamethasone drops.

Typically, epithelialization occurs in the first couple of days, but if the healing process is prolonged, artificial tears and corneal gels should be added to the treatment, the therapeutic contact lens reapplied, or a plug placed in the lacrimal canal (Fig. 34.4). If the results are still unsatisfactory, autologous serum (prepared by professionals using the patient's own blood) should be added in the form of eye drops; a temporary amniotic membrane may also be placed. In unresponsive cases photo-therapeutic keratectomy (PTK) can be performed.

The stromal edema of the cornea is usually transitory; it most often withdraws spontaneously after a few days or weeks, and during that time insight into the deeper parts of the eye is more difficult, so it is sometimes necessary to perform an ultrasound examination to determine the condition of the retina. If silicone oil or gas is placed in the vitreous body, ultrasonography is irrelevant.

Development of a 2–3 mm hyphema is not considered dangerous, but the occurrence of total hyphema following vitrectomy carries a discrete risk of corneal hemosiderosis (hematocornea). Since the risk is small unless the intraocular pressure (IOP) is also elevated, only monitoring

Z. Ignjatović (✉)
Director of Milos Clinic Eye Hospital, Belgrade, Serbia
e-mail: zora.ignjatovic@milosklinika.com

U. Spandau et al. (eds.), *Retinal Detachment Surgery and Proliferative Vitreoretinopathy*,
https://doi.org/10.1007/978-3-031-11946-0_34

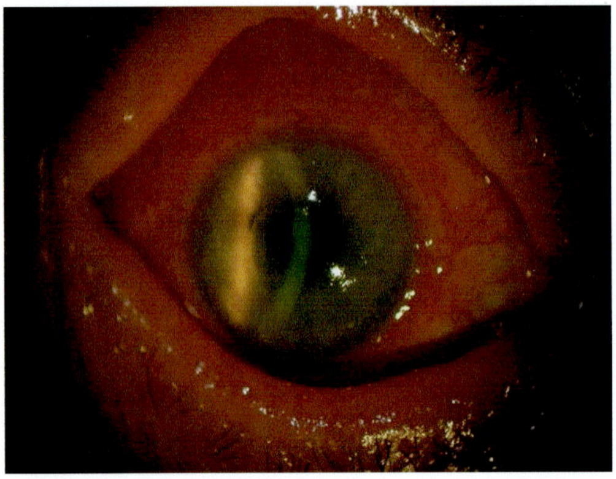

Fig. 34.1 Epithelial defect

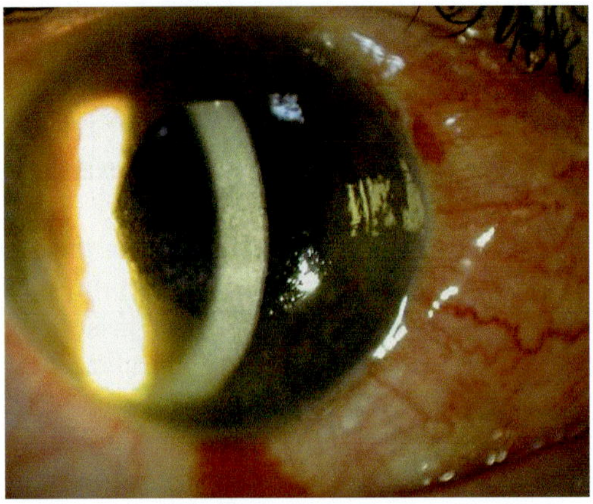

Fig. 34.2 Epitheliopathy

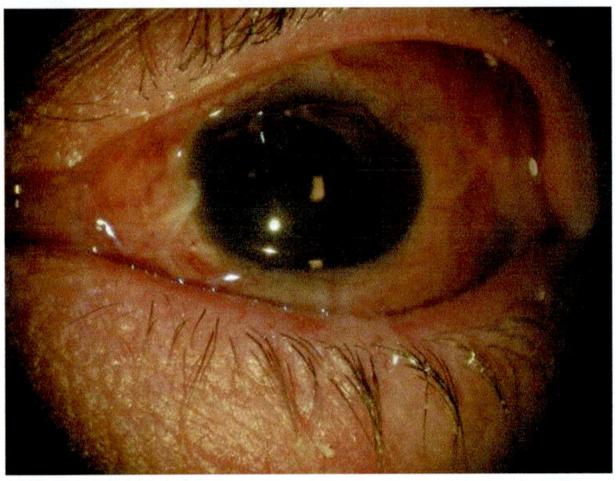

Fig. 34.3 Large erosion of the epithelium

is advised—the blood usually precipitates spontaneously. However, in cases of total hyphema with an IOP above ~30 mmHg the risk of hematocornea is very high, and it is necessary to irrigate the anterior chamber no later than 3–4 days. In the meantime aqueous (blood) can be released daily through a paracentesis and anti-glaucoma therapy applied.

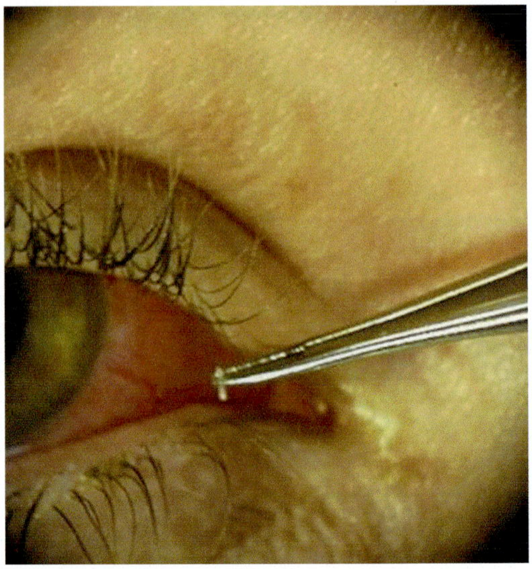

Fig. 34.4 Plug for the lacrimal canal

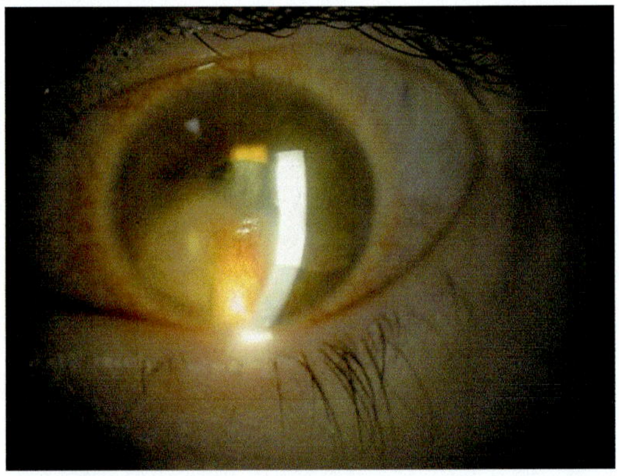

Fig. 34.5 Chronic keratopathy with scarring

There is also a risk of silicone oil keratopathy occurring if the silicone oil is in contact with the cornea for an extended period of time [17]. There is no exact time limit in terms of the duration of silicone oil-endothelium contact (an absolute risk for developing chronic keratopathy), but in most cases it is reversible in the first two months (even if corneas have been reported to recover after as long as six months). In general, the longer the period of contact between silicone and endothelium, the higher the risk. For an inexperienced ophthalmologist, it is sometimes not easy to determine the presence of silicone oil in the anterior chamber if it is completely filled with oil. It is most easily recognized by a shiny reflection from the iris surface.

Initially, the cornea remains completely transparent. After several months, however, band keratopathy develops as the first sign of trouble (Fig. 34.6). Every effort should be undertaken to allow removal of the silicone oil from the anterior chamber, before the endothelium is permanently damaged. Unfortunately, this is not always possible (the biggest problem occurs in eyes that do not produce enough aqueous humor such as following injuries or multiple surgeries).

As soon as the oil has been removed, the cornea that has long been in contact with silicone oil looks even worse: it becomes hydrated due to aqueous penetration into the stroma. If the endothelium is not permanently destroyed, this condition is transient and the resolution of keratopathy follows over the next few weeks. In cases of chronic keratopathy (Fig. 34.7) penetrating keratoplasty (Fig. 34.8) may become necessary. A small bubble of silicone in the anterior chamber (approximately up to one third of its volume) does not present a problem.

Very rarely, ischemic keratopathy can develop, caused by a very tight cerclage. It is occasionally combines with ischemia of the entire anterior segment, which represents a very serious condition with a poor prognosis.

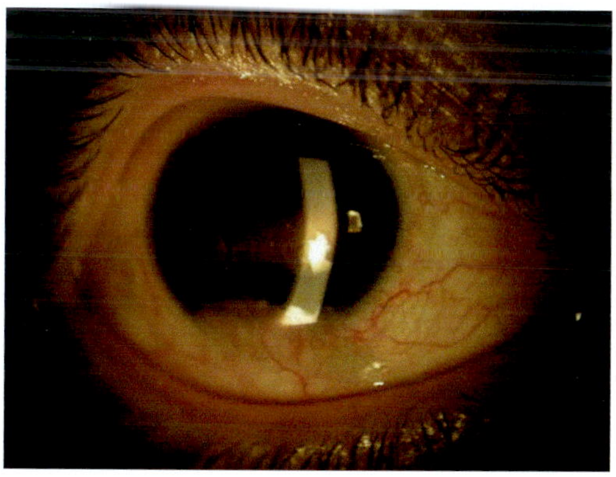

Fig. 34.6 “Band shaped” keratopathy

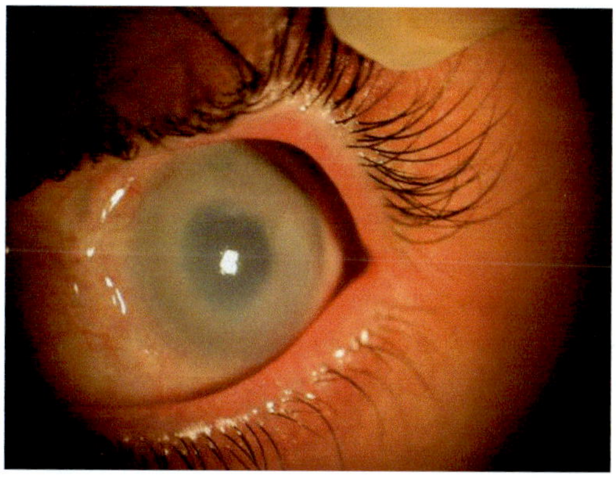

Fig. 34.7 Keratopathy due to contact with silicone oil

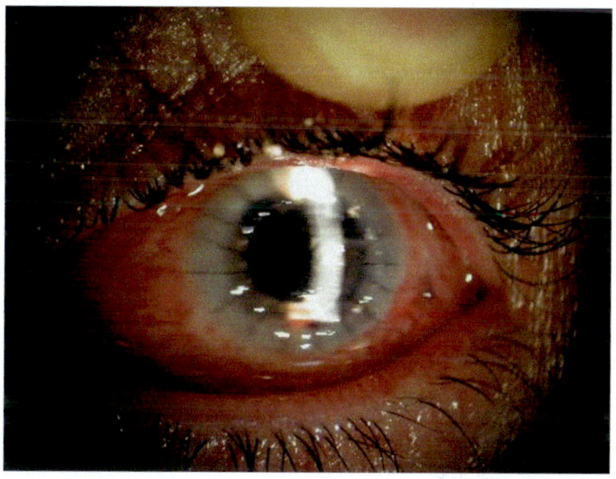

Fig. 34.8 Keratopathy due to contact with silicone oil, following penetrating keratoplasty

Finally, after multiple failed surgeries, various degenerative changes are possible, most frequently band keratopathy with calcium deposits, Salzmann degeneration or a definitive leukoma.

34.2 Complications Related to Surgical Wounds

In recent years oblique (tunnel) entries into the sclera have become the technique of choice in vitreoretinal (transconjunctival) surgery; due to the valve effect there is almost never the need to place sutures since at the end of the operation since the wound is usually well sealed after a light massage of the sclera at the incision site. If the surgeon finds that the tunnel incision leaks, a suture could be placed or diathermy used to coagulate the conjunctiva above the incision site. Sutures are particularly recommended for eyes after multiple surgeries where the sclera is very thin and damaged by many scleral scars, and also in eyes with silicone oil implantation. Use of a suture is also advised in pediatric patients where the rigidity of the sclera differs from that of adults, and in cases where the surgeon is keen to avoid potential postoperative hypotony [23].

Hypotony is the most common problem associated with surgical wounds in the postoperative period (usually after vitrectomy or removal of the silicone oil). If the eye is slightly hypotonic it should be patched, or viscoelastic can be injected through a paracentesis at the slit lamp, and the patient checked again the following day. In most patients, the IOP is restored during the following 24 h. However, in case of extreme hypotony complicated with choroidal detachment, a revision is advised, searching for the leakage site and placing a suture there. The leak may be in the cornea if intraoperatively a paracentesis has been made. Patients with a leak must be monitored the following day. The biggest risk in these eyes is an infection (endophthalmitis). Hypotony also increases the risk of hemorrhage [6].

The sutures themselves can cause itching, which can be mitigated with the use of ointments instead (or between) the usual eye drops, and the suture in the scleral tunnel incision can be removed in as short a period as one week. (Typically these sutures do not need to be removed because they degrade over time and fall out spontaneously.)

Very rarely a granuloma may form around the suture; the eye is inflamed and pretty sore so the suture should be removed as soon as possible. Another potential consequence of the suture is astigmatism, linked to the suture's tightness. Fortunately, it is almost always transitory and spontaneously resolves after several weeks.

At the incision site, immediately after the surgery and sometimes even after a longer interval, a subconjunctival bubble of gas and silicone oil can be observed. The gas will disappear by itself on the following day; the silicone oil can be easily released by incising the conjunctiva with a sharp needle (under the slit lamp) and a slight compression with a cotton-tip applicator. If this is not done, over a period of several weeks or months, encapsulation of drops of silicone oil below the conjunctiva can ensue, which makes the oil removal more difficult. Rarely, alongside a big bubble, a Dellen ulceration of the cornea can also be seen (Fig. 34.9).

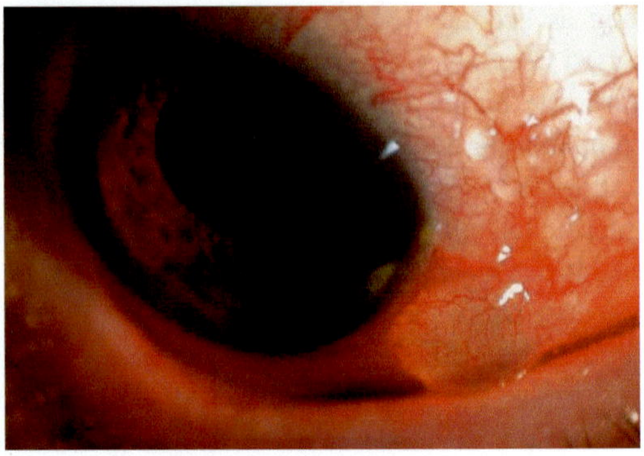

Fig. 34.9 Subconjunctival bubble, Dellen

Finally, the ophthalmologist should always keep in mind the risk of the development of a retinal tear at the sclerotomy site, caused by the incarceration of the vitreous; untreated, it may lead to a retinal detachment. The risk of this complication is dramatically reduced with the use of the tunnel incisions and trans-scleral cannulas, as opposed to the traditional 20 g surgery.

34.3 Hemorrhage

The intraocular hemorrhage occurring immediately after the surgery most commonly originates at the sclerotomy site (Fig. 34.10).

It usually develops at the time of cannula removal; sometimes it is already visible on the operating table but more often it is detected after the patch is removed on the first postoperative day. If it is not a large amount of blood, even if it is visible at the end of the surgery, its removal is not mandatory; whether to remove it or let it spontaneously reabsorb is at the surgeon's

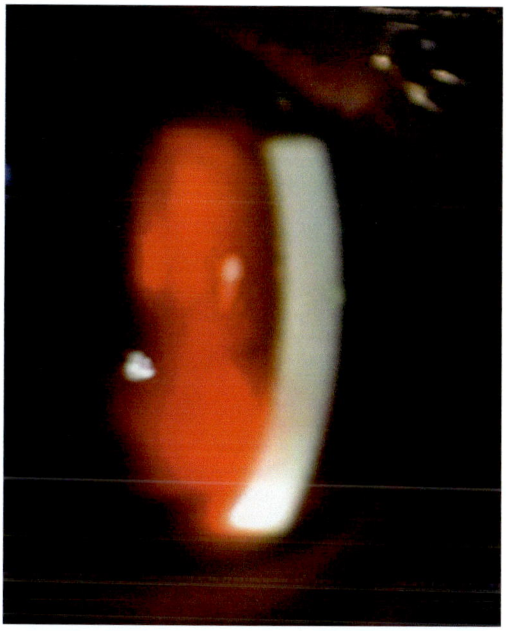

Fig. 34.10 Almost total hyphema on the first post-vitrectomy day

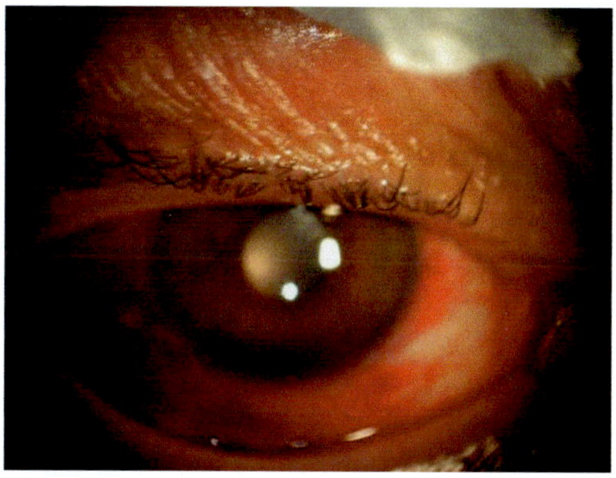

Fig. 34.11 Hyphema postoperatively

discretion. The appearance of the blood depends on the material left behind in the vitreous cavity. In fluid (BSS, aqueous), the blood is diffuse; in air/gas it typically blood that floats on the surface; in silicone oil it is usually in front or more rarely behind oil (between it and the retina as a preretinal coagulum). The blood from a sclerotomy can sometimes appear in the anterior chamber as well (some surgeons believe that this complication can be avoided with diathermy at the sclerotomy site at the end of the surgery).

Postoperative hemorrhage can also occur, usually during the night, into the fluid in the vitreous cavity or between the gas/silicone oil bubble and the retina. This bleeding originates from the retinal blood vessels themselves. The cause of this bleeding is postoperative hypotony or the elevation of the systemic blood pressure. This blood becomes visible at the first follow-up just after the patch is removed (Fig. 34.11). Even if lower, the risk is still present in the following days, especially in patients on anticoagulants.

A postoperative hemorrhage is usually an unpleasant surprise, and its treatment depends on multiple factors [14]. Smaller hemorrhages, still allowing visualization of the retina, are monitored only, and the patient should be informed that the resolution is expected in the following 2–3 weeks. Even if it is a coagulum over the posterior pole and even if it is behind the silicone oil, a hemorrhage that is not very large usually spontaneously dissolves in about 3 weeks. Their interference with the patient's vision is greater in monocular patients since they will be incapacitated during that time; therefore, in such cases the surgeon has to decide whether to intervene rather than wait for the spontaneous resolution. If reoperation for blood removal is chosen, it is still recommended to wait for at least 5–7 days for partial hemolysis because removing the fresh coagulum, which is very adherent to the retina carries a risk of causing even more serious complications, e.g., tearing the central retina.

In case of total hemophthalmos or hyphema, it is also acceptable to wait for spontaneous reabsorption for a couple of weeks, as long as regular echography checkups are performed and the IOP is not high (see earlier). A reoperation ("wash out" vitrectomy) might still be needed eventually if the blood does not start to disappear.

34.4 Inflammation

In the last decade the advancements in technology and surgical techniques have made vitreoretinal surgery much less traumatic to the eye. The concept of transconjunctival surgery with the introduction of valvulated cannulas prevents the sudden IOP drops during the surgery; the reduction of incision size to 23G, 25G, 27G helps avoiding the need for sutures almost entirely; the efficient vitrectomy machines and improved surgical techniques reduce the length of surgery and minimize tissue trauma etc. have led to fewer complications postoperatively as well as to increased convenience to the patients: less irritation, no pain or red eye.

The face-down position often leads to the accumulation of precipitates in the lower half of the cornea ("positional keratopathy") (Fig. 34.12); even (small amounts of) fibrin can occur and the eyelids may become swollen.

However, in eyes undergoing a reoperation for retinal detachment with PVR, PDR, ROP retinal detachment, or other pediatric retinal detachment, the surgery can still be a difficult, complicated, lengthy, and demanding undertaking, with a variety of inflammatory responses in the postoperative course (Fig. 34.13). Heavy oil tamponade can also often causes inflammatory response (Fig. 34.14).

Sometimes the inflammatory response is already visible on the first postoperative day but it may also take a couple of days to fully develop. Usually this is characterized by serous exudates or a limited fibrinous reaction, or, very rarely, a large amount of fibrin resembling a cake or in the form of a hypopyon can be observed.

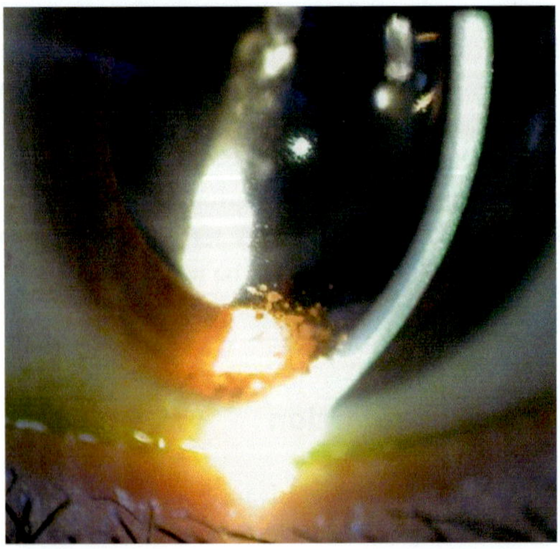

Fig. 34.12 Precipitates due to positioning

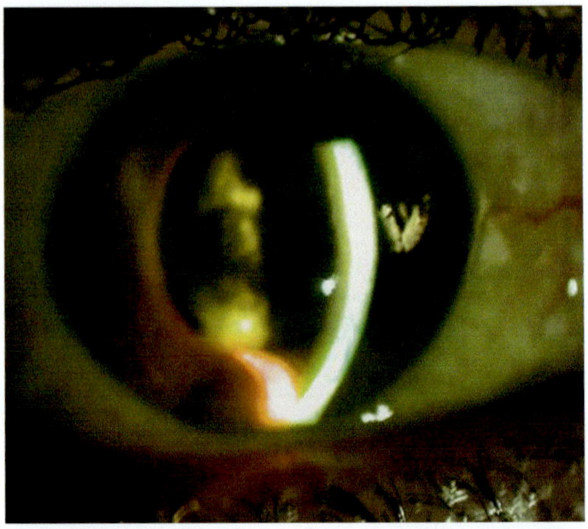

Fig. 34.13 Fibrin in the anterior chamber

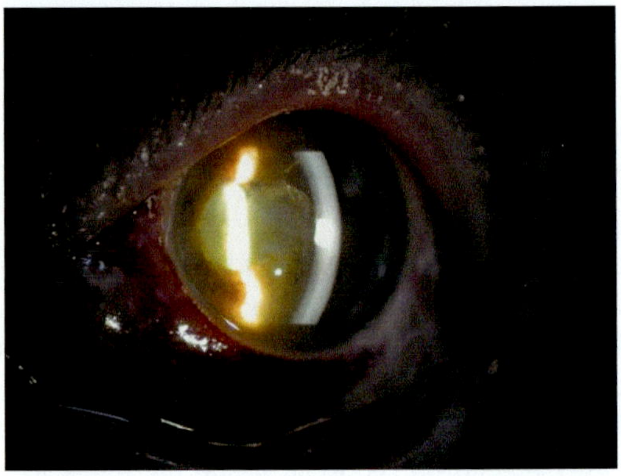

Fig. 34.14 Fibrin after vitrectomy (heavy oil)

Like after any other surgery, the most important thing is to differentiate between a sterile inflammatory response and an infectious inflammatory response (Fig. 34.15).

The rate of endophthalmitis after vitrectomy varies in the literature reports from 0.03 to 2.17% [6]. After vitrectomy, hypotony is very conducive to an infection, so these cases deserve special focus. Pain, swollen eyelids, chemosis of the conjunctiva and the presence of hypopyon are suggestive of an infection, especially in eyes undergoing combined surgery (vitrectomy plus cataract surgery). Sometimes the first signs of an infection are more easily noticed in the vitreous

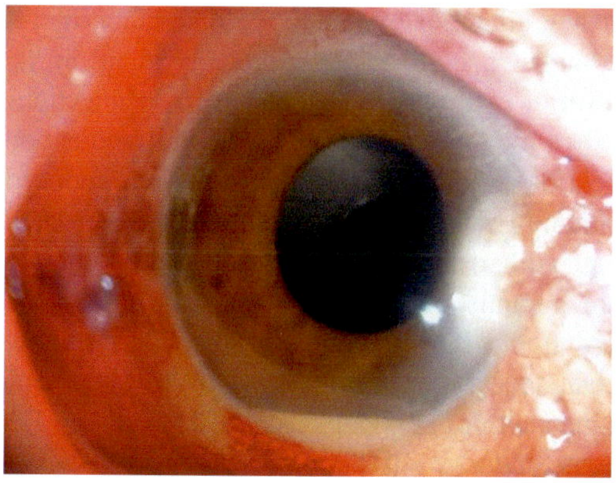

Fig. 34.15 Endophthalmitis after vitrectomy

cavity, where a fibrin thread or abscess can be found. It is necessary to take a sample for culture from the vitreous cavity and then either intravitreally administer the antibiotics, or, if the inflammation is more severe, immediately proceed to re-vitrectomy [8]. The surgery is completed with the intravitreal injection of antibiotics (vancomycin plus ceftazidime). Most commonly, dexamethasone or triamcinolone are also used, intravitreally or subconjunctivally. There is usually no need for systemic antibiotics. If all of this is done in a timely fashion (preferably on the same day that the diagnosis is made) the prognosis is typically very good.

If a sterile inflammation is diagnosed, treatment with cortisone, subconjunctivally or systemically at the dose of 1 mg of prednisolone per 1 kg of body weight (avoid systemic administration in cases of diabetics because of the risk of elevating the blood sugar) is advised. An antibiotic, most commonly vancomycin, can also be injected subconjunctivally if an infection is not definitely ruled out.

Applying TPA (tissue plasminogen activator) in the vitreous space or the anterior chamber to achieve fibrinolysis results in very quick (in just half an hour) resolution of the fibrin, but can also cause profuse bleeding, so it is relatively rare to be employed. Also, in case of masked endophthalmitis, TPA leads to drastic worsening of the infection.

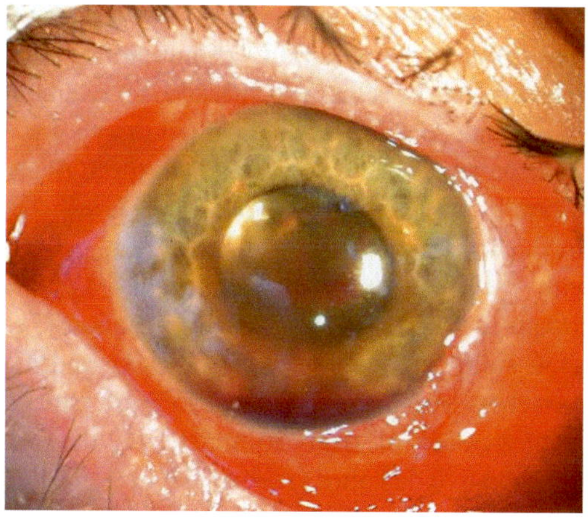

Fig. 34.16 Fibrin and blood on the first postoperative day

Sometimes blood, fibrin, or circulating erythrocytes imitate serous exudates if minor hemorrhage was present postoperatively (Fig. 34.16).

Hourly dexamethasone is prescribed, cortisone ointment before bedtime, mydriatics 2–3 times a day, and antibiotic drops regularly.

These patients should be closely monitored, as often as a few hours apart on the same day. The improvement is usually seen in just a day or two.

34.5 Secondary Glaucoma

This very serious and relatively frequent complication occurring after vitreoretinal surgery is sometimes a real enigma in terms of etiology and treatment, especially for ophthalmologists with less experience in the field of posterior segment surgery. It is very important to determine the exact etiology of the glaucoma and base the treatment on the cause. If the IOP elevation is unrecognized and untreated, the eyes may end up blind despite the anatomical success of the vitreoretinal surgery [1].

Glaucoma found in eyes with a silicone oil tamponade, where it is often thought that the silicone oil is the cause of such glaucoma even though it is usually not true, is especially intriguing.

The ophthalmologist should also take into consideration the possibility of an earlier, undiagnosed glaucoma that was masked, for example, by a retinal detachment that had led to hypotony; once the retina has been reattached, the IOP can return to its preoperative, elevated level. The prevalence of open angle glaucoma in patients with rhegmatogenous detachment is 4–5.8%, compared to 1–3.3% in general population [7].

A study carried out by Anderson and his coworkers showed that about 15% of patients have pressure of over 30 mmHg on the first postoperative day after vitreoretinal surgeries [2].

Statistics and clinical practice show that the most common type of secondary glaucoma after vitreoretinal surgery is cortisone glaucoma. It can develop after several days or up to several weeks following the operation, e.g., after the postoperative treatment with Dexamethasone eye drops was initiated.

It most commonly occurs in myopic patients after retinal detachment surgery, and more often in patients with a history of glaucoma [10]. The clinical picture is characterized by an initially moderate IOP spike, but if Dexamethasone is not withdrawn, very high values of IOP can be reached after just several days: severe pain, and pronounced hyperemia, which sometimes precedes the IOP spike by a day or two. It is believed that a diffuse swelling of the trabeculum causes the IOP spike so that drainage through the trabecular meshwork is made very difficult or completely impossible. This process is usually reversible, and immediate intervention, i.e. discontinuation of Dexamethasone and introduction of topical antiglaucoma medication, results in prompt pressure stabilization. Continuation of cortisone administration can result in permanent secondary glaucoma that is very difficult to treat.

If the anti-inflammatory treatment is still needed, in most patients it is enough to switch to Prednisolone or Fluorometholone, or NSAID drops, in order for the IOP to normalize. Although sometimes, especially after repeated surgeries or with a history of cortisone glaucoma episodes, this is not possible and we can only administer nonsteroidal anti-inflammatory drugs locally. If a patient with cortisone glaucoma has a strong inflammatory response, it is much safer to administer cortisone systemically than in the form of eye drops or subconjunctival injections. When it comes to local antiglaucoma medication, beta blockers and alpha agonists are introduced, although some patients respond well to prostaglandin drugs. Carbonic anhydrase inhibitors are administered both systemically and locally and if the IOP value is very high, as soon as glaucoma occurs, it is best to release some aqueous through a paracentesis. This can also be done under a slit lamp, following a judicious rinse of the conjunctival sac with povidone iodine; an already existing paracentesis can be utilized with a regular 25 g needle (Fig. 34.17). The tip of the needle is advanced into the anterior chamber; gentle pressure on the lower lip of the paracentesis will release the required amount of aqueous humor. If there is no paracentesis present, one can easily be created with any a 23 g or 20 g knife.

Usually, after just a few days the IOP begins to normalize and the antiglaucomatous treatment can be gradually withdrawn and in most cases stopped completely (note that both eyes should be monitored in the future because of the risk of open angle glaucoma [POAG], to which these patients are more susceptible).

If glaucoma surgery is needed in a vitrectomized eye, the most common procedures include cyclodestructive ones, although filtration surgeries are also frequently employed. Shunts, especially the Ahmed valve (Fig. 34.18), are

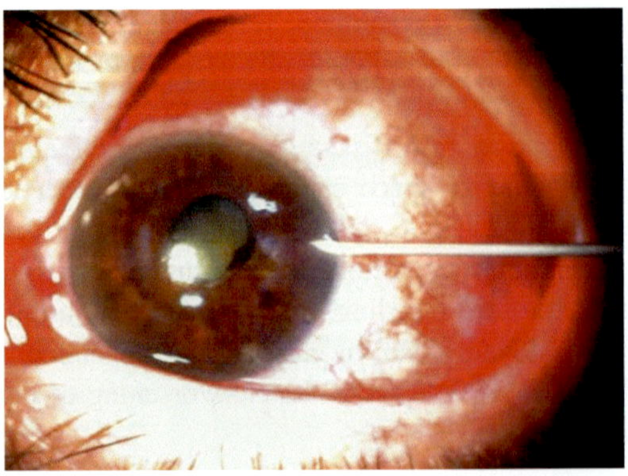

Fig. 34.17 Releasing of aqueous humor from CA

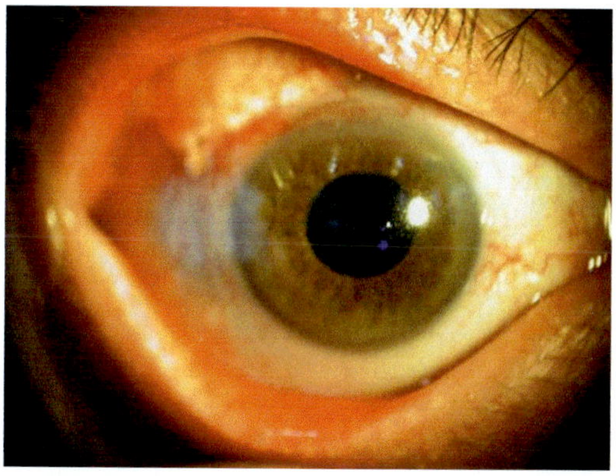

Fig. 34.18 Ahmed valve

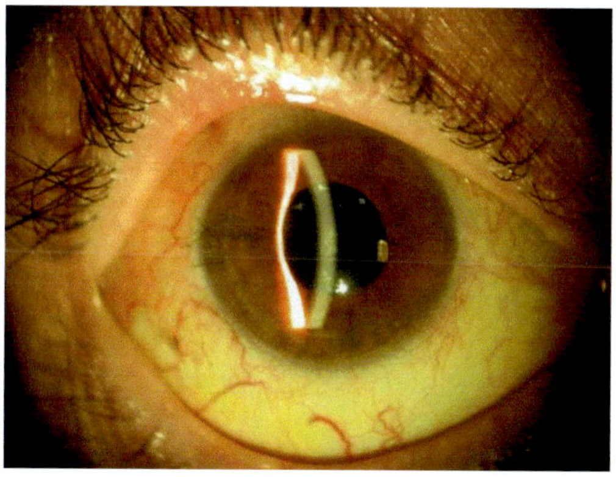

Fig. 34.20 Iris bombe

usually safer options than trabeculectomy [12]. Vitrectomized eyes are more prone to hypotony and development of choroidal detachment than nonvitrectomized eyes; if trabeculectomy is performed, for example, it is advisable to leave a bubble of about 0.5 ml of pure SF_6 gas at the end of the surgery.

Glaucoma caused by a pupillary block (Figs. 34.19 and 34.21) occurs acutely, the IOP is very high, the iris is bulging (iris bombe) (Fig. 34.20) and the eye is painful [13, 25]. In case of pupillary block glaucoma two situations can occur: iris can stick either to anterior capsule or a tiny membrane. Since the cause of synechiae formation is always some inflammation we can presume that there must be some membrane covering either pupillary edge like a ring only or

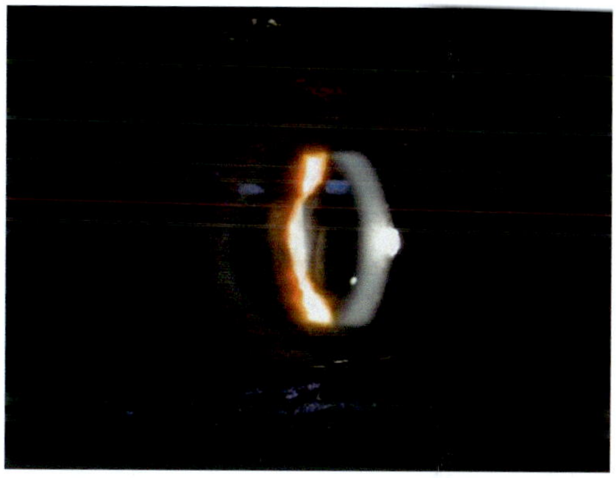

Fig. 34.21 Pupil block

the entire posterior surface of the iris. The patient should immediately undergo Nd:YAG-laser iridotomy, which usually normalizes the IOP immediately (Fig. 34.22). It is advisable to make a somewhat larger opening in the iris than usual, and in two to three places, because these iridotomies have a tendency to close fast, especially in eyes with a silicone oil tamponade. In case of a silicone tamponade, the location of the iridotomy should be chosen according to the oil's molecular weight, to allow the necessary aqueous circulation: for regular oil at the 6 o'clock position and for heavy oil at the 12 o'clock position.

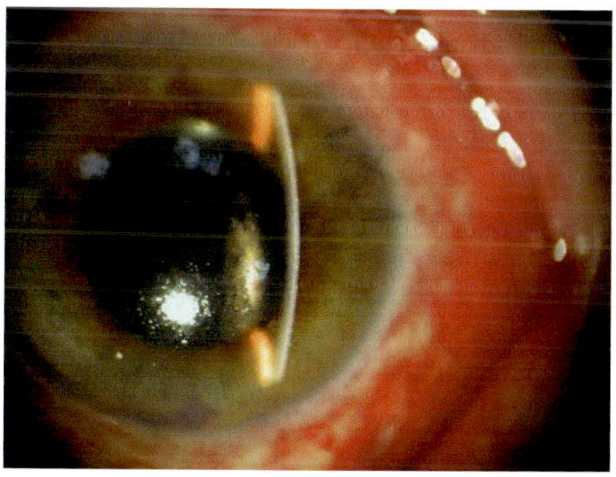

Fig. 34.19 Pupil block glaucoma

Pupillary block can also occur as a consequence of silicone oil protruding into the anterior chamber and its bubble getting stuck in the pupillary area. In such cases the oil should be drained or possibly pushed back.

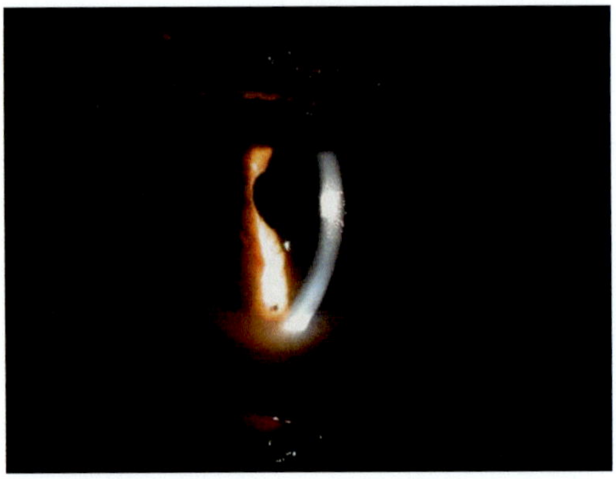

Fig. 34.22 After a Nd YAG laser iridotomy

If the iridotomy is not performed on time, goniosynechiae will develop and chronic angle-closure glaucoma can ensue. If the laser iridotomy is repeatedly closed by newly-formed fibrin, it is necessary to perform a surgical iridotomy.

Ghost-cell glaucoma (Fig. 34.23) occurs as a consequence of denaturalized erythrocytes seeping into the anterior chamber from the vitreous cavity. These erythrocytes have lost their elasticity, and have great difficulty exiting the eye through the trabecular meshwork, clogging it up and causing a spike in the IOP. A yellowish, sanguinolent liquid is typically found in the anterior chamber. The condition can be cured with medications and rinsing of the anterior chamber (or the vitreous cavity itself). Sometimes it is necessary to rinse the chamber multiple times because the erythrocytes often stick to the backside of the iris, making their definite removal difficult [14].

Glaucoma caused by emulsification of the silicone oil occurs after the oil has stayed in the eye for a certain period of time; this period can vary extensively, from 2–3 months to several years [11]. Emulsification is considered a consequence of "shaking", which is mixing the oil with water. The vitreous cavity can never be completely filled with silicone so initially the (normal weight) oil bubble actually floats on the water surface, and then these two substances start to mix. If the tamponade is not complete, the meniscus of the water is larger so there is more mixing and the emulsification occurs faster. However, that is not the only risk factor; sometimes we cannot explain why in some eyes the oil emulsification occurs faster, while in other patients significant emulsification occurs only after several months or years; purity of the oil certainly plays a role.

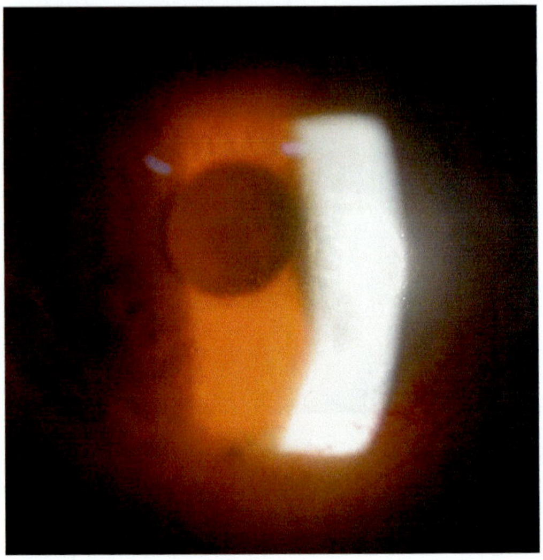

Fig. 34.23 Ghost cell glaucoma

The emulsified oil droplets are tiny and move easily into the anterior chamber where, initially, they accumulate in the upper half of the chamber angle (where they can be found by gonioscopy); later they can be seen floating in the aqueous humor ("magnified Tyndall phenomenon"). As time goes by, they increase in number more and more and take up the upper part of the anterior chamber (so called "inverse hypopyon") (Fig. 34.24) [11, 24]. The diagnosis is established when we find emulsified drops in the aqueous humor and the chamber angle. Such a glaucoma can, at the onset, be treated with topical antiglaucoma medication for a short time, until evacuation or silicone oil exchange is performed. Recurrence is possible even after the oil has been removed as the remaining drops keep emulsifying, breaking apart, and entering the anterior chamber; repeated anterior chamber irrigations may be necessary.

Glaucoma caused by too large of an oil tamponade—"overfill" glaucoma—is encountered

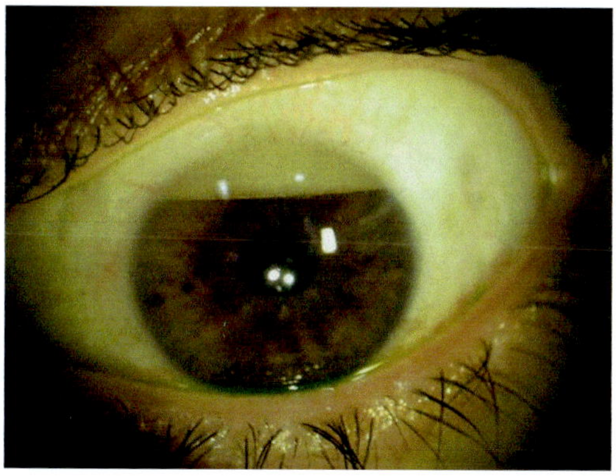

Fig. 34.24 Emulsified oil, inverse hypopyon

very rarely because the surgeon, at the end of the surgery, must check the IOP. Conversely, tamponade-related IOP elevation is not uncommon in cases of implanting an inappropriate mixture of gas. The gas expands and leads to a sudden spike in IOP [3]. The condition can be treated with medications, but sometimes the gas must be released from the vitreous space (the simplest way is by placing a cannula with no valves or by completely replacing the gas.) If the sclerotomies are not sutured properly, an expulsion of a small amount of oil or gas under the conjunctiva can easily occur when external pressure is exerted on the eye.

Sometimes glaucoma in the vitrectomized eye cannot be placed into any of these categories so we can consider that it is of unknown etiology. These cases should best be treated with antiglaucoma medication (usually, just in case, we also stop using cortisone, as it is the most common cause of glaucoma). Close monitoring is recommended because after a while the true etiology of the glaucoma becomes obvious.

In case the IOP cannot be controlled medically and it persists, surgical treatment is needed. Glaucoma surgery in a vitrectomized eye has its peculiarities and, not surprisingly, a higher risk of early and late postoperative complications [5]. Filtration surgeries can be associated with hyperfiltration and choroidal detachment—this is why, at the conclusion of the trabeculectomy, we often leave an air or pure gas bubble in the vitreous cavity. In patients with already scarred conjunctiva, or following cyclodestructive procedures, a shunt such as the Ahmed or Molteno valve is the surgeons' best choice [12]. Cyclocryo-coagulation is still a useful option in recalcitrant cases, as are transscleral laser cyclophotocoagulation and repeat vitrectomy with silicone oil removal, combined with endo-cyclophotocoagulation (using the standard endolaser probe).

34.6 More Complications Related to Silicone Oil Tamponade

The silicone oil is very conducive to the development of cataract, so much so that even after just a few months it is rare that the crystalline lens is completely clear. In the presence of cataract, viewing of the retina obviously difficult or impossible and ultrasound examination is of no use, since the resulting echo of the silicone oil is seen as an elongated globe [21, 26].

The silicone oil also causes a strong fibrosis of the posterior lens capsule. Therefore, in eyes undergoing silicone oil tamponade either a primary posterior capsulotomy should be performed during the initial surgery, or a Nd:YAG laser posterior capsulotomy done at a later date (after silicone oil removal—the disadvantage here is the interference of the capsule with visualization until the capsulotomy takes place: laser application on the posterior capsule is not possible in the presence of oil in the vitreous cavity.

Heavy oil is also susceptible to emulsification (Figs. 34.25 and 34.26), similarly to 1000 and 1300 oils, and compared to these oils it carries a somewhat higher risk of inflammatory response [19].

The presence of silicone oil in the anterior chamber (Fig. 34.27) also risks the development of keratopathy (Fig. 34.28).

The oil can also be partially released from the anterior chamber under the slit lamp through a paracentesis at the 12 o'clock position (with the patient looking down). If that does not work and the patient is brought to the operating room where he/she lays on the table, the oil tends to always keep coming from the back (because it

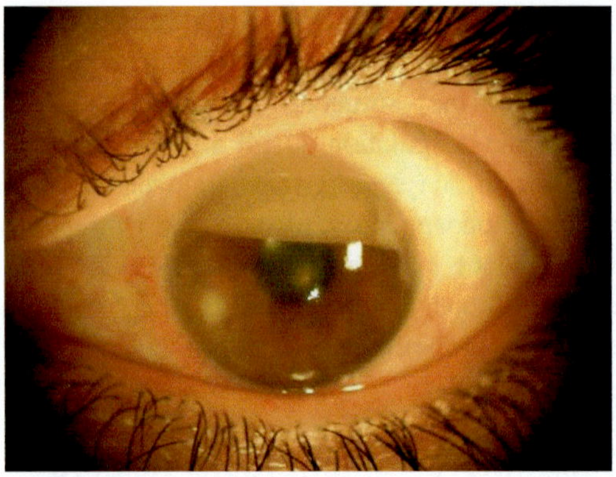

Fig. 34.25 Extreme emulsification

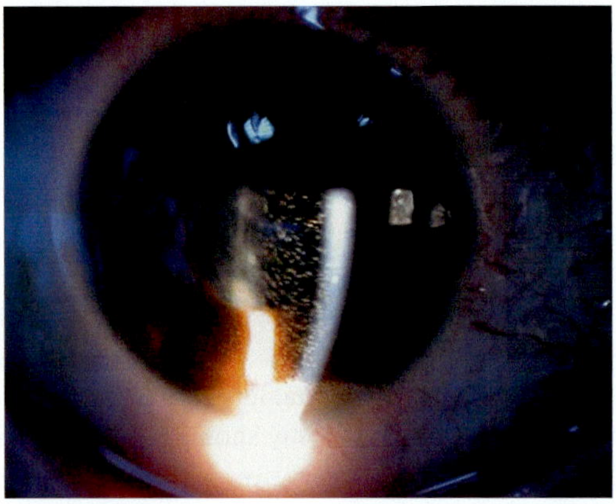

Fig. 34.26 Emulsified heavy oil (Oxane HD)

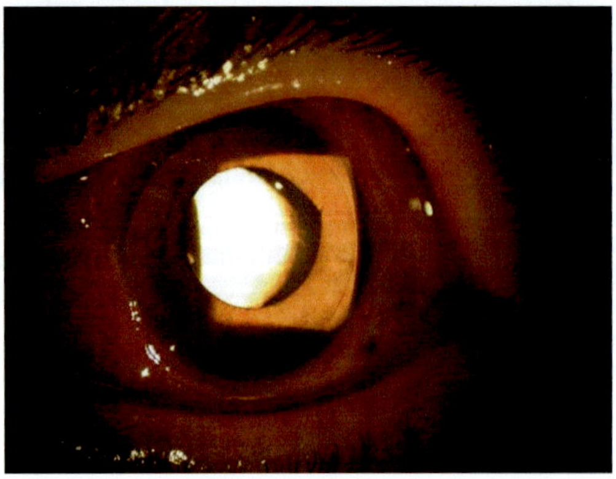

Fig. 34.27 AC filled with oil

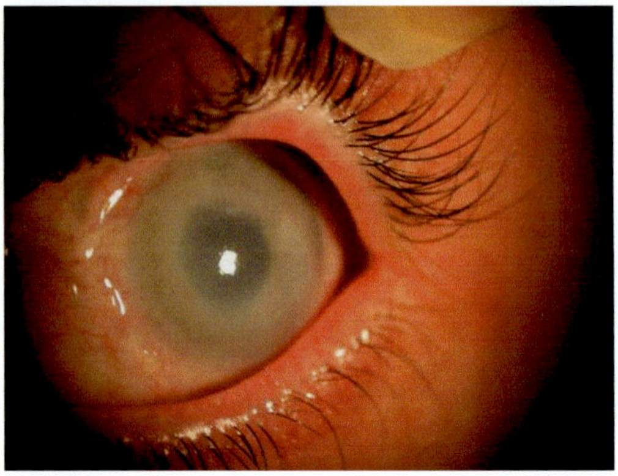

Fig. 34.28 Keratopathy, Silicone

"finds the way", either somewhere between the zonules or near the larger defects of the posterior capsule in pseudophakic eyes), and therefore the anterior chamber usually needs to be filled with viscoelastic to prevent, at least temporarily, the reappearance of the oil.

In eyes in which the oil tends to prolapse into the anterior chamber it is advised not to dilate the pupil, at least in the first couple of days, as that the iridolenticular barrier may keep the silicone in the vitreous humor. This warning should be mentioned in the discharge summary to the ophthalmologist into whose care the patient is released for follow-ups. In case of total aniridia or lack of iris in the lower half, the contact between silicone oil and the cornea is often inevitable in aphakic eyes (Fig. 34.30), especially if the eyes in question are hypotonic with low production of aqueous humor. If the oil cannot be removed, chronic keratopathy occurs, along with band shaped deposits; there is also a risk of thinning and even perforation (Fig. 34.29) over the long term.

A pupillary block is a rare but possible complication (Fig. 34.31) caused by a bubble of oil that got stuck in the pupillary area, while moving into the anterior chamber. In that case, the oil should be released or removed immediately, because the patient has all symptoms of acute glaucoma.

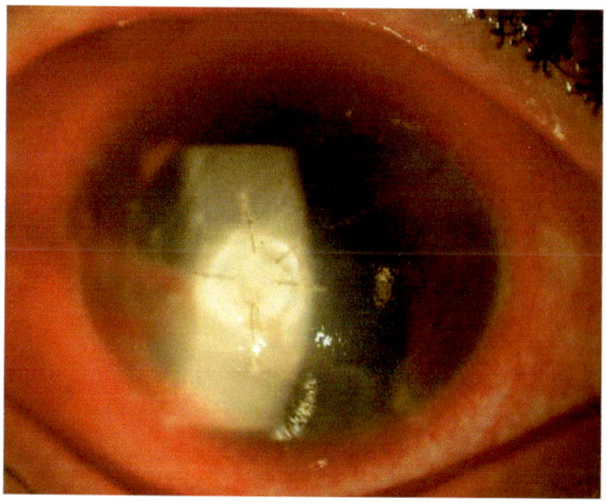

Fig. 34.29 Mini graft at the perforation site

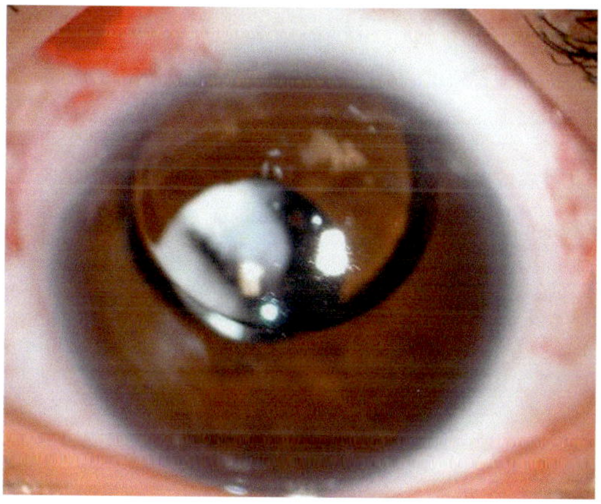

Fig. 34.30 Large silicone drop in AC, posterior capsule defect

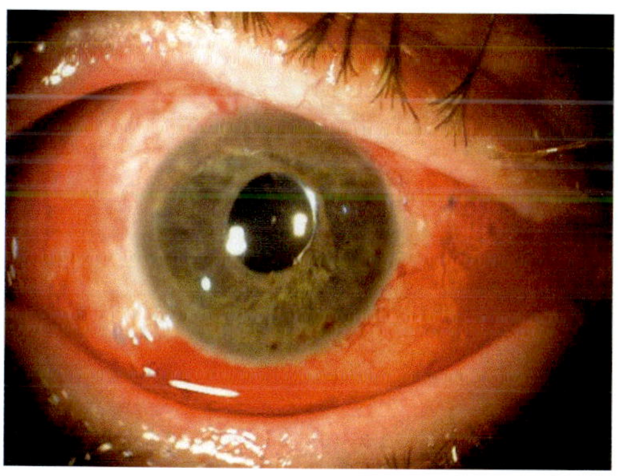

Fig. 34.31 Silicon oil causing pupillary block

Silicone oil is generally translucent, and patients can see through it immediately after the surgery, but it also changes the eye's refractive power, usually requiring and extra ~+5D lens for correction. If the patient has monocular vision, he/she should be given prescription eyeglasses as soon as possible. In patients whose other eye is emmetropic or myopic, this refractive anomaly may be unacceptable and should be corrected with a contact lens, either on the eye operated or on the other one, depending on the situation. In eyes undergoing combined cataract and vitrectomy surgery, the IOL calculation is most often made for the condition after the oil has been removed, which means that a temporary anisometropia is inevitable.

34.7 Residual Perfluorocarbon

If residual perfluorocarbon is present in small amounts in the vitreous cavity, it is not a major problem, but if it is present in the anterior chamber or under the macula, it must be removed because of the associated toxicity [18]. It can be recognized postoperatively because unlike a bubble of air, gas or silicone oil, it can always be found at the bottom of the vitreous cavity or the anterior chamber (Fig. 34.32).

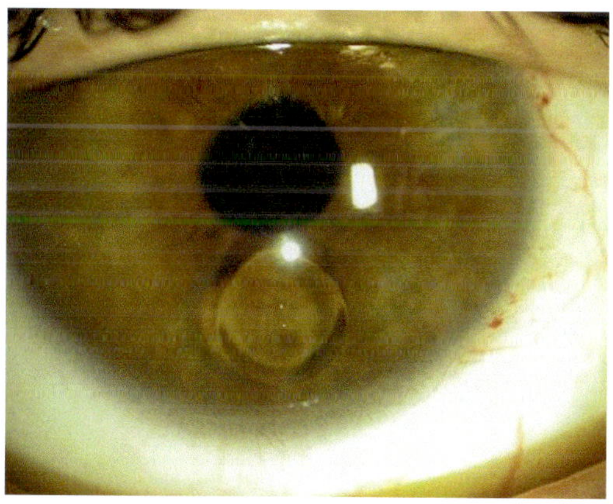

Fig. 34.32 Perfuorocarbon in AC

34.8 Buckling Procedure Complications

Following an encircling band ("cerclage"), the most serious complication is anterior segment ischemia, caused by a too tight band blocking blood flow in the posterior ciliary arteries. The conditions is characterized by severe keratopathy, uveitis, glaucoma and even loss of the eye, if the cerclage is not loosened (cut).

Cerclage (in case it is set in front of the equator) can also apply pressure on the vortex veins, compromising venous drainage, which may lead to the enlargement and forward rotation of the ciliary body, and glaucoma [20].

Glaucoma can also occur via narrowing the angle; the suppression of the iridolenticular diaphragm, caused by a buckle that is too anterior; or shallow detachment of the ciliary body, which may also move forward and close the angle (typically between the second and the seventh postoperative day). In these cases, cycloplegics and cortisone should be locally administered, because miotics can cause further movement of the iridolenticular diaphragm forward and cause the glaucoma to worsen [9]. As a last resort, the buckle should be removed (Figs. 34.33, 34.34 and 34.35).

Deeply embedded radial buckles can deform the eyeball, cause a feeling of localized pressure on the eye, as well as pain; it can with time, erode the sclera (Fig. 34.36) and even result in the

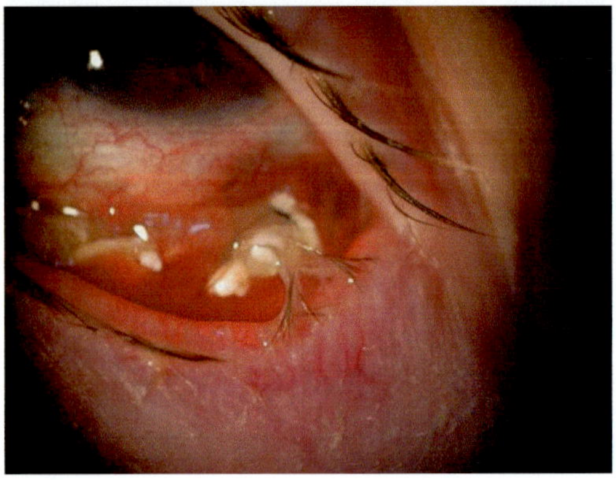

Fig. 34.33 Protrusion of the buckle

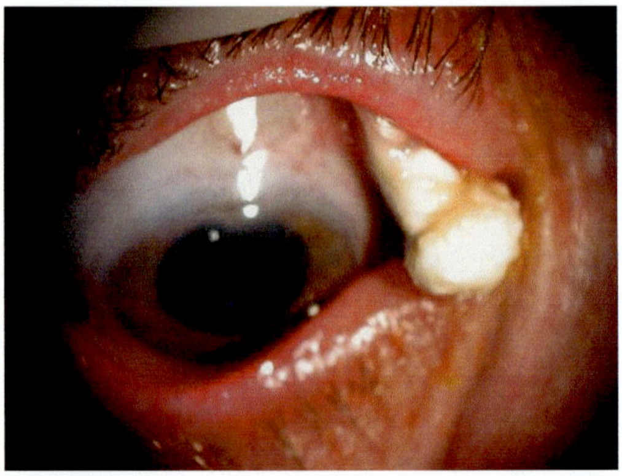

Fig. 34.34 Buckle protrusion

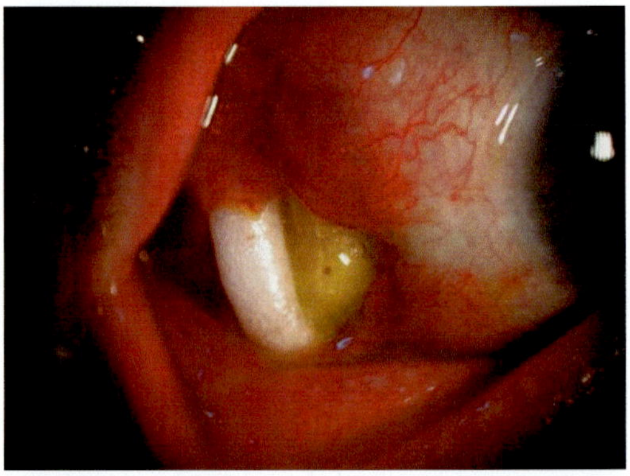

Fig. 34.35 Buckle protrusion with infection

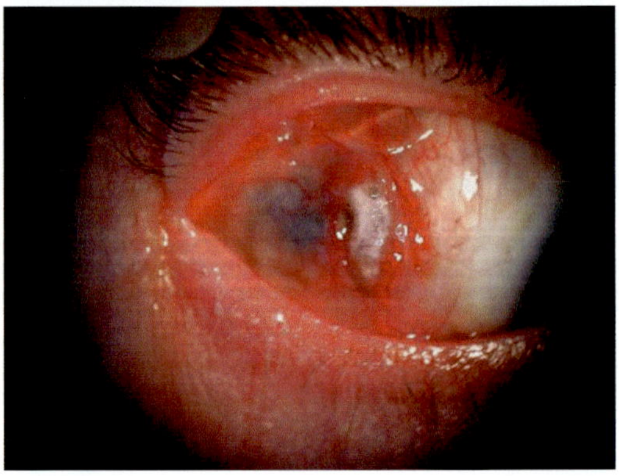

Fig. 34.36 Buckle protrusion with scleral necrosis

buckle being inside the vitreous cavity. If the buckle is underneath an extraocular muscle, diplopia is a common occurrence. These phenomena can spontaneously disappear over time.

Excessive cryocoagulation is one of the risk factors for the development of PVR, and it also leads to significant pain and swollen eyelids.

A buckle can be displaced immediately after the surgery (Fig. 34.33), in which case it loses its purpose to achieve retinal reattachment. Subsequently, even as late as after several years, buckle protrusion (Fig. 34.34) may occur, complicated with the conjunctival erosion, and an infection (Fig. 34.35). Such a buckle must be removed or, at least, shortened. After irrigating the subconjunctival space with antibiotics, the conjunctiva also needs to be sutured once its edge has been refreshened.

References

1. Abrams TM, Van Horn D. Late complications of pars plana vitreous surgery. Ohthalmology. 1978;85:126–40.
2. Anderson NG, Finemand MS, Brown GC. Incidence of intraocular pressure spike and other adverse events after vitreoretinal surgery. Ophthalmology. 2006;113:42–7.
3. Benz MS, Escalona Benz EM, Murray TG, et al. Immediate postoperative use of a topical agent to prevent intraocular pressure elevation after pars plana vitrectomy with gas tamponade. Arch Ophthalmol. 2004;122:705–9.
4. Brightbill, Myers FL, Bresnick GH. Postvitrectomy keratopathy. Am J Ophthalmol. 1978;85(5):651–5
5. Budenz DI, Taba KE, FeuerWJ, et al. Surgical management of secondary glaucoma after pars plana vitrectomy and silicon oil injection for complex retinal detachment. Ophthalmology. 2001;108:1623–32
6. Chen JK, Khurana RN, Do DV. The incidence of edophthalmitis following transconjunctival sutureless 25- vs 20-gauge vitrectomy. Eye. 2009;23:780–4.
7. Desai UR, Alhalell AA, Schiffman RM, et al. Intraocular pressure elevation after simple pars plana vitrectomy. Ophthalmology. 1997;104:781–5.
8. Eifrig CW, Scott IU, Flynn HW. Endophthalmitis after pars plana vitrectomy: incidence, causative organisms and visual outcomes. Am J Ophthalmol. 2004;138:799–802.
9. Gedde SJ. Management of glaucoma after retinal detachment surgery. Curr Opin Ophthalmol. 2002;13:103–9.
10. Han DP, Lewis H, Lambrou RM, et al. Mechanisms of intraocular pressure elevation after pars plana vitrectomy. Ophthalmology. 1989;96:1357–62.
11. Honavar SC, Goyal M, Majji AB, et al. Glaucoma after pars plana vitrectomy and silicon oil injection for complicated retinal detachments. Ophthalmology. 1999;106:169–76.
12. Ishida K, Ahmed I, Netland PA. Ahmed Glaucoma Valve surgical outcomes in eyes with and without silicon oil endotamponade. J Glaucoma. 2009;18:325–30.
13. Jackson TL, Thiagarajan M, Murthy R, et al. Pupil block glaucoma in phacic and pseudophacic patients after vitrectomy with sillicon oil injection. Am J Ophthalmol. 2001;132(3):414–6.
14. Jamli AL. Managing patients after retinal surgery. Rev Ophthalmol., Ophthalmic Product Guide; 2013.
15. Kim SJFlach AJ, Jampol LM. Nonsteroidal anti-inflammatory drugs in ophthalmology. Surv Ophthalmol. 2010;5(2):108–33.
16. Lakhanpal RR, Humayun MS, et al. Outcames of 140 consecutive cases of 25-gauge transconjunctival surgery for posterior segment desease. Ophthalmology. 2005;112:817–24.
17. Lemmen KD, Moter H, et al. Keratopathy following vitrectomy with silicone oil injection. Fortschr Ophthalmol. 1989;86(6):570–3.
18. Lesnoni G, Rossi T, Gelso A. Subfoveal liquid perfluorocarbon. Retina. 2004;24:172–6.
19. Li W, Zheng J, Zheng Q, Wu R, et al. Clinical complications of Densiron 68 intraocular tamponada for complicated retinal detachment. Eye 2010;24 (1):21–8.
20. Perez RN, Phelps CD, Burton TC. Angle closure glaucoma following sclera buckling operations. Trans Am Academy Ophthalmol Otolaryngol. 1976;81:247–52.
21. Reidel KG, Gabel VP, Neuberger L, et al. Intravitreal silicon oil injection: complications and treatment of 415 consecutive patients. Graefes Arch Clin Exp Ophthalmol. 1990;228(1):19–23
22. Shimada H, Nakashizuka H, et al. Incidence of endophthalmitis after 20 and 25-gauge vitrectomy. Ophthalmology. 2008;115:2215–20.
23. Spandau U, Heimann H. Practical handbook for small-gauge vitrectomy. Springer;2012.
24. Valone J, McCarthy M. Emulsified anterior chamber silicon oil and glaucoma. Ophthalmology. 1994;101:1908–12.
25. Zalta AH, Boyle NS, Zalta AK. Silicon oil pupillary block. Arch Ophthalmol. 2007;125(7):883–8.
26. Živojnović R. Silicon oil in vitreoretinal surgery. Martinus Nijhoff/Dr W. Junk Publish, Dordrecht;1987.

35 Tipps and Tricks for Retinal Detachment Surgery

Zoran Tomic and Ulrich Spandau

35.1 Anterior Chamber

35.1.1 Surgical Pearls No. 1

35.1.1.1 Insertion of a Synergetics Chandelier Light

(1) The insertion of the chandelier light is easier using hands rather than with the trocar forceps. But the surgeon must exert a relatively strong pressure to insert the tip of the chandelier through the sclera. If this does not succeed, the surgeon can expand the sclerotomy with a 25G trocar stiletto. The insertion is now easier, but the chandelier sits a little loose in the sclerotomy.

(2) Conjunctival chemosis or hemorrhage may make it difficult to identify the sclerotomy. In such cases use a pressure plate (DORC, no. 2117) or open the conjunctiva focally with scissors and forceps in order to visualize the sclerotomy.

Z. Tomic
Milos Klinika, Belgrade, Serbia

U. Spandau (✉)
St. Eriks Hospital, University of Stockholm, Stockholm, Sweden
e-mail: ulrich_spandau@yahoo.de

Surgical Pearls No. 2

When working with *27G*, insert the superotemporal trocar towards the superior pole. This upward position of the trocar reduces the bending of the instruments and allows in the most eyes a complete trimming of the vitreous at the superior pole.

Surgical Pearls No. 3

BSS damages the phakic lens: In pseudophakic eyes BSS is used as irrigation fluid but in phakic eyes BSS Plus® (Alcon) is required to avoid a lens damage. BSS Plus® contains also glutathione, glucose and sodium bicarbonate.

Surgical Pearls No. 4

Corneal lubrication; A major problem during vitrectomy, especially in combined surgeries with a duration of over 1 h, is corneal epithelial oedema. With the application of methylcellulose (Celoftal®, Alcon or Ocucoat®, Bausch & Lomb) on the cornea the cornea can remain clear for many hours. A debridement of the epithelium is rarely necessary, but if needed use a broad blade (crescent knife).

Surgical Pearls No. 5

Posterior capsular defect during anterior vitrectomy: This is no catastrophe and if the defect is circular you don't need to do anything. Otherwise cut a round capsular rhexis with the vitreous cutter (e.g. 500 cuts/min). The rhexis will not go out and the IOL remains stable in the bag.

U. Spandau et al. (eds.), *Retinal Detachment Surgery and Proliferative Vitreoretinopathy*,
https://doi.org/10.1007/978-3-031-11946-0_35

Surgical Pearls No. 6

Small pupil: If the pupil constricts during surgery, inject 0.01% Adrenalin into the anterior chamber. The pupil should enlarge within seconds. If the small pupil is caused by posterior synechiae, use stretching instruments such as a push–pull instrument (Sinskey hook) or insert iris hooks to enlarge the pupil.

Surgical Pearls No. 7

Posterior dislocated IOL: An IOL-in-the-bag luxated onto the posterior pole is not easy to grasp. It is usually enclosed inside the lens capsule. The lens capsule, however, is difficult to grasp. Lift the IOL up together with the light fiber and a forceps and then grasp the IOL from the side. As forceps we prefer a 27G endgripping forceps (DORC) with sharp edges.

Surgical Pearls No. 8

Difficult IOL extraction from posterior pole: Try the following manoeuvres: (1) Grab the haptic or rhexis edge with an intravitreal forceps. (2) Insert a chandelier light and work bimanual with one intravitreal forceps and one 27G membrane pic (DORC) to elevate the IOL. (3) Inject a small bubble of PFCL to elevate the IOL and to protect the macula. Grab the IOL. (4) Inject a small bubble of PFCL to elevate the IOL. Then remove the lens capsule around the haptic with the vitreous cutter (Fig. 35.1). If the haptic is freed from the lens capsule, it is easy to grasp with a forceps. Remark: The fourth method is always successful.

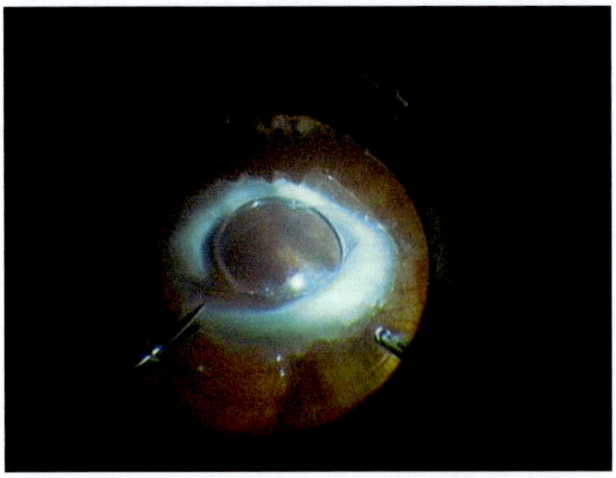

Fig. 35.1 A luxated in-the-bag IOL. In case of a big Soemmering ring it may be difficult to grasp the IOL

Surgical Pearls No. 9

Enclavation of iris-claw IOL: Instead of enclavating the IOL from both paracentesis you can enclavate the IOL from one paracentesis. The tip of the enclavation spatula is long enough to reach both iris-claws.

Surgical Pearls No. 10

Do not enclavate too much iris tissue during iris-claw implantation: It may cause ocular pain. In order to avoid this side effect use the thin Sekundo enclavation spatula from Geuder.

Surgical Pearls No. 11

Fibrin or clotted blood in the anterior chamber can be extracted easily with Eckardt forceps via a paracentesis.

Surgical Pearls No. 12

Do not open the *pars plana infusion* without visualizing it first. If you are unable to see the internal opening of the infusions port, start the vitrectomy using an infusion via an anterior chamber maintainer. This is especially the case for ocular hypotony with choroidal detachment.

Surgical Pearls No. 13

Corneal suture: In case of an unstable anterior chamber, place a single 10-0 nylon suture at the end of the phaco & IOL. This avoids accidental opening of the corneal wound during indentation, which may lead to flattening of the anterior chamber and even dislocation of the IOL. The suture can be removed 1 week postoperative.

Surgical Pearls No. 14

Capsular tension ring: A good idea is the insertion of a capsular tension ring after aspiration of the cortex. The capsular tension ring stretches the capsular bag so that the posterior capsule does not sag or dip. This reduces the risk of injury to the lens capsule during vitrectomy. If you are using a capsular tension ring, make sure that it is in the right place, as removing a capsular tension ring from the vitreous base is not an easy task.

Surgical Pearls No. 15
6 o'clock iridectomy for light silicone oils: If aphakia or zonular lysis is present, create an Ando-iridectomy (6 o'clock) to prevent an increase in intraocular pressure. An Ando iridectomy prevents a secondary angle-closure, because the aqueous can flow through the iridectomy at 6 o'clock into the anterior chamber and presses the oil bubble back into the vitreous cavity. Work bimanually: Draw the pupillary edge at 6 o'clock with an intravitreal forceps. Place the vitreous cutter (low cut rate: about 200 cuts/min) with the opening forward behind the iris at 6 o'clock, aspirate the iris and then cut a hole.

Surgical Pearls No. 16
12 o'clock iridectomy for heavy silicone oils: Densiron 68® (Geuder) is a heavy silicone oil and tamponades the inferior retina. If an iridectomy is needed, it must be performed at 12 o'clock. Perform the iridectomy optimally in a perfluorocarbon liquid (PFCL) or water filled eye, i.e. before silicone oil injection.

Surgical Pearls No. 17
Methylcellulose in anterior chamber: If a large zonular lysis is present, inject methyl cellulose into the anterior chamber; it can be left there postoperatively. It holds the anterior chamber silicone oil free. There will be only a slight postoperative rise of IOP.

Surgical Pearls No. 18
Silicone oil in the anterior chamber: Remove the silicone oil bubble with I/A hand pieces (Figs. 35.2 and 35.3). The removal is simple, if the vitreous cavity is filled with BSS. Usually the vitreous cavity is filled with silicone oil and the risk is that after removal of the silicone oil bubble a new bubble comes into the anterior chamber. The reasons for this is overfill of silicone oil in the vitreous cavity and a zonular defect. If a new bubble comes into the anterior

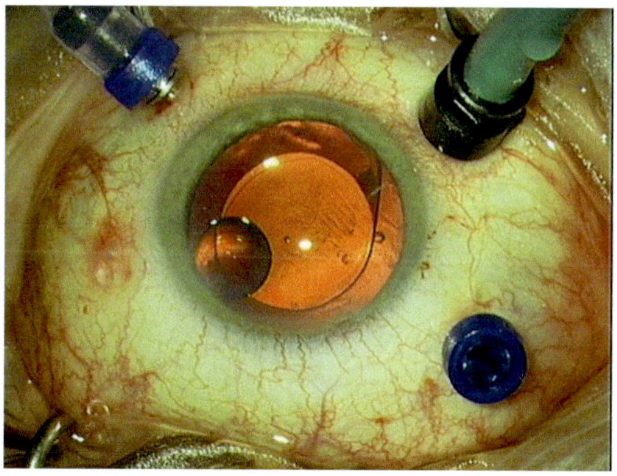

Fig. 35.2 A silicone oil bubble in the anterior chamber

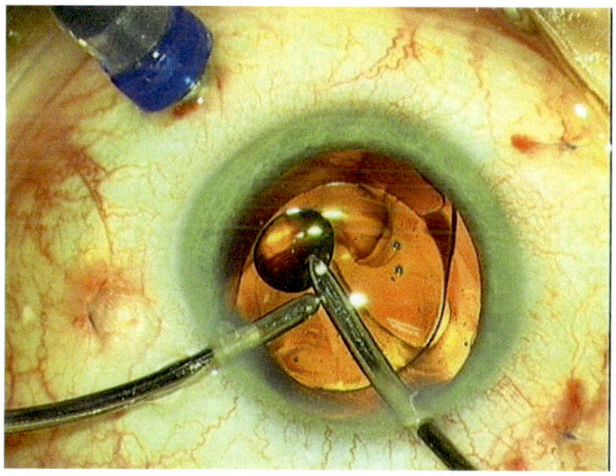

Fig. 35.3 Remove the silicone oil bubble with I/A. Inject at the end methylcellulose into the anterior chamber

chamber, then remove first the silicone oil bubble with I/A. Then remove the aspiration handpiece but leave the irrigation in the anterior chamber. Then inject with the second hand methylcellulose into the anterior chamber and slowly retrace the irrigation handpiece. The methylcellulose causes no ocular hypertension.

Surgical Pearls No. 19
1-piece IOL versus 3-piece IOL: Do not implant a 1-piece IOL into the sulcus because the haptics cause a focal depigmentation of the iris resulting in a secondary pigment glaucoma. This does not happen with a 3-piece IOL. The reason for this is that a 1-piece IOL has big haptics with sharp edges whereas a 3-piece IOL has small round haptics.

Surgical Pearls No. 20
Posterior synechiae: How do you remove posterior synechiae? (1) Simultaneous injection of viscoelastics and delamination with the viscoelastics cannula. (2) If the adhesions are too strong you can cut them with a (curved) vitreous scissors.

Surgical Pearls No. 21
Cyclocryopexy: 3–5 cryopexy effects on the inferior half of the ciliary body with approximately 30 s duration. Be careful with the dosage of cryopexy because too much may result in an irreversible hypotony. It is advisable to perform one cryopexy treatment with 3 effects, wait 4 weeks for the effect and then repeat the cryopexy if necessary.

Surgical Pearls No. 22
An *anterior chamber maintainer* can be used for a vitrectomy instead of a pars plana infusion, if there is sufficient flow between anterior and posterior chamber, e.g. aphakia. It cannot be used in a phakic eye because there is no sufficient flow from the anterior to the posterior chamber.

Surgical Pearls No. 23
Seidel test after closure of a corneal wound. In order to test if the globe is watertight perform a Seidel test. Perform a paracentesis and inject BSS into the anterior chamber. If the globe is normotensive you can close the case. If the globe is hypotensive search for the leakage and close it.

Surgical Pearls No. 24
Anterior chamber haemorrhage: A fresh ACH is not easy to remove, because the fibrin is difficult to aspirate. Inject rtPA at the beginning, wait 2–3 min and then the blood can be removed easier.

Surgical Pearls No. 25
Scleral perforation: Measure the distance of the traumatic *scleral defect* from the limbus with a *caliper*. If the distance is longer than 4.0 mm than a retinal defect is likely. Add in this case a retinal cryopexy.

Surgical Pearls No. 26
If the same *scleral defect* is located >4 mm behind the limbus then perform a (blind) retinal cryopexy around the wound edges and, if you want to be absolutely safe, suture a *silicone sponge* above the scleral defect.

Surgical Pearls No. 27
Air bubbles behind IOL: Beware of a posterior capsulotomy and a fluid-air exchange in pseudophakic patients. During a fluid-air exchange the water condenses at the posterior surface of the IOL in the area of the capsulotomy, thereby greatly impairing the view of the posterior pole. It can either be removed with a flute instrument or injection of viscoelastics onto the posterior surface of the IOL (Figs. 35.4 and 35.5).

Surgical Pearls No. 28
I think that the implantation of a foldable iris prosthesis and a *combo iris-IOL prosthesis* with an IOL injector is the method of choice because it is easy and because the main incision is only 2.4 mm wide.

Surgical Pearls No. 29
The ultimate surgery would be to fasten the *IOL-iris prosthesis* with the *Scharioth* method (Fig. 35.6).

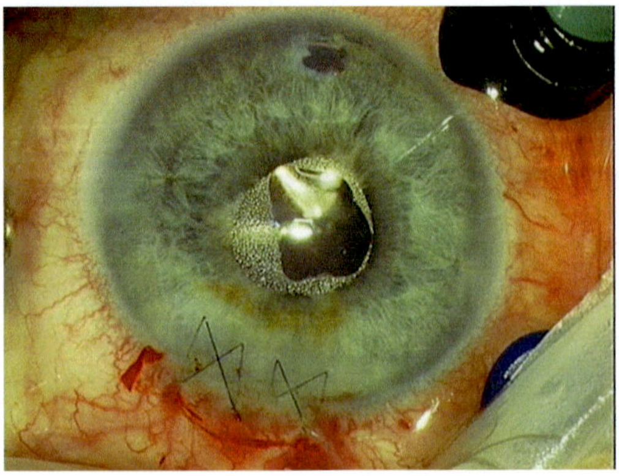

Fig. 35.4 Condensed air behind the IOL

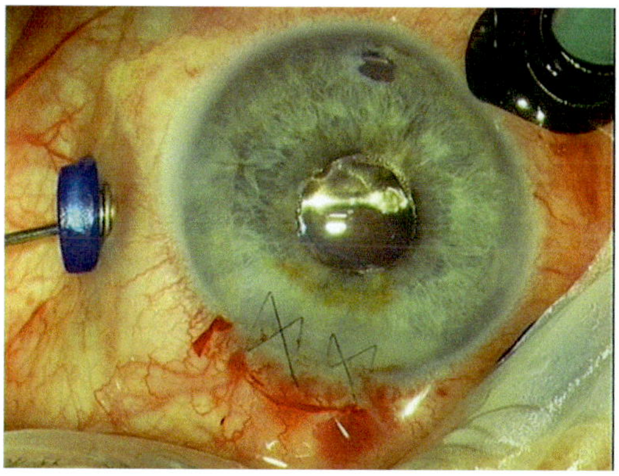

Fig. 35.5 Remove the air bubbles with an instrument or inject methylcellulose on the backside of the IOL

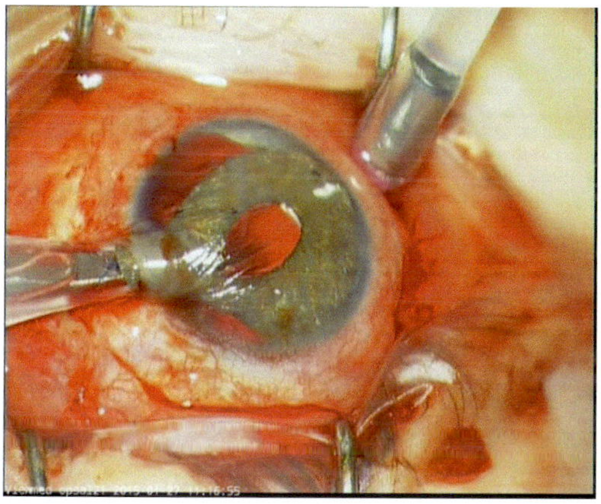

Fig. 35.6 The combo iris-IOL prosthesis is inserted with an IOL injector. The iris prosthesis is from Human Optics, Germany and the IOL from Alcon

35.2 Posterior Chamber

Surgical Pearls No. 30

BIOM and air: When filling air into the vitreous cavity the image is out of focus due to the different refractive index. If you move the BIOM-lens a little bit up, the image becomes focussed again.

Surgical Pearls No. 31

PFCL injection: Try to inject one bubble only. Start very slowly, and then keep the tip of your cannula always in touch with the bubble. This avoids splitting the stream into multiple bubbles, which can then displace into the subretinal space.

Complications of PFCL Injection

Subretinal PFCL: (1) Do not inject PFCL in direction of a retinal break; the PFCL may flow subretinal. (2) Use trocars with valves to avoid/reduce PFCL bubbles.

Surgical Pearls No. 32

Trypane blue: Staining may become difficult if you use the syringe of the company. If too much force is applied during injection, a sudden jet of dye can be injected into the eye which will obscure the view and is cumbersome to remove. We recommend therefore to change the syringes. We use a regular 3 cc syringe instead, which is predictable in its behaviour (Fig. 35.7).

Surgical Pearls No. 33

The location of fluids in the vitreous cavity during retinal detachment surgery is shown in Table 35.1. Note the changes of intraocular fluids during and after surgery.

Surgical Pearls No. 34

PVD: If you plan to stain with trypane blue then use it also for PVD instead of triamcinolone. It makes surgery so much easier. But if you stain the vitreous you need to restain for the membrane.

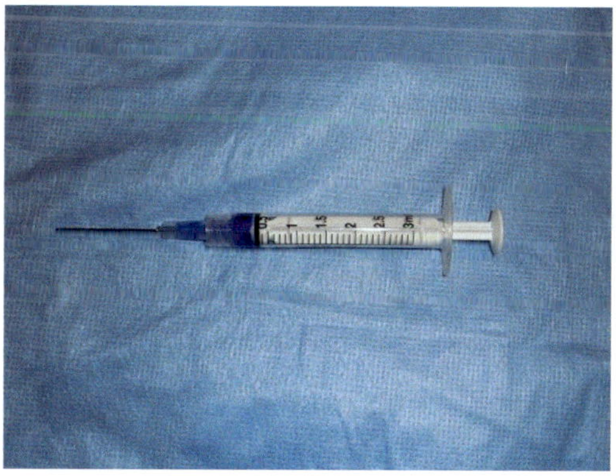

Fig. 35.7 A 3 cc syringe with trypane blue

Table 35.1 Location of fluids in the vitreous cavity during and after retinal detachment surgery

Intraoperatively	Postoperatively	
Silicone oil	Silicone oil	Vitreous cavity
BSS		
Perfluorocarbon	Aqueous	

Surgical Pearls No. 35

Membrane & dye: Stain the membrane repeatedly, as there are often several membranes present. You can only exclude a residual membrane, if staining was negative. And the better the membrane is made visible, the easier it can be peeled.

Surgical Pearls No. 36

In cases of ERM, you can try a "two in one" *peeling of ERM and ILM* by starting your peeling more peripheral than usual (for example, at the major vessel arcades). If you manage to grasp the ILM, continue your peeling towards the centre. The ERM should sit on top of the ILM and both layers can be removed with one peeling.

Surgical Pearls No. 37

Staining in air filled eye: This method achieves a much higher concentration of the dye; you need less dye and staining is faster. Perform a fluid x air exchange and leave a small puddle of water on the central pole. Use a 3 cc syringe with a backflush needle for injection. Inject 2–3 drops of Brilliant Blue G into the puddle, wait 15 s (Fig. 35.8), position the flute tip in the puddle and remove the dye (Fig. 35.9). Then perform an air x fluid exchange. The advantage here is: The dye acts only in the water puddle, and the surgeon can remove it more quickly than if the dye is distributed throughout the vitreous cavity.

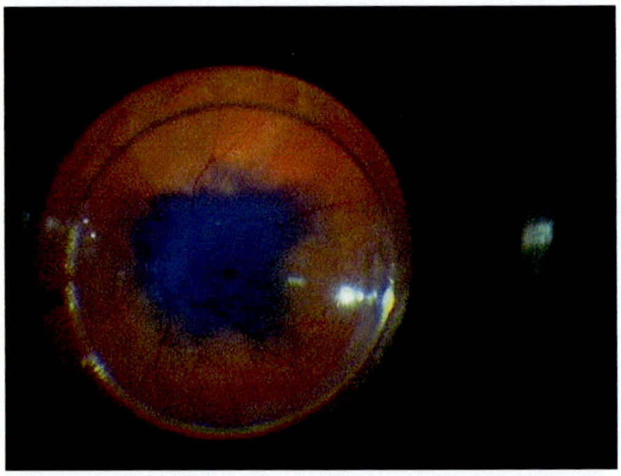

Fig. 35.8 Inject Brillant Blue G onto the posterior pole in an air filled vitreous cavity

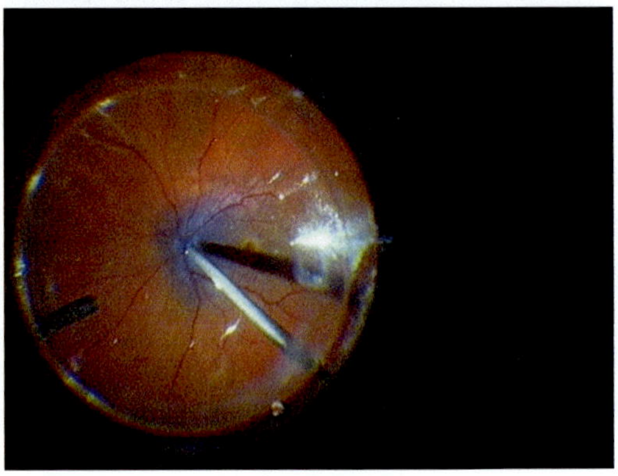

Fig. 35.9 Then aspirate the dye and switch to air x fluid exchange

Surgical Pearls No. 38

ILM peeling and dot-hemorrhages: Small dot-hemorrhages occur only during ILM-peeling and do not appear with ERM peeling (Fig. 35.10).

Surgical Pearls No. 39

Peeling with chandelier light: Insert a chandelier light. Assist the dominant hand under peeling, you will be surprised how calm your hand is and without tremor. If you have a hand without tremor take a Charles flute needle in the non-dominant hand and aspirate the pieces of membrane or ILM. If you use a vacuum cleaner you can even lift up the edges of the membrane and then remove them with the forceps.

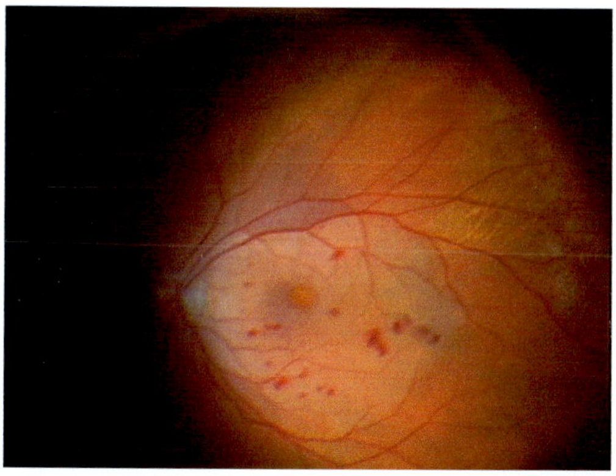

Fig. 35.10 Dot-haemorrhages occur only during ILM-peeling

Surgical Pearls No. 40

Backflush instrument: When working with 27G you should perform an active fluid aspiration. Use the backflush instrument with active suction or alternatively the vitrector. Be cautious when coming close to the retina. It is not possible to aspirate the water completely with the vitrector due to the position of the opening.

Surgical Pearls No. 41

Treat the retinal tears and not the detachment: This sounds simple but often an overtreatment is performed. If you mend a hole in a bicycle tyre then you only mend the hole and not the complete tyre. The same principle applies to a hole in the retina. Treat only the hole edges and not the complete retina.

Surgical Pearls No. 42

Retinal tear under a muscle: Alternatively to a limbal sponge you can apply a radial sponge. If you want to apply a radial sponge under the muscle, then remove the muscle, suture the sponge and suture the muscle back to place. Or suture the sponge onto the muscle. If the patient experiences diplopia after surgery you can remove the sponge after approximately 2–4 weeks.

Surgical Pearls No. 43

Bulbar hypotony: (1) Especially in vitrectomized eyes the globe may be hypotensive with scleral folds. Inject BSS with a 30G needle via pars plana until the globe is normotensive. (2) The risk for subretinal placement of trocars is high in bulbar hypotony. Use 6 mm trocars from Alcon (and not 4 mm trocars) and insert them perpendicular (and not lamellar).

Surgical Pearls No. 44

PVD

(1) The correct assessment of the relationship between the posterior vitreous face and the retina/optic disc is one of the key steps to master pars plana vitrectomy. Always check if a PVD is present or not. Even in cases when you expect a PVD to be present (for example, retinal detachments), you will sometimes be surprised by an attached vitreous face.

(2) The freshly detached posterior vitreous face has a "beaten metal" appearance. You know that you have induced a PVD if you see this appear on the posterior surface of the vitreous. When a PVD is induced, suddenly, a lot more vitreous, which must be removed, will appear in the vitreous cavity.

Surgical Pearls No. 45

PVD and Dye

(1) We recommend beginners to stain the vitreous at the beginning of vitrectomy for the first 10–20 vitrectomies. The vitreous is much easier to recognize and vitrectomy and especially the induction of a posterior vitreous detachment becomes considerably easier.

(2) To stain the posterior vitreous face with triamcinolone: Perform a core vitrectomy and a peripheral vitrectomy in front of your ports. Induce the cannula into the mid vitreous (be careful not to inject peripherally, or you will inject in to the vitreous base and exert traction). Inject a small amount of triamcinolone that will drop down onto the posterior pole. This will very nicely stain the bursa praemacularis of the vitreous. Do not inject too much triamcinolone for vitreous staining. It will only obscure your

view and will be cumbersome to remove later on during the surgery. Few drops are sufficient for staining the posterior vitreous.

(3) Once the bursa praemacularis is stained with triamcinolone, try to engage the posterior vitreous face at the optic disc. Try to cut a small break in the posterior vitreous face nasal to the disc, then "pick up" the posterior vitreous phase with the cutter and suction only. Pull anterior towards the lens. Try to keep an eye on the advancing posterior vitreous face in the mid-periphery. This looks like a tidal wave. It is where breaks will develop during induction of a PVD.

Surgical Pearls No. 46 (Figs. 35.10, 35.11 and 35.12)

Difficult PVD: If you are not able to induce a PVD try the following: (1) Increase the vacuum to 600 mmHg and try again. (2) Stain the vitreous with trypane blue or triamcinolone and try again. (3) Insert a 60D lens and mobilize the posterior hyaloid membrane with an Eckardt forceps. If you have created a hole, try to aspirate this part with a vitreous cutter and provoke a PVD. (4) Create a hole in the posterior hyaloid with a 27G Atkinson cannula (Beaver-Visitec). Then mobilize the hole edges with a forceps (Figs. 35.11, 35.12 and 35.13).

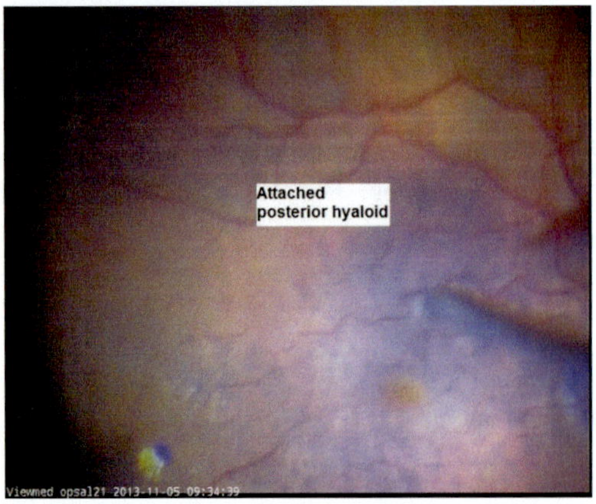

Fig. 35.11 Attached posterior hyaloid

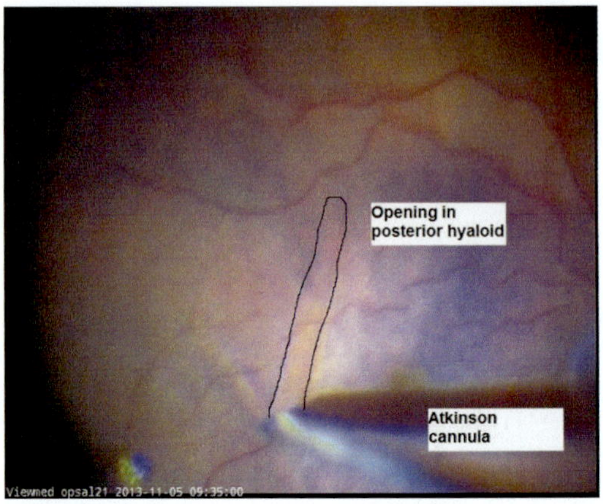

Fig. 35.12 Create an opening in the posterior hyaloid with a sharp instrument

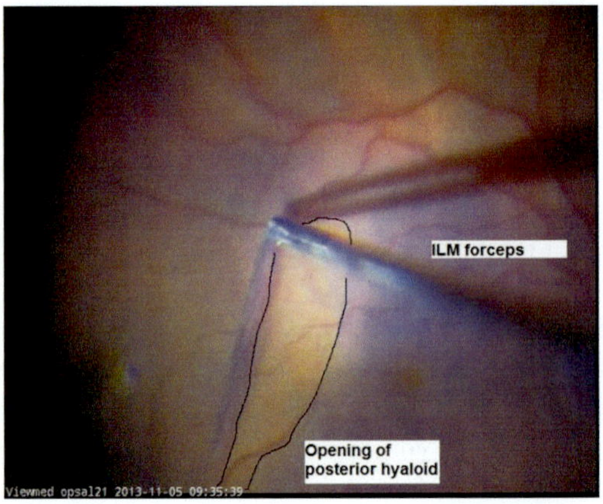

Fig. 35.13 Then grasp an edge of posterior hyaloid and create a PVD

Surgical Pearls No. 47

PVD in RRD: In about 15% of patients with RRD, the vitreous is still attached at the posterior pole. One group at risk is myopic patients below the age of 50 years with multiple small round breaks. The vitreous may be very adherent to the retina in such cases and trying to induce a PVD can lead to multiple iatrogenic breaks. These cases usually do very well with scleral buckling surgery. If in doubt, check the status of vitreous attachment/detachment with preoperative ultrasound before deciding to perform a vitrectomy.

Surgical Pearls No. 48

Triamcinolone and RRD: Many cases of RRD are caused by strong vitreoretinal adhesion. It may not be possible to separate vitreous and retina simply by engaging the vitreous with the vitreous cutter and pulling it off the retina—you may enlarge pre-existing breaks or induce iatrogenic breaks in some cases. If you find very strong vitreoretinal adhesions, it is advisable to "stop pulling" and start "shaving" the vitreous of the retina. This is facilitated by staining the adherent vitreous with triamcinolone. When staining the vitreous with triamcinolone, use minimal amounts and direct the injection to the area of interest. Injecting too much triamcinolone may interfere with your view and it can be cumbersome to remove this later on in the procedure.

Surgical Pearls No. 49

Unseen breaks and Schlieren phenomenon: Inject PFCL slowly and watch for the "Schlieren-phenomenon". In particular in long-standing RRD, the subretinal fluid appears like a muddy stream when entering the vitreous cavity. This "Schlieren phenomenon" may point to the location of the retinal break at the entry site of the Schlieren in cases of "unseen breaks".

Surgical Pearls No. 50

PFCL is quite expensive. In more complicated cases, it may be necessary to perform multiple manipulations under PFCL, occasionally removing and then again adding PFCL at a later stage. If PFCL needs to be removed, one can easily aspirate it back into the injection syringe for re-injection at a later stage of the procedure.

Surgical Pearls No. 51

Iatrogenic break: If the break and the bullous detachment are far apart from each other it is difficult to drain the subretinal fluid from the break. In the first case one can try to massage the subretinal fluid with a scleral depressor to the break. Or perform an iatrogenic break in the area of trapped fluid. Mark the inferior retina close to the ora serrata with endodiathermy. Then cut a hole with the vitreous cutter (setting: approx. 300 cuts/min) by suctioning the retina and then cutting it cautiously. Drain the subretinal fluid from this break.

Surgical Pearls No. 52

Laser: Be careful with your laser energy. Only a mild whitening of the RPE is necessary. Burns which are too strong will weaken the retina and are a predilection site for the formation of new retinal breaks. They may also cause contraction of the choroid or even choroidal hemorrhage s. A typical beginner's mistake is to perform too much laser or cryotherapy as an extra safety measure that then may turn out to have exactly the opposite effect.

Surgical Pearls No. 53

Lasercerclage: A circumferential 360° laser is not recommended. It is essential to identify and treat all retinal breaks. A circumferential laser has the big disadvantage that in case of a redetachment the breaks are difficult to find within the patches of chorioretinal atrophy.

Surgical Pearls No. 54

Laser necrosis: Another complication of laser is a retinal necrosis. Too high laser intensity may cause a necrosis of the retina and small, difficult-to-find holes. These tears occur often at the outer edge of the laser treatment. The same applies for cryopexy.

Surgical Pearls No. 55

Iatrogenic break: When a small break is located within the vascular arcades, a laser treatment is not necessary as the pigment epithelium in the central area has sufficient pumping function so that no detachment occurs. If the break is large, however, we recommend lasering the break with one row of laser burns. Even if you create a peripheral break this is not a problem as long as you also recognize the break. Surround the tear with three rows of laser burns and perform a gas tamponade.

Surgical Pearls No. 56

Laser therapy:

(1) A laser treatment can be carried out in a water-(BSS)-filled, silicone oil filled and PFCL-filled eye. In an air-filled eye it is difficult to laser due to a poor visibility.
(2) It is easiest to laser breaks under heavy liquid, as you have a good apposition of retina and retinal pigment epithelium. One of the disadvantages of this technique is that the margins of the break are more difficult to see. Mark the location of breaks with endodiathermy or laser spots before covering it with heavy liquid. This way it is easy to identify them under heavy liquid.
(3) Beware of the "continuous" function of the laser. You can easily overtreat. This may result in mini-explosions, choroidal hemorrhage, retinal breaks or predispose to postoperative tears. Pigmentation increases towards the periphery. Less energy is needed for peripheral laser spots.
(4) The further you move the laser probe away from the retina, the larger the resulting spot size on the retina (and the more energy you need to create a burn). This can be quite useful if you want to treat larger areas as the resulting burns have softer edges and do not cut the retina like a knife.
(5) Use 360° prophylactic laser with caution. It may not be necessary, may result in anterior segment ischemia and will make it very difficult to identify small breaks in cases of postoperative retinal detachments. Treat only the visible tears instead.

Surgical Pearls No. 57

Trimming of vitreous base: There are various ways to trim the vitreous base. (a) Bimanual technique using a scleral indentor, (b) removal under coaxial light (only with microscope illumination) by using a cotton wool swab or a scleral depressor to indent the sclera or (c) using the light fiber as an external scleral depressor (this gives you a focussed beam of light transsclerally to illuminate the vitreous base).

Surgical Pearls No. 58

Active aspiration: In 25G and 27G the aspiration of subretinal fluid is easier and faster with active (than passive) aspiration. If you do not want to use PFCL, e.g. because only a focal retinal detachment is present, then you should aspirate subretinal fluid with active aspiration.

Surgical Pearls No. 59

Removal of PFCL: Two pearls for PFCL removal: (1) When using a silicone tip-flute needle, the risk of retinal or optic disc touch is much lower. (2) If you are not sure whether you aspirated the entire PFCL: Instil a little water into the air-filled vitreous cavity (with a brief water–air exchange) and then completely remove the residual PFCL-water puddle.

Surgical Pearls No. 60

B-scan: In cases with vitreous hemorrhage, always perform a detailed preoperative ultrasound examination. Try to determine the state of the posterior vitreous face (attached, partially attached or detached) and the retina.

Surgical Pearls No. 61

Blocked infusion: The hemorrhagic vitreous blocks sometimes the infusion. Check the infusion trocar before vitrectomy and if in doubt then cut the hemorrhagic vitreous around the infusion trocar.

Surgical Pearls No. 62

Removal of anterior hyaloid: In case of a hemorrhage directly behind the lens it may be necessary to remove the anterior hyaloid. This is an easy procedure in pseudophakic patients but a lens threatening procedure in phakic patients. We perform 2 techniques: Work at the edge of the lens (i.e. behind the zonules) in order to avoid a lens touch. (1) With help of a serrated jaws forceps grab the anterior hyaloid/vitreous and pull it towards the center of the globe. Work from both sides. (2) With help of a vitreous cutter suck the anterior hyaloid/vitreous (only aspiration) and pull the vitreous cutter towards the center of the globe. Cut the vitreous there. Work from both sides.

Surgical Pearls No. 63

How should epiretinal blood be removed? 1. Aspirate epiretinal blood by sweeping with a silicone tip flute needle over the retina. 2. By pressing several times on the side opening/tubing of the backflush instrument, water is ejected from the tip of the flute needle and blows the epiretinal blood upward. The blood can then be easily aspirated at the same time with the vitreous cutter. 3. Clotted blood can be grasped with an ILM forceps and be removed with the vitreous cutter.

Surgical Pearls No. 64

Recurrent vitreous hemorrhage: After a vitrectomy for a vitreous hemorrhage, bleeding may reoccur after surgery. If the recurrence is associated with a hyphema then check if the patient takes anticoagulants, i.e. aspirin. The patient should stop taking blood thinning medication for approximately 1 month. In most cases the hyphema resolves. If the hyphema resolved spontaneously, then continue waiting until the haemorrhage in the vitreous cavity has resorbed.

Surgical Pearls No. 65

Clogged infusion line in the beginning of silicone oil removal: The reason of the clogged infusion line is silicone oil within the infusion. (1) Do not press with the syringe onto the globe. You press otherwise the silicone oil into the infusion line. (2) Increase the IOP to 40–50 mmHg until the BSS comes. Then reduce again to 25 mmHg.

Surgical Pearls No. 66

Peeling and choroidal hemorrhage: Do not pull a diabetic membrane forwards to the lens – you may cause a choroidal hemorrhage. Pull the membrane parallel to the retina.

Surgical Pearls No. 67

Intraoperative hemorrhage and adrenaline: If there is constant bleeding from several vessels under surgery then add adrenaline to the BSS bottle. Adrenaline will constrict the vessels and reduce the bleeding.

Surgical Pearls No. 68

Postoperative vitreous hemorrhages are the number one problem following vitrectomy for proliferative diabetic retinopathy. In order to lower the rate of this complication, be meticulous with hemostasis. Watch out for small oozing bleeding sites after PRP has been performed. Even small collections of blood point at continuous bleeding sites that should be treated before closing up.

Surgical Pearls No. 69

Lens sparing vitrectomy: In young diabetic patients we experienced good results with a lens sparing vitrectomy and then a SF_6 gas or 1000 cSt silicone oil tamponade. Even after 10–20 years, the lens hardly opacifies.

Surgical Pearls No. 70

The most patients who underwent a *complicated cataract surgery* do not complain about the complication but about the painful procedure. Why? The cataract surgery was started with drop anaesthesia and when the complication occurred the surgery was continued with the same anaesthesia. Our recommendation: If you experience a complication, decide if you continue or delay the surgery. If you decide to continue, then add a subtenonal or retrobulbar anaesthesia before continuing surgery. You will have a happy patient.

Surgical Pearls No. 71

Dropped nucleus: The difficulty of this step is that the nucleus is located on the posterior pole so that a damage of the retina is easily induced. Three advices: (1) Inject a PFCL bubble to (a) protect the macula and (b) elevate the nucleus. (2) Work bimanual so that one hand can fixate the nucleus and the other hand can remove it. (3) If the posterior vitreous is attached, then the vitreous cortex is like a cushion for the nucleus making its removal difficult, In this case induce a PVD to free the access to the nucleus.

Surgical Pearls No. 72

The trimming of the vitreous base is an important step because a *residual nuclear fragment* will cause a postoperative sterile uveitis. Conclusion: Do not be satisfied after removal of the large nucleus but after complete removal of all small fragments.

Surgical Pearls No. 73
Removal of PVR-membranes: After silicone oil tamponade, peripherally located membranes in particular are very difficult to mobilize from the retina. A retinal scraper such as a 25G/27G Atkinson blunt cannula can be very helpful. With its help you can elevate the membrane of the retina. Then you can grasp the membrane with a forceps and cut the adhesions with a scissors (Fig. 35.14).

Surgical Pearls No. 74
The conventional *Eckardt ILM forceps* is often *not* sufficient for removal of PVR membranes. Try more powerful forceps such as a serrated jaws forceps or an Eckardt power forceps.

Surgical Pearls No. 75
Doughnut shape of anterior retina: One of the major risks of a retinectomy is cutting into the choroid. This will cause a significant hemorrhage and may be difficult to control. It usually happens if the retina is too close to the choroid in the area of the retinectomy. To detach it from the choroid, fill the eye with PFCL. The subretinal fluid will be pushed anteriorly in a doughnut shape and will detach the anterior retina. It is now easier to perform a retinectomy and the anterior edge of the retina is easily identified.

Surgical Pearls No. 76
Laser cerclage ≠ encircling band: Both, an encircling band and a laser cerclage, create a barrier for subretinal fluid originating from tears located anterior to the cerclage. An encircling band creates an indentation of the retina which results in a relaxation of the shortened retina. In addition, a laser cerclage along the indentation of the encircling band is safe against laser necrosis (Fig. 35.15).

Surgical Pearls No. 77
Avoid if possible an inferior *laser cerclage* (Fig. 35.16) Why? There is always more traction on the inferior pole because the gas or silicone oil presses against the superior pole. In case of an inferior laser cerclage the laser weakens the retina and may cause a detachment along the laser cerclage. Exception: Heavy silicone oil as tamponade or an encircling band (Fig. 35.15).

Surgical Pearls No. 78
Choroidal detachment: Use 6 mm trauma trocars from Alcon (23G). The risk for a subepithelial location is low.

Surgical Pearls No. 79
Difficult removal of suprachoroidal blood: If only little blood can be extracted although a highly bullous choroidal detachment persists,

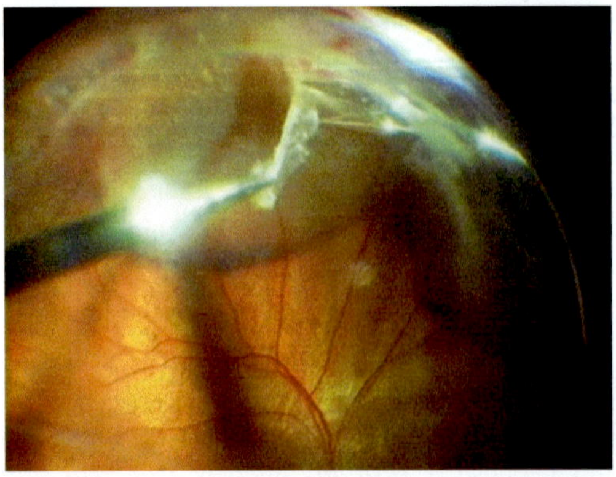

Fig. 35.14 Bimanual removal of peripheral membranes with straight scissors and forceps

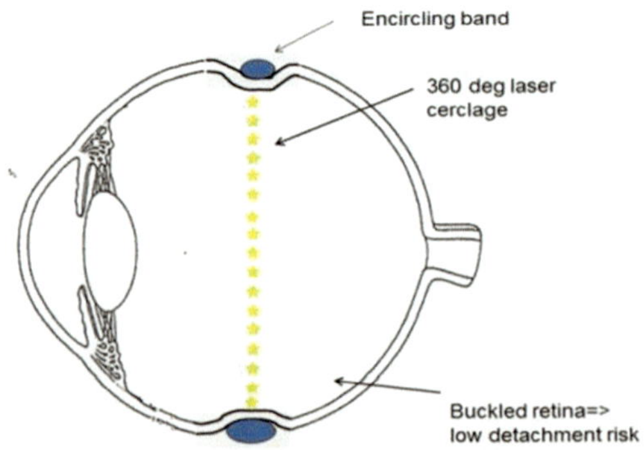

Fig. 35.15 A laser cerclage on the indentation of an encircling band is safe for lasernecrosis

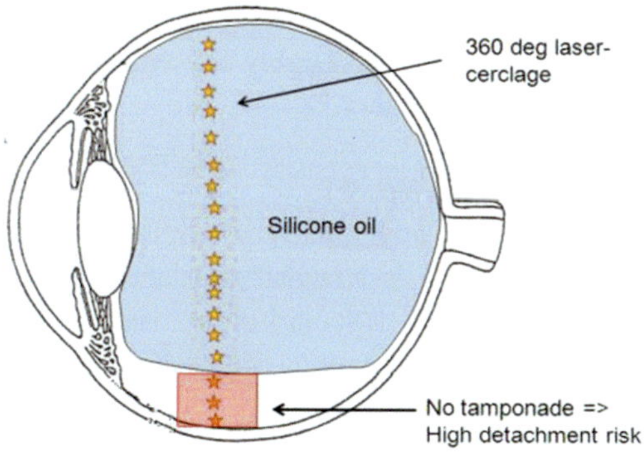

Fig. 35.16 A 360° laser cerclage may cause a laser necrosis at the inferior pole

then you should enlarge the sclerotomies to 4 mm. The reason is that the subchoroidal blood is clotted and cannot be extracted through 3 mm large sclerotomies.

Surgical Pearls No. 80

Subepithelial location of trocars: Especially in eyes with choroidal hemorrhage an initially correctly placed trocar cannula may move subepithelially during a later stage of the operation. Double-check the trocars several times during surgery.

Surgical Pearls No. 81

Chandelier light for choroidal detachment: It is advisable to use a trocar based chandelier light. Insert a 6 mm trauma trocar and then the light fiber (e.g. DORC).

Surgical Pearls No. 82

A *hypotony* is present if the IOP <6 mmHg. If a silicone oil filled eye has an IOP <6 mmHg, you cannot remove the silicone oil because the eye would fall into a hypotony and finally into a phthisis bulbi.

Surgical Pearls No. 83

PFCL injection: Work bimanual with Charles flute needle and fluid cannula. Hold the tip of the PFCL needle always first centrally in the PFCL bubble and then move it forward as the bubble gets larger.

Surgical Pearls No. 84

Residual PFCL? Perform a short fluid x air exchange (2–3 s) and remove the BSS together with the PFCL.

Surgical Pearls No. 85

Residual PFCL? Aspirate it with a 41G needle.

Subretinal fluid? Aspirate it with a 41G needle (Fig. 35.17). A laser treatment of the hole is not necessary

Surgical Pearls No. 86

Peeling in *diabetic* eyes: Peel from periphery to posterior pole.

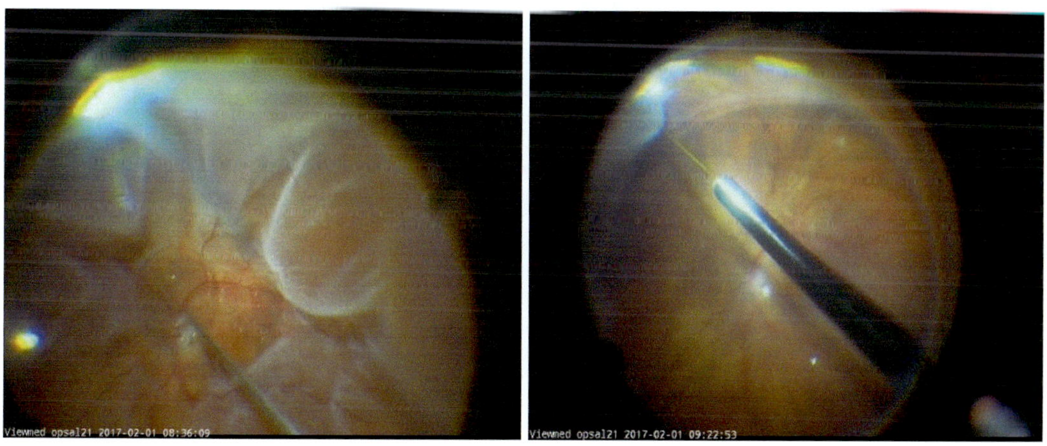

Fig. 35.17 Aspiration of subretinal fluid with 41G needle

Peeling in *PVR* eyes: Peel from posterior pole to periphery.

Surgical Pearls No. 87

Subretinal located trocar? Check distance to limbus! If it is correct, then an anterior retinal displacement is likely. Remove the retina around the trocar, cauterize the edges and then laser treat.

Surgical Pearls No. 89 (Fig. 35.18)

Marking of retinal breaks: If you do not have an endodiathermy, then mark the ora serrata posterior to the rupture with a laser burn.

Surgical Pearls No. 88

A rhegmatogenous retinal detachment with pigment line: A pigment line is an excellent marker for the presence of a retinal break (Fig. 35.19).

Surgical Pearls No. 90

Cyclitic membranes: If the vitreous base is not removed during vitrectomy and silicone oil used as a tamponade, then the silicone oil will press the vitreous base against the ciliary body resulting in cyclitic membranes and hypotony. It is almost impossible to remove these membranes. It is therefore essential to prevent them. This can be done by trimming thoroughly the vitreous base during the first surgery.

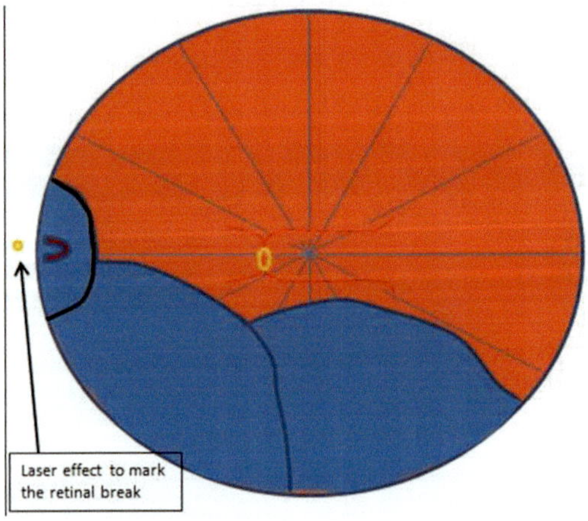

Fig. 35.18 If diathermy is not possible you can mark the retinal break with a laser spot above the ora serrata

Surgical Pearls No. 91

Avoid operating an *inflamed or vascularly active eye*. If the retina is attached wait and treat the inflammation and vascularisation; use steroids and anti-VEGF. If the retina is detached you have to operate.

Surgical Pearls No. 92

Open globe injury: In case of a scleral defect posterior to the pars plana, measure the distance between limbus and scleral defect with the caliper. If the distance <4 mm then a retinal incarceration in the wound is unlikely. If the distance >4 mm then a retinal incarceration is likely. Schedule a vitrectomy 2 weeks after the primary closure; see Diagram 35.1.

35.3 Tamponade

Surgical Pearls No. 93

Gas tamponade: Hold the flute needle behind the lens or close to the trocar. Do not hold the flute needle in the middle of the vitreous body. The injected gas is heavier than air and flows to the bottom of the globe. You can only extract the air if you hold the flute needle in the front part of the eye (behind the IOL).

Surgical Pearls No. 94

Gas filling with 27G: The main advantage of 27G is the tight sclerotomy. A 27G sclerotomy has less leakage than a 23G sclerotomy and the gas filling is therefore much better and longer. This feature is important for detachment surgery. In 27G we use often only an air tamponade in superior detachments.

Surgical Pearls No. 95

Physics of a gas tamponade (exchange of air against gas): See Fig. 35.20 and Table 35.2.

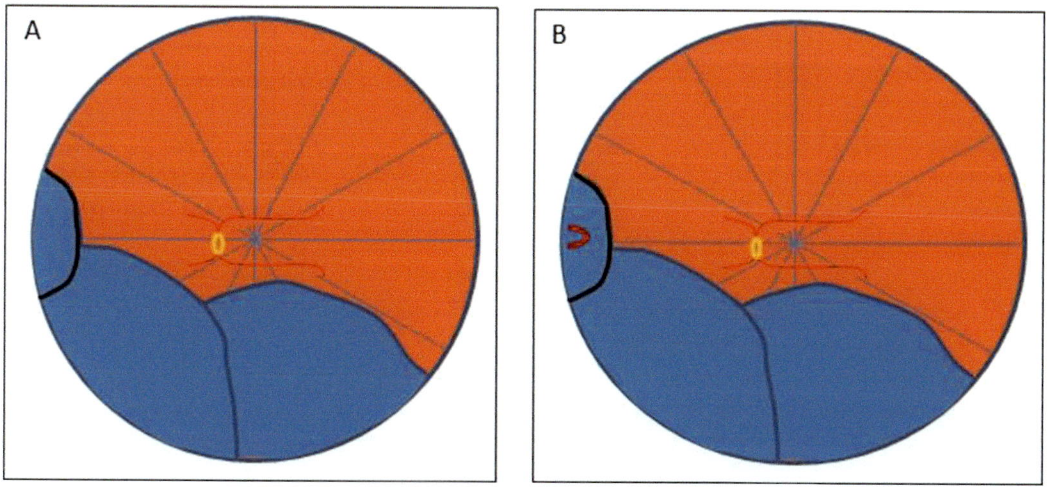

Fig. 35.19 An inferior retinal detachment with unclear hole situation (**A**). Note the pigment line at 8:30–9:30 (**A**). A pigment line points to a retinal break (**B**)

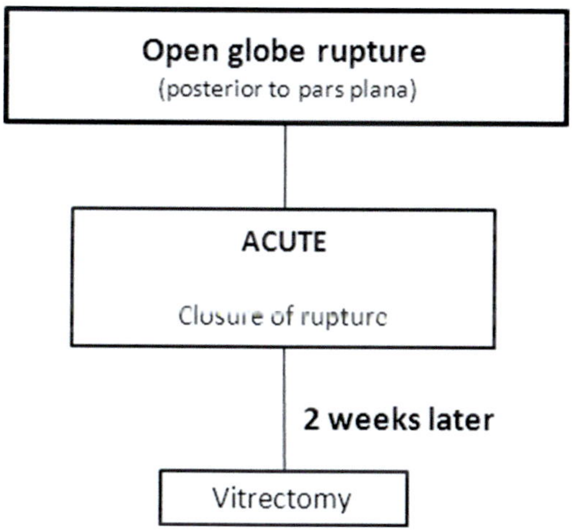

Diagram 35.1 Our treatment algorithm for open globe injuries

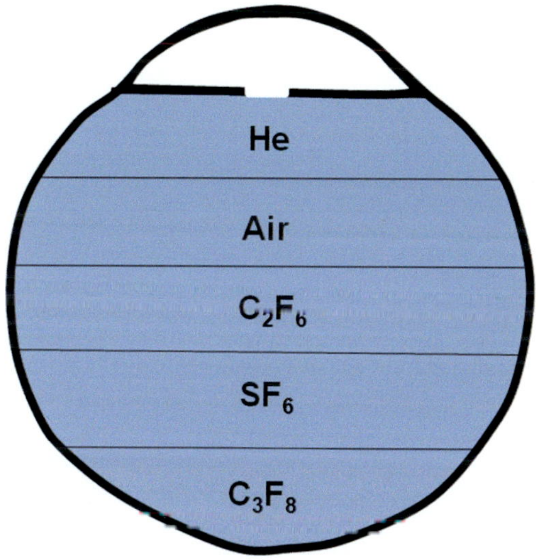

Fig. 35.20 Relative location of gases within the eye according to their molecular weight (g/mol). He = Helium (SG = 2.016); Air (SG = 29); C_2F_6 (SG = 138); SF_6 (SG = 146); C_3F_8 (SG = 188)

Surgical Pearls No. 96

Shake the 50cc gas syringe before injection because the gas sinks to the bottom of the syringe resulting in a wrong concentration of the gas in the eye.

Surgical Pearls No. 97

Air travel with gas: An airplane travels at a height of 10 km, the cabin is regarding the air pressure at a height of 2 km. An air travel with a gas filled eye is safe if the distance between the optic disc and the lower apex of the air bubble is more than 4 disc diameter (see Fig. 35.21).

Surgical Pearls No. 98 (Figs. 35.22 and 35.23)

Infusion line and silicone oil: An infusion line with metal cannula (e.g. Alcon) falls off when injecting silicone oil. Use instead a DORC

Table 35.2 Our normogram for tamponades in regard to the specific pathology. We use rarely 5000 csts silicone oil and C_3F_8

	Easy retinal detachment	Easy retinal detachment with residual submacular fluid	PVR detachment
Postoperative tamponade	SF_6	SF_6	1000 csts silicone oil; in case of inferior detachment: Densiron 68
Duration of tamponade	2–4 weeks	2–4 weeks	Silicone oil and Densiron 68: 6–12 weeks
Postoperative posture	5 days on the opposite cheek of the retinal hole	3 h supine position and then face down position	7 days depending on position of retinal rupture

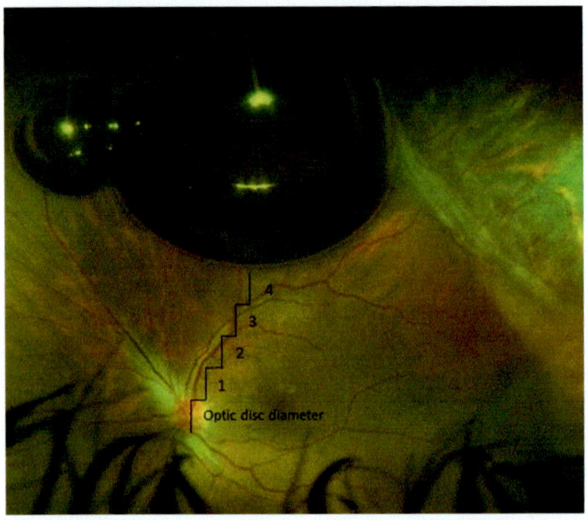

Fig. 35.21 An ora dialysis operated with cryopexy and scleral buckling and air injection. This patient can air travel because a distance of 4 optic disc diameter between optic disc and gas bubble is present

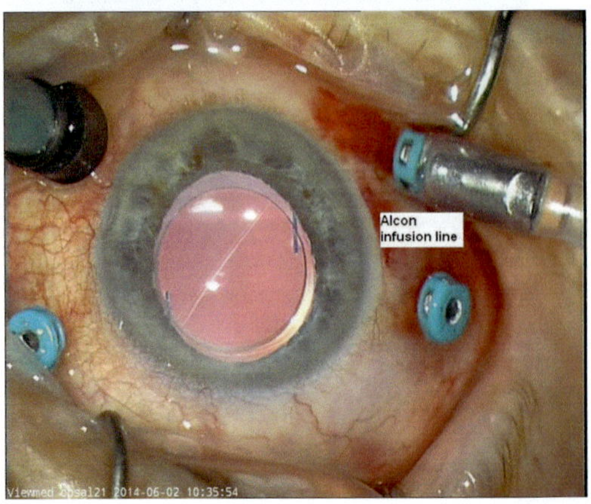

Fig. 35.22 An infusion line with metal cannula (e.g. Alcon) falls off when injecting silicone oil

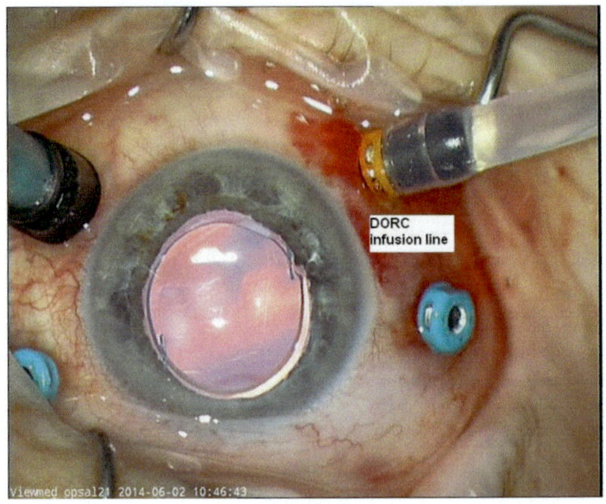

Fig. 35.23 Use instead a DORC infusion line which has a plastic cannula. It remains stable under silicone oil injection

infusion line which has a plastic cannula with a special shape. This infusion will remain stable in the infusion trocar when injecting silicone oil.

Surgical Pearls No. 99

Most vitreoretinal clinics use 20% SF_6 as *tamponade for macular hole*. However, some clinics prefer 15% C_2F_6, 14% C_3F_8 or even 1000 csts silicone oil. Silicone oil is also a good choice for patients who are unable to position themselves in the prone position.

Surgical Pearls No. 100

Air as tamponade in 27G: In case of a superior detachment with a break between 11 o'clock and 1 o'clock we use often only air as tamponade.

27G sclerotomies leak very little. There is an excellent tamponade present for 7–10 days and laser treatment is effective after 3–4 days.

Why does it matter? Especially professionally active patients will appreciate to regain their visual acuity after 1 week. In comparison, C_3F_8 makes an eye blind and the patient earthbound for 2 months.

Surgical Pearls No. 101 (Fig. 35.24)

Air test for detachment: When the retina is completely attached under air, you have drained the subretinal fluid completely. Air presses the entire subretinal fluid from the periphery to the optic disc, where it is easy to spot. This is only partly true for PFCL because PFCL pushes the subretinal fluid from the posterior pole to the periphery, where the "trapped fluid " is hard to detect. **Remark**: PFCL attaches the retina by its specific gravity. (Specific gravity of PFCL = 1.75, Densiron 68 = 1.06). Air, in contrast, attaches the retina due to its high surface tension pressure.

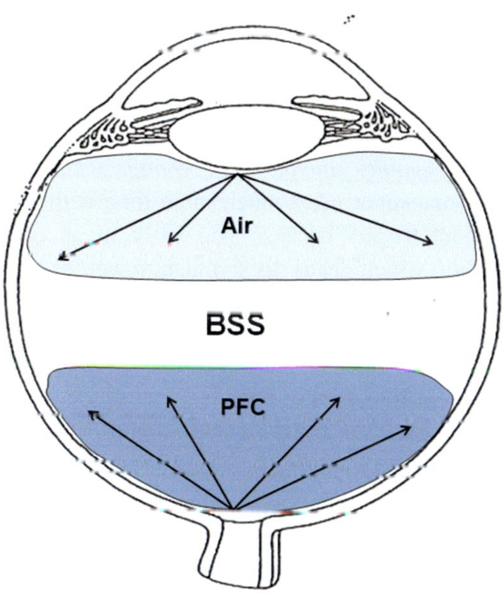

Fig. 35.24 Opposite mechanisms of action of PFCL and air in a BSS-filled eye. Air fills the globe from anterior to posterior. PFC fills the globe from posterior to anterior

Surgical Pearls No. 102 (Fig. 35.25)

Gas versus silicone oil: If the retina is attached under air in detachment surgery, then it will also be attached under gas but that's not necessarily the case for silicone oil. Why? The surface tension pressure of the gas/water interface is the greatest and therefore is the most effective in closing retinal breaks (70 mN/N). So when the retina is attached under air then it is also attached under gas. The same statement is not true for silicone oil. Why? Because the surface tension of silicone oil/water with 50 mN/N is less than that of air/water. So when the retina is attached under air it might not be attached under silicone oil.

Surgical Pearls No. 103

Location of liquids during an air/silicone oil exchange.

Intraoperatively	Postoperatively	
Air	Silicone oil	Vitreous cavity
Silicone oil	Water	

Surgical Pearls No. 104

PFCL against silicone oil exchange: Do not confuse this method with air against silicone oil exchange (Fig. 35.25). If you disconnect the infusion line with air and connect it to the silicone oil syringe then the eye will collapse. An air filled eye needs constant air infusion in order not to collapse. This is not the case in a PFCL filled eye. The eye is stable even if you disconnect the infusion line.

Surgical Pearls No. 105 (Fig. 35.26)

Physics of a silicone oil tamponade.

Surgical Pearls No. 106

PFCL against silicone oil exchange:

(1) If unsure whether there still is some heavy liquid left behind, pause and wait. The heavy liquid will collect and the interface will be clearly visible after approximately 20 s.

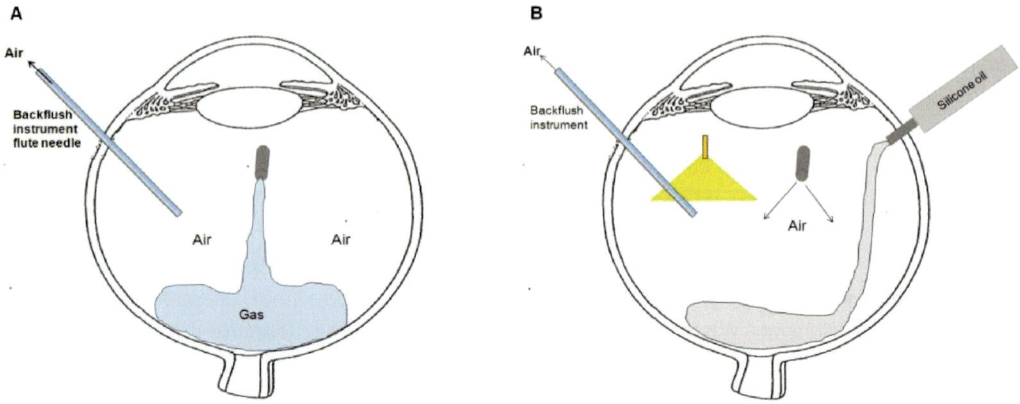

Fig. 35.25 The left eye **A** shows the injection of gas and the right eye **B** shows the injection of silicone oil. The gas sinks on the posterior pole because the Fluor atoms make the gas heavier than air (**A**). And silicone oil flows onto the posterior pole because it is heavier than air (**B**)

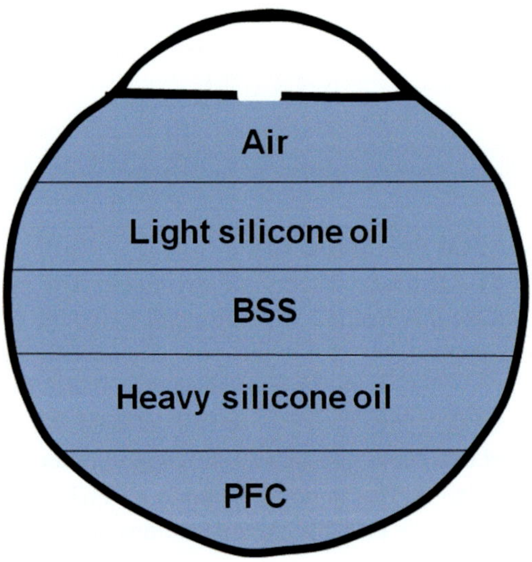

Fig. 35.26 Relative location of fluids within the eye according to their specific gravity. Air (SG = 0.001); Light silicone oil (SG = 0.97); Water (SG = 1); Heavy silicone oil (SG = 1.06); PFC (SG = 1.75)

(2) Removing the final puddle of heavy liquid is not an easy step. The danger is to aspirate retina into the flute needle at the posterior pole or to damage the optic disc. Either try to remove the final bubble "in one go" or let it collect over the optic disc. Then increase the pressure with the silicone oil injection and touch the bubble with the opening of the backflush instrument. For small remnant bubbles, indent the eye with your ring finger. This will give you a much better pressure control than the injection of silicone oil with the foot pedal. Aspirate the heavy liquid bubble and immediately cover the opening of your backflush instrument before withdrawing it from the eye, otherwise the heavy liquid bubble will drop back onto the posterior pole.

Surgical Pearls No. 107

PFCL against silicone oil exchange with 20G: This maneuver takes much more time with 20G without trocars because you work in an open system which leads to a much lower counter pressure. In contrary, a trocar system with valve creates a much higher counter pressure.

Surgical Pearls No. 108

When removing Densiron 68® with a short cannula, it is important not to lose contact with the bubble before it starts "floating up" towards the cannula. In order to guarantee uninterrupted suction, check the residual volume that is left to be aspirated in your suction line just before you are about to "pick up" the residual bubble. If only a few ml are left in your syringe, remove the oil from the syringe by switching to injection mode outside the eye, then go back in to remove the residual bubble with uninterrupted suction. If you lose contact with the bubble and it is too small to be reached with the short cannula, you need to proceed with a backflush cannula (which takes a long time). A special Densiron 68 removal cannula (23G) is available from the company DORC.

Surgical Pearls No. 109 (Fig. 35.27)

View to retina during gas or silicone oil tamponade: An instillation of gas is done without view to retina. An injection of silicone oil is usually done under view to retina. If you want to have a view to retina during the injection than a chandelier light is required. If you exchange air against silicone oil you inject the silicone oil with one hand and remove the air with the other hand. In order to view the fundus you need a chandelier light.

Surgical Pearls No. 110

Caution: During air x fluid exchange the instreaming fluid may damage the retina: Use Charles flute needle with passive aspiration, DO NOT use active aspiration.

Surgical Pearls No. 111 (Fig. 35.28)

Scleral perforation: If you use a 25G or 23G cannula you may perforate the globe during retrobulbar anaesthesia. Use a blunt 25G retrobulbar cannula from Atkinson instead. The blunt tip prevents a scleral perforation.

Surgical Pearls No. 112

What is the mechanism for trocar induced retinal tear? This occurs during trocar insertion. The reason is anterior PVR with anterior displacement of the retina. A very difficult pathological and surgical situation.

Practical management:

Avoid to place a trocar in an area with anterior displacement.
If it happened, check first that the distance from the limbus is correct.
If you find an area in the eye without retinal displacement then replace the trocar there.
Then cauterize the retinal tear around the trocar and treat it as a retinal break.
Often you need to do a focal retinotomy at this area.

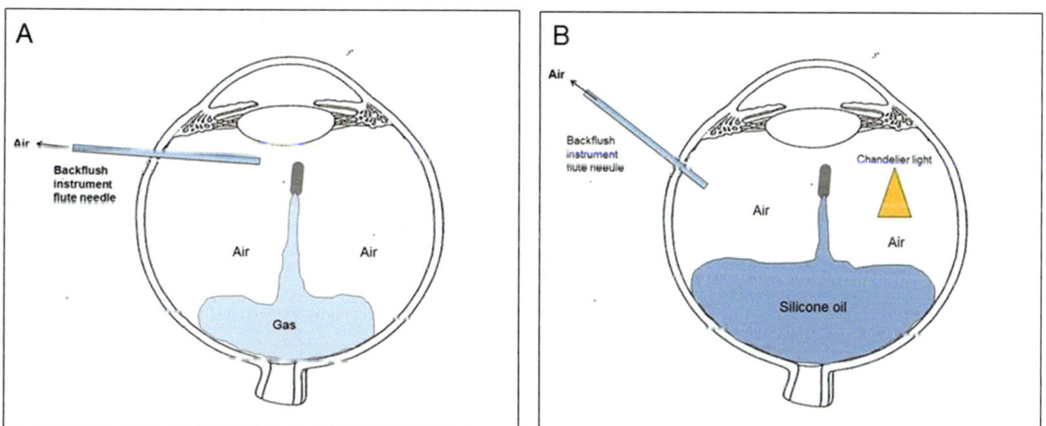

Fig. 35.27 Gas tamponade without view to retina (**A**). Silicone oil tamponade with view to retina (**B**). A chandelier light is required

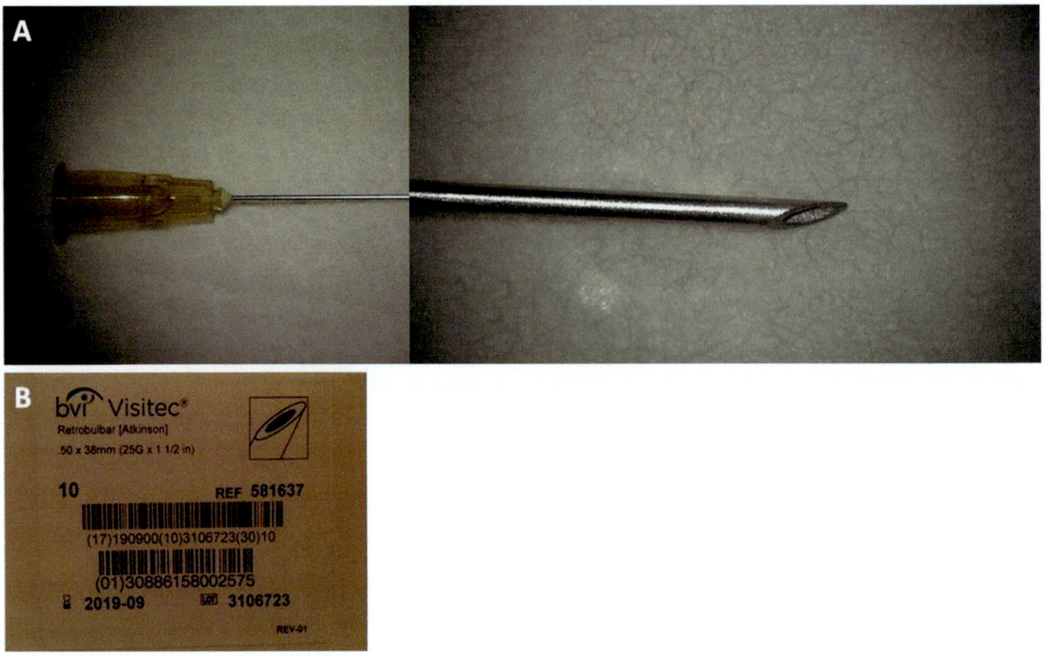

Fig. 35.28 A retrobulbar cannula from Atkinson. The blunt tip prevents a scleral perforation

Surgical Pearls No. 113

Pars plana detachment: The main problem with pars plana detachment is the insertion of trocar cannulas. They may dislocate under the pars plana epithelium. Surgical solution: Use 6mm trocars (Alcon) and insert trocars perpendicular or inject heavy water to attach the pars plana.

Companies Addresses

Alcon

Alcon Laboratories (U.K.) Ltd.
Pentagon Park
Boundary Way
Hemel Hempstead
Herts HP2 7UD, England
Phone: 44 + 1442.341.234
www.alcon.com

Arcadophta

293, route de Seysses
F-31100 Toulouse
Phone: 0033/561/405235
Fax: 0033/5617 408 466
info@arcadophta.com
www.arcadophta.com

Bausch & Lomb

United Kingdom
Europe, Middle East & Africa Division
European Headquarters
Bausch & Lomb House
106-114 London Road
Kingston-Upon-Thames
Surrey KT2 6QJ, England
Phone: 44-20-8781-5500
Fax: 44-20-8781-2989
www.bausch.com

Beaver Visitec

http://www.beaver-visitec.com/

DORC

Dutch Ophthalmic Research
Center International BV
Scheijdelveweg 2
3214 VN Zuidland
The Netherlands
Phone: +31 181 458080
Fax: +31 181 458090
www.dorc.nl

Eye Technology Ltd.

19 Totman Crescent
Brook Road Industrial Estate
Rayleigh
Essex SS6 7UY
United Kingdom
sales@eye-tech.co.uk

Fluoron GmbH

Magirus-Deutz-Strasse 10
89077 Ulm
Phone: 0731/20,559,970
Fax: 0731/205 599 728
info@fluoron.de
www.fluoron.de

Germa AB

Box 2127,
SE-291 02 Kristianstad, Sweden
Industrigatan 54–56,
SE-291 36 Kristianstad, Sweden

U. Spandau et al. (eds.), *Retinal Detachment Surgery and Proliferative Vitreoretinopathy*,
https://doi.org/10.1007/978-3-031-11946-0

+46 (0)44 12 30 30
+46 (0)44 10 31 79
info@germa.se.
www.germa.se

Geuder AG

Hertzstr. 4
69126 Heidelberg,
Phone: 06221/3066
Fax: 06221/303 122
info@geuder.de
www.geuder.de

IRIDEX Corporation

1212 Terra Bella Avenue
Mountain View, CA 94043, USA
www.iridex.com

Labitician Ophthalmics

2140 Winston Park Drive, Unit 6
Oakville, Ontaria LgH 5V5
Canada

Medilens

Medilens Nordic AB
Box 1347
251 13 HELSINGBORG
www.medilens.se

MedOne Surgical Inc.

Sarasota, FL USA 34 243
www.MedOne.com

Ophtec BV

Schweitzerlaan 15
9728 NR Groningen,
Netherlands
www.ophtec.com

Serag Wiessner GmbH

Zum Kugelfang, 8–12
95119 Naila
Germany

Sooft Italia SP A.

Contrada Molino, 17
63833 Montegiorgio Fermo
Italy
Phone: +39 0734 964096
www.oogroup.it/sooft/en/gruppo_gruppo.html

Synergetics France GmbH

Synergetics France SARL
6 Place de la Madeleine
75008 Paris
France
Phone: 825 825 250
Fax: 1 64 11 16 99
E-mail: plecharpentier@synergeticsusa.com
www.synergeticsusa.com

Retinal implants:

DORC (Netherlands)
http://www.dorc.eu/

FCI (France)
http://www.fci-ophthalmics.com/retina

Labtician (Canada)
http://www.labtician.com/
http://www.labtician.com/International/retina-home.html

MIX
Papier aus verantwortungsvollen Quellen
Paper from responsible sources
FSC® C105338

If you have any concerns about our products,
you can contact us on
ProductSafety@springernature.com

In case Publisher is established outside the EU,
the EU authorized representative is:
Springer Nature Customer Service Center GmbH
Europaplatz 3, 69115 Heidelberg, Germany

Printed by Libri Plureos GmbH
in Hamburg, Germany